ESSENTIALS FROM THE GOLDEN CABINET

Translation and Annotation of Jin Gui Yao Lue

金匮要略

ESSENTIALS FROM THE GOLDEN CABINET

Translation and Annotation of Jin Gui Yao Lue

金匮要略

By **Zhongjing Zhang**
Eastern Han Dynasty, China

Edited by **Aiyun Liu**
Shanghai University of Traditional Chinese Medicine, China

Translated by **Chouping Han**
Shanghai University of Traditional Chinese Medicine, China

World Century

Published by

World Century Publishing Corporation
27 Warren Street, Suite 401-402, Hackensack, NJ 07601

Library of Congress Control Number: 2020938724

British Library Cataloguing-in-Publication Data
A catalogue record for this book is available from the British Library.

Supported by the Chinese Fund for the Humanities and Social Sciences

《金匮要略译注》
Originally published in Chinese by Shanghai Chinese Classics Publishing House

English translation rights arranged with Shanghai Chinese Classics Publishing House

ESSENTIALS FROM THE GOLDEN CABINET
Translation and Annotation of Jin Gui Yao Lue 金匮要略

ISBN 978-1-945552-06-9 (hardcover)
ISBN 978-1-945552-07-6 (ebook for institutions)
ISBN 978-1-945552-08-3 (ebook for individuals)

For any available supplementary material, please visit
https://www.worldscienti ic.com/worldscibooks/10.1142/U034#t=suppl

Preface

The *Jin Gui Yao Lüe* (Essentials from the Golden Cabinet) is a classic book of traditional Chinese Medicine. It is the oldest clinical book dedicated to internal, external, gynecological and obstetrical diseases. It is also the first medical book on differential diagnosis of diseases and symptoms, along with treatment and prescriptions.

This classic book was originally written by Zhang Zhongjing (formal name Zhang Ji) (150–219), an eminent Chinese physician in the Eastern Han dynasty (25–220). The original *Shang Han Za Bing Lun* (Treatise on Cold Damage and Miscellaneous Diseases) was lost during wars that ravaged China during the period of the Three Kingdoms. The book was collected and organized later into two books, namely for the former, the *Shang Han Lun* (Treatise on Cold Damage), which was mainly a discourse on how to treat epidemic infectious diseases during his era, and the latter, the *Jin Gui Yao Lüe* (Essentials from the Golden Cabinet), a compendium of various clinical experiences which was regarded as a main discourse on internal diseases. The word *Jin Gui* literally means golden cabinet and shows great respect for Zhang Zhongjing's work—the book deserves to be kept in a cabinet-like storage box made of gold, i.e., a place to store one's most valuable items.

The *Jin Gui Yao Lüe* consists of 25 chapters. The first chapter serves as an introduction. It explains the disease onset, progression and transmission from the zang-fu organs/meridians (space) and sequence (time). This chapter also presents a general guideline that "great doctors treat the early stages of a disease". Chapters 2–22 discuss the diagnosis and treatment of sixty diseases, involving internal medicine, external medicine, and gynecology & obstetrics. Chapter 23 discusses emergency treatments. Chapters 24 and 25 discuss food contraindications (fowls, beasts, fruits, vegetables and grains) and treatment.

Despite the differences in disease names, the categorization of each chapter is quite similar to that of modern medicine. For example, the *Lung Decline, Lung Abscess, and Coughing with Panting* (chapter 7) is similar to respiratory diseases; the *Chest-Bi Impediment, Chest Pain and Shortness of Breath* (chapter 9) is similar to circulatory system diseases; the *Abdominal Fullness, Cold-Induced Abdominal Pain and Retained Food in the Stomach* (chapter 10) is similar to the acute abdomen (surgical); the *Retching, Vomiting, Hiccups and Diarrhea* (chapter 17) is similar to gastrointestinal diseases; the *Pregnancy-Related Problems* (chapter 20) and *Postpartum Diseases* (chapter 21) are similar to obstetrical diseases; and the *Women's Miscellaneous Diseases* (chapter 22) is similar to gynecological diseases. The classification of diseases recorded in this classical text helps with differential diagnosis.

The record and treatment of some diseases in the text are pioneering in the world, such as *Hu Huo Bing* (Behçet's syndrome) and malaria. This text presented a set of treatment methods for Behçet's syndrome, including orally administered decoctions/powder and externally used fumigant and washing lotion. Malaria was recorded in inscriptions on bones or tortoise shells and classified in *Huang Di Nei Jing Su Wen* (The Yellow Emperor's Internal Classic—Basic Questions); however, this text first mentioned that recurrent attacks of malaria may result in splenomegaly. In addition, chapter 24 (Food Contraindications and Treatment of Poultry, Fowl, Fish and Insects) mentioned on several occasions that ingestion of raw or undercooked meat (beef or pork) can cause intestinal tapeworm infection.

All eight treatment methods—sweating, vomiting, draining downward, warming, clearing, harmonizing, eliminating and reinforcing, are included in this text. The formulas share the similar functions as antipyretics, emetics, laxatives, diuretics, sedatives, stomachic, antimalarial drugs, pain killers, anti-dysenteric, anti-asthmatics, anti-shock drugs and antidotes. The text recorded a total of 205 formulas (excluding the annex ones). Orally administered dosage forms include decoction, pill, and powder, and medicinal liquor. Externally used dosage forms include fumigant, washing lotion, ointment/plaster/powder for topical application and suppository. As for weights and measures in the formula, 1 *dòu* = 10 *shēng* (2,045 milliliters); 1 *shēng* = 10 *gě* (204.5 milliliters); 1 *jīn* = 220 grams; 1 *liǎng* = 13.8 grams; 1 square inch spoon = 1–2 grams; 1 qian-spoon = 2 grams; and 1 *chǐ* = 23 centimeters. Chapter 23 (Miscellaneous Formulas) recorded the artificial respiration method for suicide by hanging, "Have one person to press the chest continuously and rhythmically and have another person to flex the patient's arms and legs with gradually increased force".

This text also elaborated treating the same disease with different methods and treating different diseases with the same method. For example, there are nine different formulas for chest-*Bi* impediment according to its severity and urgency. Another example is vomiting. There are three different formulas—*Da Huang Gan Cao Tang* (Rhubarb and Licorice Decoction) for vomiting immediately after eating food due to excess heat (similar to acute gastritis); *Da Ban Xia Tang* (Major Pinellia Decoction) for eating in the morning and vomiting in the late afternoon due to deficiency cold (similar to pyloric obstruction); and *Si Ni Tang* (Frigid Extremities Decoction) for vomiting with a faint pulse due to depletion of yang (similar to shock). In addition, *Ba Wei Shen Qi Wan* (Eight Ingredients Kidney Qi Pill) in this text is indicated for general deficiency, phlegm-fluid retention, wasting & thirsting, and difficult urination.

Many formulas in the *Jin Gui Yao Lüe* have been widely used in clinical practice for thousands of years as the "origins of medical formulas". For example, as the original formula to tonify the kidney, *Ba Wei Shen Qi Wan* (Eight Ingredients Kidney Qi Pill) has later been modified into hundreds of formulas including *Liu Wei Di Huang Wan* (Six Ingredients Rehmannia Pill), *Zhi Bai Di Huang Wan* (Anemarrhena, Phellodendron and Rehmannia Pill), *Qi Ju Di Huang Wan* (Lycium Berry, Chrysanthemum and Rehmannia Pill), *Qi Wei Du Qi Wan* (Seven Ingredients Qi-Restraining Pill), and *Ba Xian Chang Shou Wan* (Eight Ingredients Longevity Pill); *Zhi Gan Cao Tang* (Honey-Fried Licorice Decoction), as the original formula to nourish yin, has later been modified into formulas including *Yi Jia Fu Mai Tang* (Single Shell Pulse-Restoring Decoction), *Er Jia Fu Mai Tang* (Double Shells Pulse-Restoring Decoction), *San Jia Fu Mai Tang* (Triple Shells Pulse-Restoring Decoction), *Jia Jian Fu Mai Tang* (Pulse-Restoring Variant Decoction) and *Da Ding Feng Zhu* (Major Wind-Stabilizing Pill); the well-known qi-supplementing formula *Si Jun Zi Tang* (Four Gentlemen Decoction) and blood-nourishing formula *Si Wu Tang* (Four Ingredients Decoction) are both modified from *Shu Yu Wan* (Dioscorea Pill); and *Xiao Yao San* (Free Wanderer Powder) is modified from *Dang Gui Shao Yao San* (Chinese Angelica and Peony Powder). These classic formulas, either developed by Zhang Zhongjing himself or collected from previous generations, have been passed on to later generations in China and other countries, especially in Japanese Kampo medicine.

To fully understand this ancient medical text, it's essential to know its grammar, explanation and rhetoric. For example, one single word "烦(fán)" can mean "feverish sensations", "severe", "stirring", "upset" or "stuffiness" in different contexts; the word "不(bù)" originally means "no or not"; however, it sometimes means "very" because "不(bù)" and "丕(pī)" are interchangeable. On many occasions, words need to be best explained according to literature and medicine. The most difficult part is the figures of speech. For example, 面目乍赤乍黑乍白(miàn mù zhà chì zhà hēi zhà bái) was used to describe the symptoms of *Hu Huo Bing* (Behçet's syndrome); the first two words 面目(miàn mù) mean face and eyes; however, they focus on the eyes only. The eyes can be red with black or white (pus-filled) sockets. The pathologic process includes red eyes like the eyes of a turtle dove (similar to iridocyclitis) during the first 3–4 days, black sockets during the 7th or 8th day and white (pus-filled) sockets (similar to retained pus in the anterior chamber of the eye). Apparently, the involvement of "face" with the intention to say "eyes" only is a figure of speech in ancient Chinese. Other figures of speech in the text included intertextuality, metonymy, pun, comparison, avoiding repetition, intricacy, combination of two or more things in one sentence, inverted sentences, elliptical sentences, synecdoche, anadiplosis, hyperbole, metaphor and descriptions. It is therefore important to read the sentences and paragraphs as a whole.

The past 1800 years have witnessed numerous editions (Deng Zhen, Yu Qiao, Xu Rong, Zhao Kaimei and Wu Qian) and annotations of *Jin Gui Yao Lüe*. The author of this edition corrected the errors in different editions, summarized their quintessence and made annotations from the perspective of literature and medicine.

The book (Chinese version) was first published by Shanghai Classics Publishing House in 2010 and served as a reference for education, research and clinical practice. Financially supported by Chinese Fund for the Humanities and Social Sciences and recommended by Prof. Chen Kaixian, an academician of Chinese Academy of Sciences and former President, Shanghai University of Traditional Chinese Medicine and Prof. Cai Gan, a tenured professor at Shanghai University of Traditional Chinese Medicine, the English version of this book will be published by World Scientific Publishing. I believe it will be beneficial to people from around the world to better study the treasure house of traditional Chinese medicine.

LIU Aiyun

About the Translator

Prof. Chouping Han is a senior translator at the International Education College, Shanghai University of Traditional Chinese Medicine, China.

Having dedicated to the translation and intercultural studies for the past twenty years, she has translated more than 30 books on traditional Chinese medicine, including *Acupuncture for Cosmetology*, *Acupuncture for Weight Loss*, *Collateral Disease Theory in Practice*, *Illustrations of Guasha Therapy*, *Illustrations of Cupping Therapy*, *Chinese Internal Medicine*, *Chinese External Medicine*, *Dictionary of Common Qigong Glossary*, *Non-surgical Treatment for Avascular Necrosis of the Femoral Head*, *Guidelines of Diagnosis and Therapy in Oncology with Traditional Chinese Medicine*, *Chinese Medicine Told in Pictures*.

Contents

脏腑经络先后病脉证第一
Chapter 1 Diseases of the Zang-Fu Organs, Meridians and Collaterals—Sequences, Pulses and Patterns

Overview

This chapter serves as an overall introduction of the book. It covers a wide range of contents—the disease location, timing, etiological factors, prevention and treatment strategies, categorization, diagnosis, treatment steps and prognosis. The zang-fu organs and meridians here refer to the depth of disease locations—the former is deeper and interior, while the latter is superficial and exterior. The sequence here refers to the time of disease onset or the process of disease occurrence, development and transmission. Generally, pathogenic factors attack meridians first and then affect the zang-fu organs. In summary, there are two essential principles for disease diagnosis and treatment: one is to identify the depth of disease location; the other is to determine the time sequence of disease onset.

*****

[01] 问曰：上工〔1〕治未病〔2〕，何也？师曰：夫治未病者，见肝之病，知肝传脾，当先实脾，四季脾王〔3〕不受邪，即勿补之；中工不晓相传，见肝之病，不解实脾，惟治肝也。

夫肝之病，补用酸，助用焦苦，益用甘味之药调之。酸入肝，焦苦入心，甘入脾。脾能伤肾，肾气微弱，则水不行；水不行，则心火气盛，则伤肺；肺被伤，则金气不行；金气不行，则肝气盛，则肝自愈。此治肝补脾之要妙也。肝虚则用此法。实则不在用之。

经曰：虚虚实实，补不足，损有余，是其义也。余藏准此。

Annotations

[1] *Shang Gong*: Great doctors. The second word '*gong*' is a general term for technical workers. In ancient times, doctors were categorized as great (*Shang Gong*), average (*Zhong Gong*) and below the average (*Xia Gong*) according to their skills in diagnosis and treatment. The *Huang Di Nei Jing Ling Shu Xie Qi Zang Fu Bing Xing Pian* (Chapter 4, Spiritual Pivot, Yellow Emperor's Inner Classic) records, "Doctors who are good at feeling the skin in the *Chi* position do not feel the pulse in *Cunkou* (radial artery); doctors who are good at feeling the pulse do not observe the five colors. Great doctors combine the three (skin in the *Chi* position, pulse and colors) and obtain a cure rate of 90%. Average doctors combine two of the three and obtain a cure rate of 70%. Below-the-average doctors only use one of the three and obtain a cure rate of 60%.

[2] *Zhi Wei Bing*: Intervention in early stages of disease. Disease is known as *Ji Bing* in Chinese—the first word *Ji* means the early stages of disease; and the second word *Bing* means further disease development and aggravation. Therefore, "*Shang Gong Zhi Wei Bing*" means great doctors treat early stages [germination stages recorded in *Su Wen Ba Zheng Shen Ming Lun* (chapter 26, Basis Questions)] of disease before further development and transmission.

[3] *Pi Wang*: Spleen qi is abundant.

Interpretations

Question: "Great doctor treat the early stages of a disease". What does it mean?

Answer: This is how they do it: while treating liver problems, since they know liver problems may affect the spleen, they prescribe formulas to reinforce spleen qi to protect qi from being affected. However, it's not necessary to do so when spleen qi is abundant in the last 18 days of each season. Average doctors may treat the liver alone without the knowledge of disease transmission.

For disorders due to liver deficiency, it's essential to use herbs that are sour in taste to directly tonify the liver, herbs that are bitter in taste to assist the heart and herbs that are sweet in taste to harmonize the spleen, because the sour enters the liver, the bitter enters the heart and the sweet enters the spleen. Hyperactivity of the spleen may affect the kidney and kidney qi weakness may slow down the flow of water, which in turn, may cause hyperactivity of heart fire. Hyperactive heart fire may affect the lung and result in failure of lung qi to disperse, which in turn, may lead to flourishing of liver qi, and the liver problems resolve accordingly. This is the subtlety of treating liver problems by fortifying the spleen. This method for liver deficiency does not apply to liver excess syndrome.

According to the *Yi Jing* (Medical Classics), reducing method aggravates a deficiency syndrome and reinforcing method aggravates an excess syndrome (both methods are wrong). The correct way is to reinforce deficiency and reduce excess. This principle also applies to the diagnosis and treatment of problems involving other zang-fu organs.

*****

[02] 夫人禀五常〔1〕，因风气〔2〕而生长，风气虽能生万物，亦能害万物，如水能浮舟，亦能覆舟。若五脏元真〔3〕通畅，人即安和。客气邪风〔4〕，中人多死。千般疢〔5〕难，不越三条。一者，经络受邪，入脏腑，为内所因也；二者，四肢九窍〔6〕，血脉相传，壅塞不通，为外皮肤所中也；三者，房室、金刃、虫兽所伤。以此详之，病由都尽。若人能养慎，不令邪风干忤经络；适中经络，未流传腑脏，即医治之。四肢才觉重滞，即导引〔7〕、吐纳〔8〕、针灸、膏摩〔9〕，勿令九窍闭塞；更能无犯王法、禽兽灾伤、房室勿令竭乏；服食节其冷、热、苦、酸、辛、甘，不遣形体有衰，病则无由入其腠理。腠〔10〕者，是三焦通会元真之处，为血气所注；理者，是皮肤脏腑之文理也。

Annotations

[1] *Wu Chang*: Normal qi of five elements.

[2] *Feng Qi*: Generalization of five qi: wind, summer-heat, dryness, damp and cold. Five qi (*Wu Qi*) is used interchangeably with normal qi of five elements (*Wu Chang*).

[3] *Wu Zang Yuan Zhen*: Qi activities of the whole body.

[4] *Ke Qi Xie Feng*: *Ke Qi* refers to external pathogenic factors; *Xie Feng* refers to deficiency coupled with extraction of pathogenic wind. When used in combination, they both refer to pathogenic qi in four seasons.

[5] *Chen*: Febrile (heat) disease. Here, it refers to 'disease'.

[6] *Jiu Qiao*: Nine orifices, namely, two ears, two noses, two eyes, mouth, urethra and anus.

[7] *Dao Yin*: A series of exercises involving tendons, bones and joints.

[8] *Tu Na*: Breathing out the turbid qi and breathing in the clean qi. It is a health preservation method to regulate one's breathing.

[9] *Gao Mo*: An external therapy to rub the surface of the body with medicated ointment.

[10] *Zou*: The place where qi and blood flow into; *Li*: streaks of the skin or zang-fu organs. *Sanjiao*: the entire body; *Yuan Zhen*: qi, blood, *ying*-nutrients and *wei*-defense.

Interpretations

Human body receives qi of five elements from the nature. Human growth depends on five qi. Just like the water can float a boat, it can also sink it, five qi enable all things in the universe to grow; however, they may also harm these things. One is healthy when qi flows freely over the body. One becomes sick when attacked by exogenous pathogenic factors.

Despite the disease varieties, there are three major routes. First, pathogenic factors attack the meridian first and then enter the zang-fu organs. Second, pathogenic factors obstruct the blood flow in four limbs and nine orifices and manifest on the surface of the body. Third, sexual indulgence, metallic wounds and insects/animal bites. These three aspects have covered all etiological factors.

It's advisable to have healthy lifestyles (nourish anti-pathogenic qi internally and avoid wind cold externally) to prevent meridians from being attacked by pathogenic factors. It's essential to remove pathogenic factors before they transmit to internal organs. To prevent obstruction of blood flow in (four limbs) and nine orifices, it's important to perform *Dao Yin* (physical exercise) *or Tu Na* (breathing exercise), acupuncture, moxibustion or rubbing the surface of the body with medicated ointment. In addition, it's advisable not to illegally kill animals or consume essential qi by sexual indulgence. What's more, it's important to adapt to weather changes and have a well-balanced diet. With a strong anti-pathogenic qi, there is no way for pathogenic factors to enter the *Zou* and *Li*: the former refers to places where qi and blood flow into; and the latter refers to the streaks of the skin or zang-fu organs.

*****

[03] 问曰：病人有气色见于面部，愿闻其说。师曰：鼻[1]头色青，腹中痛，苦冷者死；一云腹中冷，苦痛者死。鼻头色微黑者，有水气；色黄者，胸上有寒；色白者，亡血[2]也，设微赤，非时者死。其目正圆者痉，不治。又色青为痛，色黑为劳，色赤为风，色黄者便难。色鲜明者有留饮。

Annotations

[1] *Bi*: face.
[2] *Wang Xue*: loss of blood.

Interpretations

Question: Patients with different illnesses may manifest differently in their face. I'd like to hear more of it.

Answer: A bluish complexion indicates abdominal pain. Cold hands and feet may indicate a critical condition. Alternatively, severe abdominal pain with a cold sensation also indicates a life-threatening condition. A dark-gray complexion indicates edema. A sallow complexion indicates cold-dampness in the abdomen. A pale complexion indicates anemia. A pale complexion with flushed cheeks (not in a hot season) may indicate a superficial yang syndrome (yin rejecting yin in an extremely deficient syndrome), which is life-threatening (it's necessary to observe five sense organs such as the eyes in addition to facial complexion). The eyes are wide open but unable to move may indicate a febrile convulsion. (In summary), a bluish complexion indicates an acute abdominal pain. A dark complexion indicates chronic consumption. A red complexion indicates extraction of wind cold. A sallow complexion indicates (jaundice) dysuria. A shiny and stretched skin indicates (edema) water retention.

*****

[04] 师曰：病人语声寂然，喜惊呼者，骨节间病；语声喑喑然〔1〕不彻者，心膈间病；语声啾啾然〔2〕细而长者，头中病一作痛。

Annotations

[1] *Yin Yin Ran*: a low weak voice.
[2] *Jiu Jiu Ra*n: a thready, long voice.

Interpretations

The Master said, "Sudden cry of pain in quietness (due to change in posture) indicates injuries of bones or tendons (such as bone fracture or joint pain). A low, faint voice (due to obstructed airway) indicates chest disorders involving the heart and lung (such as chronic bronchitis, emphysema or respiratory failure). A thready, long voice indicates problems of the head; alternatively, this can be explained by headache (patients are scared of talking loudly in order not to aggravate the headache).

*****

[05] 师曰：息〔1〕摇肩〔2〕者，心中坚；息引胸中，上气〔3〕者，咳；息张口短气〔4〕者，肺痿〔5〕唾沫。

Annotations

[1] *Xi*: breathing.

[2] *Yao Jia*n: breathing with lifted shoulders, difficulty breathing due to lung qi obstruction.

[3] *Shang Qi*: panting or gasping, inability to lie flat due to adverse flow of lung qi, coupled with phlegm sounds in the throat.

[4] *Duan Qi:* rapid breathing or shortness of breath, breathing with an open mouth due to lung qi deficiency (another manifestation of difficulty breathing)

[5] *Fei Wei:* Lung decline (chronic consumptive lung conditions).

Interpretations

The Master said, "Patients who breathe with lifted shoulders often have epigastric hardness and fullness. Patients who experience panting often suffer from coughing. Patients who breathe with an open mouth often have thin, foamy phlegm due to chronic consumptive lung conditions".

*****

[06] 师曰：吸而微数，其病在中焦〔1〕，实也，当下之即愈，虚者不治。在上焦者，其吸促；在下焦者，其吸远，此皆难治，呼吸动摇振振者〔2〕，不治。

Annotations

[1] *Zhong Jiao*: upper part of the three jiao, i.e., the place where the spleen and stomach are located. Here it refers to intestines and stomach.

[2] *Hu Xi Dong Yao Zhen Zhen Zhe:* Breathing with shaking of the entire body, more severe (difficulty breathing) than breathing with lifted shoulders.

Interpretations

The Master said, "Mild rapid breathing due to disorders of the intestines and stomach indicate an excess syndrome. The treatment strategy is to reduce heat to restore normal breathing. A deficiency syndrome (spleen qi collapse) is more difficult to treat, so are rapid or prolonged breathing due to disorders of the upper *jiao* or lower *jiao*. Panting with shaking of the entire body indicates an incurable condition".

*****

[07] 师曰：寸口脉[1]动者，因其王时而动，假令肝王色青，四时各随其色。肝色青而反色白，非其时色脉，皆当病。

Annotations

[1] *Cun Kou Mai:* a place to feel the pulse, located in the medial side of the radius where the radial artery pulsation can be felt.

Interpretations

The Master said, "The pulsation of the radial artery varies in seasons. For example, the liver is prosperous in spring and its color is green. Presence of white rather than green and non-wiry pulse in spring may indicate a pathological state".

*****

[08] 问曰：有未至而至，有至而不至，有至而不去，有至而太过。何谓也？师曰：冬至[1]之后，甲子[2]夜半[3]，少阳[4]起少阴之时，阳始生，天得温和。以未得甲子，天因温和，此为未至而至也；以得甲子，而天未温和，此为至而不至也；以得甲子，而天大寒不解，此为至而不去也；以得甲子，而天温如盛夏五、六月时，此为至而太过也。

Annotations

[1] *Dong Zhi:* winter solstice, one of the 24 solar terms. It often falls on November in Chinese lunar calendar.

[2] *Jia Zi*: an ancient method to calculate the date, month and year using heavenly stems and earthly branches. There are 10 heavenly stems (*Jia, Yi, Bing, Ding, Wu, Ji, Geng, Xin, Ren* and *Gui*) and 12 earthly branches (*Zi, Chou, Yin, Mao, Chen, Si, Wu, Wei, Shen, You, Xu* and *Hai*). There are a total of 66 results, starting from *Jia Zi* and ending at *Gui Hai.* Here it refers to 60 days after the winter solstice.

[3] *Ye Ban*: midnight (*Zi Shi*), one of the 12 *Shi Chen* (2-hour periods) in ancient China, i.e., 11:00 pm—1:00 am.

[4] *Shao Yang*: one of the time seasons in a year. In ancient China, one year is divided into six stages: *Shao Yang*, *Yang Ming*, *Tai Yang*, *Tai Yin*, *Shao Yin* and *Jue Yin*.

Interpretations

Question: Sometimes the climate changes before the season arrives; sometimes the climate changes after the season arrives; sometimes climate does not change when the new season arrives; and sometimes climate changes too fast when the season arrives. How do we understand these exceptions?

Answer: *Shao Yang* becomes active on the first day of the first *Jia Zi* cycle (60 days) after the winter solstice. In the meantime, yang qi starts to grow and the weather gradually becomes warm (this is the normal weather). If the weather becomes warm before the day of *Jia Zi*, this is called "the climate changes before the season arrived". If the weather has not become warm after the day of *Jia Zi*, this is called "the climate changes after the season arrives". If the weather remains cold after the day of *Jia Zi*, this is known as "climate does not change when the new season arrives". If the weather is as hot as summer (May or June) after the day of *Jia Zi*, this is called "climate changes too fast when the season arrives" (all these are abnormal climates).

*****

[09] 师曰：病人脉浮者在前[1]，其病在表；浮者在后[2]，其病在里。腰痛背强不能行，必短气而极也。

Annotations

[1] *Qian:* the pulse-feeling location in front of the *Guan* position, i.e., the *Cun* position. There are three positions around the radial artery: *Cun* (closest to the wrist), *Guan* (styloid process) and *Chi* (distal to the wrist).

[2] *Hou*: the *Chi* position of feeling the pulse.

Interpretations

The Master said, "A superficial pulse in the *Cun* position, coupled with stiffness of the low back and difficulty walking often indicates problems involving the surface of the body (exterior). A superficial pulse in the *Chi* position, coupled with shortness of breath and fatigue often indicates problems of internal organs (interior)".

*****

[10] 问曰：经云"厥阳[1]独行"，何谓也？师曰：此为有阳无阴，故称厥阳。

Annotations

[1] *Jue Yang:* according to *Shuo Wen Jie Zi* (Explaining and Analyzing Characters), the first word *Jue* means stones, which later referred to a sudden onset.

Interpretations

Question: The *Classic* mentions "*Jue Yang* travels alone", what does it mean?

Answer: When yang qi becomes overwhelming, there is no yin. Yang without yin is called *Jue Yang*.

*****

[11] 问曰：寸脉沉大而滑，沉则为实，滑则为气，实气相搏〔1〕，血气入脏即死，入腑即愈〔2〕，此为卒厥〔3〕，何谓也？师曰：唇口青，身冷，为入脏即死；知身和，汗自出，为入腑即愈。

Annotations

[1] *Chen Ze Wei Shi...Shi Qi Xiang Bo*: This explains the underlying principle of a sudden syncope. The *Jin Gui Yao Lüè Xin Dian* (Personal Standards for the 'Essentials from the Golden Cabinet') states, "*Shi* (excess) here refers to blood excess, and *qi* here mean qi excess. *Shi Qi Xiang Bo* means intertwined excess of both blood and qi".

[2] *Xue Qi Ru Zang Ji Si, Ru Fu Ji Yu*: This refers to the prognosis of a medical problem. The *Jin Gui Yao Lüè Bian Zhu* (Editor's Notes to the "Essentials from the Golden Chamber) states, "Blood qi entering the zang-organs means pathogenic qi entering the zang-organs". Pathogenic qi entering the deep-located zang-organs often indicates an unfavorable prognosis, whereas pathogenic qi entering the superficial fu-organs often indicates a favorable prognosis.

[3] *Cu Jue*: a condition of sudden syncope in Chinese medicine. Here it refers to all conditions with a sudden onset. The first word *Cu* means sudden and the second word *Jue* means onset.

Interpretations

Question: As for a deep, large and slippery pulse in the *Cunkou* region, "deep" indicates blood excess, and "slippery" indicates qi excess. Intertwined excess of both blood and qi may result in a sudden syncope. Pathogenic qi entering the zang-organs indicates a severe condition, whereas pathogenic qi entering the fu-organs indicates a mild condition. How do we evaluate the prognosis of conditions with a sudden onset such as syncope?

Answer: The evaluation is based on the presenting signs and symptoms. Cyanosis of the lips (due to qi stagnation and blood stasis) and extremely cold hands and feet (due to sudden collapse of yang qi) are signs indicative of a critical condition with pathogenic qi entering the zang-organs, along with an unfavorable prognosis. A warm sensation of the body and spontaneous sweating (because of smooth flow of qi and blood) are signs indicative of a mild condition with pathogenic qi entering the fu-organs, along with a favorable prognosis.

*****

[12] 问曰：脉脱〔1〕入脏即死、入腑即愈，何谓也？师曰：非为一病，百病皆然。譬如浸淫疮〔2〕，从口起流向四肢者，可治；从四肢流来入口者，不可治。病在外者可治，入里者即死。

Annotations

[1] *Mai Tuo*: The first word *Mai* refers to blood qi (i.e., pathogenic qi), not the pulse felt at the radial artery; and the second word *Tuo* means "or". The *Jin Gui Yu Han Yao Lüè Shu Yi* (Elaborations on Essentials from the Jade Case Classic of the Golden Cabinet) states, "the word *Mai*

refers to *Xue Mai* (blood vessels), an abbreviation of blood qi, whereas *Tuo* is a modal adverb, meaning "or". The *Huang Di Nei Jing Su Wen Fang Sheng Shuai Lun* (Chapter 80 of the Basic Questions) states, "*Mai Tuo* probably means that the pulse cannot be felt for a short moment due to pathogenic factors blocking the flow of blood and qi".

[2] *Jin Yin Chuang*: a gradually spreading skin condition in Chinese medicine. Here it refers to all types of gradually developed conditions. *Jin Yin* means gradual progression.

Interpretations

Question: How do we understand that pathogenic qi entering the zang-organs has an unfavorable prognosis, whereas pathogenic qi entering the fu-organs has a favorable prognosis?

Answer: This applies not just to one single condition, but to all medical conditions. As for gradually developed conditions like *Jin Yin Chuang* (Wet Spreading Sores, similar to universal eczema in modern medicine), spreading from the mouth toward the four limbs indicates a favorable prognosis, whereas spreading from the four limbs toward the mouth indicates an unfavorable prognosis. It's easier to manage problems affecting the exterior (superficial location) and more difficult to manage problems affecting the interior (deeper location).

*****

[13] 问曰：阳病十八〔1〕，何谓也？师曰：头痛、项、腰、脊、臂、脚掣痛。阴病十八〔2〕，何谓也？师曰：咳、上气、喘、哕、咽〔3〕、肠鸣、胀满、心痛、拘急。五脏病各有十八，合为九十病〔4〕。人又有六微〔5〕，微有十八病，合为一百八病〔6〕。五劳、七伤、六极〔7〕、妇人三十六病〔8〕，不在其中。清邪〔9〕居上，浊邪〔10〕居下，大邪〔11〕中表，小邪〔12〕中里，槃饪之邪〔13〕，从口入者，宿食也。五邪中人，各有法度。风中于前，寒中于暮。湿伤于下，雾伤于上。风令脉浮，寒令脉急，雾伤皮腠，湿流关节，食伤脾胃。极寒伤经，极热伤络。〔14〕

Annotations

[1] *Yang Bing Shi Ba*: Eighteen disorders of the three yang meridians: Taiyang, Yangming and Shaoyang. Yang meridians run on the back and surface of the body. Yang disorders refer to problems affecting the exterior and meridians. The text records six syndromes. Since each syndrome is subcategorized into *Ying*-nutrients syndrome, *Wei*-defense syndrome and combined *Ying*-nutrients and *Wei*-defense syndrome, there are a total of 18 yang disorders.

[2] *Yang Bing Shi Ba*: Eighteen disorders of the three yin meridians: Taiyin, Shaoyin and Jueyin. Yin meridians run on the front of the body and are connected with internal zang-fu organs. Yin disorders refer to problems affecting the interior and zang-fu organs. The text records nine syndromes. Since each syndrome is subcategorized into deficiency and excess, there are a total of 18 yin disorders.

[3] *Yan*: A sense of obstruction in the throat.

[4] *Wu Zang Bing Ge You Shi Ba, He Wei Jiu Shi Bing*: Disorders of the five-zang organs (heart, liver, spleen, lung and kidney) are subcategorized into six pathogenic factors (wind, cold, summer heat, dampness, dryness and fire), qi problem, blood problem and combined qi and blood problem, there are a total of 90 conditions of the five-zang organs.

[5] *Liu Wei*: Disorder of the six-fu organs. The first word *Liu* means six fu organs. The second word *Wei* means mild conditions, as opposed to zang-organ problems.

[6] *Wei You Shi Ba Bing, He Wei Yi Bai Ba Bing*: Disorders of the six-fu organs (gallbladder, stomach, large intestine, small intestine, Sanjiao and urinary bladder) are subcategorized into six pathogenic factors, qi problem, blood problem and combined qi and blood problem, there are a total of 108 conditions of the six-fu organs. The above categorization was based on etiological factors, syndrome patterns, locations and pathology mechanisms. It is no longer used today.

[7] *Wu Lao*, *Qi Shang* and *Liu Ji*: Three categories of difficult and complicated disorders. *Wu Lao* means chronic deficiencies of the five-zang organs (due to consumption of qi, blood, yin or yang). *Qi Shang* means seven injuries, which include yin cold, yin flaccidity, a frequently recurring or continuous sense of desire to empty the bowels, seminal emissions, thin, clear semen, frequent but scanty urination, and a low concentration

of sperm. *Liu Ji* means six extremes, which include extreme deficiencies of qi, blood, tendons, bones, muscles and essence.

[8] *Fu Ren San Shi Liu Bing*: According to the *Bei Ji Qian Jin Yao Fang* (Important Formulas Worth a Thousand Gold Pieces for Emergency), "The twelve gynecological symptoms include irregular periods and vaginal discharges that resemble thick cheese, dark blood, purple juice, red meat, pus-filled scab, fermented mung bean juice, okra soup, coagulated blood, clear (watery) blood, rice-washed water, and menstrual blood. The nine types of pain include vaginal pain, pain coupled with dribbling of urine, pain during urination, cold pain, dysmenorrhea, distending pain, insect-gnawed pain coupled with vaginal discharge, subcostal pain, and low back and hip pain. The seven disorders include pain and obstruction of orifices, pain due to cold/heat, acute, persistent (lower) abdominal pain, numbness, cervix pain that radiates toward the back, heavy or scanty menstruation and morning sickness. The five injuries include subcostal fullness and pain, chest pain that radiates toward the subcostal region, pain due to qi stagnation, diarrhea and pain with a cold sensation. The three chronic conditions include weight loss, lactation failure and amenorrhea".

[9] *Qing Xie*: Pathogenic wind.

[10] *Zhuo Xie*: Pathogenic dampness (the word *Zhuo* means heavy and turbid).

[11] *Da Xie*: Six pathogenic factors (wind, cold, summer heat, dampness, dryness and fire).

[12] *Xiao Xie*: Seven emotions (joy, anger, melancholy, worry, grief, fear and fright).

[13] *Gu Ren Zhi Xie*: Improper diet.

[14] *Ji Han Shang Jing, Ji Re Shang Luo*: Extreme cold or heat damages meridians and collaterals.

Interpretations

Question: What are the eighteen problems of the Yang meridians?

The Master said, "Headache, and pain in the back of the neck, low back, spine, arm and foot".

Question: What are the eighteen problems of the Yin meridians?

The Master said, "Coughing, shortness of breath, panting, hiccups, a sensation of obstruction in the throat, bowel sounds, distension/fullness, chest pain and contracture/spasm.

Each of the five zang-organs has 18 disorders, and there are 90 in total. Each of the fu-organs has 18 disorders, and there are 108 disorders in total. In addition, there are chronic deficiencies of the five-zang organs, the seven injuries, the six extremes and the thirsty-six gynecological conditions.

When attacking the body, pathogenic qi follows a specific pattern. For example, wind tends to affect the upper part of the body, whereas dampness tends to affect the lower part of the body. Six exogenous pathogenic factors affect the exterior first, whereas seven emotions affect the interior first. Improper diet may cause food retention. There is also a specific pattern for the invasion time of pathogenic qi. For example, wind tends to affect the body in the morning, whereas cold tends to affect the body at night; water dampness tends to affect the lower part of the body, whereas foggy dew tends to affect the upper part of the body. In addition, wind often causes the pulse to be sluggish, whereas cold often causes the pulse to be tight; fog often affects the surface of the body, dampness often affects the joints and improper diet often damages the spleen and stomach. Extreme cold or heat damages meridians and collaterals.

*****

[14] 问曰：病[1]有急当救[2]里救表者，何谓也？师曰：病[3]，医下之，续得下利，清谷[4]不止，身体疼痛[5]者，急当救里；后身体疼痛，清便自调者，急当救表也。

Annotations

[1] *Bing*: Presence of combined exterior syndrome and interior syndrome.

[2] *Jiu*: Treatment.

[3] *Bing*: Exterior syndrome.

[4] *Qing Gu*: Undigested food in stool. Here it refers to interior syndrome.

[5] *Shen Ti Teng Tong*: Body ache. Here it refers to exterior syndrome.

Interpretations

Question: When exterior syndrome and interior syndrome are present simultaneously, sometimes it's necessary to treat the interior syndrome first, but sometimes it's necessary to treat the exterior syndrome first. How do we differentiate the treatment sequence?

The Master said, "Purging method is indicated for an interior syndrome; however, when used for an exterior syndrome, it may cause persistent diarrhea with undigested food in stools. Despite the complaint of body ache (a sign of exterior syndrome), it's important to treat the interior syndrome (diarrhea) first and address the body ache when the bowel movements restored normal.

*****

[15] 夫病痼疾〔1〕，加以卒病〔2〕，当先治其卒病，后乃治其痼疾也。

Annotations

[1] *Gu Ji*: Chronic illnesses. The word *Gu* means persistent illnesses.

[2] *Cu Bing*: Sudden, acute illnesses. The word *Cu* means sudden.

Interpretations

When patients who have chronic medical conditions develop a new illness, it's important to treat the new illness first and then address the previous conditions.

*****

[16] 师曰：五脏病各有得〔1〕者愈，五脏病各有所恶〔2〕，各随其所不喜〔3〕者为病。病者素不应食，而反暴思〔4〕之，必发热也〔5〕。

Annotations

[1] *You De*: Appropriate food.
[2] *You Suo E*: Improper food.
[3] *Suo Bu Xi*: Inappropriate food (food to avoid).
[4] *Bao Si*: Binge eating.
[5] *Bi Fa Re Ye*: Fever, suggesting a worsened condition.

Interpretations

The Master said, "It's important for patients with five-zang disorders to select appropriate food, because appropriate food help to speed up the recovery. Patients having five-zang disorders should avoid specific food, because these food may trigger dysfunctions of the zang organs. Binge eating of food that should be avoided can aggravate the preexisting medical conditions".

*****

[17] 夫诸病在脏〔1〕，欲攻〔2〕之，当随其所得而攻之，如渴者，与猪苓汤〔3〕。余皆仿此。

Annotations

[1] *Zai Zang:* In the interior.
[2] *Gong*: To treat.
[3] *Zhu Ling Tang* (Polyporus Decoction): Ingredients: *Zhu Ling* (Polyporus), *Fu Ling* (Poria), *E Jiao* (Colla Corii Asini), *Hua Shi* (Talcum) and *Ze Xie* (Rhizoma Alismatis). Actions: Nourishes yin and promotes urination.

Interpretations

The treatment of internal organ problems should be based on the root cause. For example, prescribing *Zhu Ling Tang* for patients with thirst (Besides damage to yin, thirst can be caused by many etiological factors. As a result, the treatment strategy varies—sometimes nourishing yin and sometimes resolving water retention by promoting urination). This principle also applies to other internal problems.

痓湿暍病脉证治第二
Chapter 2 Tetany, Dampness and Heat Stroke—Pulses, Patterns and Treatment

Overview

This chapter discusses three disorders—tetany, dampness and heat stroke. All three disorders result from external contraction of pathogenic factors and share the common symptoms (fever, chills, etc.) in exterior syndrome. As a result, the three are discussed together. The Chinese character "痓" (z*hi*) in this chapter should be written as "痉" (*jing*).

According to *Shuo Wen Jie Zi* (Explaining and Analyzing Characters), the *jing* means spasm. The *Guang Yun* (Revised Tone Rhymes) states, "Wind causes spasm or rigidity". Spasm is often caused by contraction of wind-cold.

Dampness affects the muscles and joints. It is often caused by external contraction of dampness. Dampness is liable to associate itself with wind, cold and heat. Dampness can be contracted externally or produced as a result of internal dysfunctions. This chapter addresses external dampness (also known as dampness stroke).

According to *Shuo Wen Jie Zi* (Explaining and Analyzing Characters), the *ye* means heat stroke. It often occurs as a result of contracting summer heat or summer heat combined with dampness.

*****

[01] 太阳病〔1〕，发热、无汗，反恶寒者，名曰刚痉〔2〕。

Annotations

[1] *Tai Yang Bing:* A syndrome name in Chinese medicine according to syndrome differentiation of the six meridians in the *Shang Han Lun* (Treatise on Cold Damage). The six meridians are Taiyang meridian, Yangming meridian, Shaoyang meridian, Taiyin meridian, Shaoyin meridian and Jueyin meridian. Taiyang disease is the initial stage of exogenous febrile conditions. The *Shang Han Lun* states, "Taiyang syndrome is characterized by a superficial pulse, headache, neck stiffness and aversion to cold".

[2] *Gang Jing*: Hard tetany. Patients may present with signs and symptoms due to excessive exterior cold syndrome (fever, absence of sweating, and aversion to cold), neck rigidity, lockjaw and opisthotonus.

Interpretations

Taiyang syndrome that is characterized by fever, sweating and aversion to cold, coupled with spasm/convulsions is called a hard tetany.

*****

[02] 太阳病，发热、汗出，而不恶寒，名曰柔痉〔1〕。

Annotations

[1] *Rou Jing*: Soft tetany. Patients may present with signs and symptoms due to exterior deficiency syndrome (fever, sweating, and aversion to wind), neck rigidity, lockjaw and opisthotonus. According to the *Jin Gui Yu Han Yao Lüè Ji Yi* (Explanations and Annotations of *Jin Gui Yao Lüè*), "Hard and soft are based on the principles of yin and yang, and yin and yang on the principles of deficiency and excess. Exterior excess syndrome is known as hard, whereas exterior excess syndrome is known as soft".

Interpretations

Taiyang syndrome that is characterized by fever, sweating and aversion to cold, coupled with spasm is called a soft tetany.

*****

[03] 太阳病，发热、脉沉而细〔1〕者，名曰痉，为难治。

Annotations

[1] *Mai Chen Er Xi*: A deep and thready pulse. Here it is used to predict the prognosis. Since pathogenic factors affect the exterior in Taiyang syndrome, the pulse is supposed to be superficial. A deep and thready pulse indicates retention of pathogenic factors in the exterior but deficiency in the interior. In addition, patients also present with major symptoms of spasticity (headache, neck stiffness, lockjaw and opisthotonus). According to the *Yi Zong Jin Jian* (Golden Mirror of the Medical Tradition), "Fever is a sign indicative of Taiyang syndrome. A deep, thready pulse is a sign indicative of Shaoyin syndrome. Patients with a spasticity syndrome present with either hard tetany or soft tetany. Taiyang spasm syndrome with a pulse of Shaoyin indicates a combined exterior and interior syndrome".

Interpretations

Taiyang syndrome that is characterized by concurrent fever and a deep, thready pulse, coupled with spasm is difficult to cure.

*****

[04] 太阳病，发汗太多，因致痉〔1〕。

Annotations

[1] *Jing*: Spasms or convulsions of the four limbs due to damage to fluids and malnourishment of the tendons and vessels, resulting from inappropriate treatment of other conditions.

Interpretations

Excessive sweating in Taiyang syndrome may cause tetany.

*****

[05] 夫风病，下之则痉，复发汗，必拘急。

Interpretations

For wind syndrome, the purgation method causes spasm. If it's further treated by inducing sweating, contractures may occur.

*****

[06] 疮家[1]虽身疼痛，不可发汗，汗出则痉。

Annotations

[1] *Chuang Jia*: Patients with skin sores/ulcers such as carbuncles, boils or furuncles.

Interpretations

For body ache (or fever) in patients with chronic skin sores/ulcers, inducing sweating cannot be used, or it may cause spasm.

*****

[07] 病者，身热，足寒，颈项强急〔1〕，恶寒，时头热、面赤、目赤〔2〕，独头动摇〔3〕，卒口噤〔4〕，背反张〔5〕者，痓病[6]也。若发其汗者，寒湿相得，其表益虚，即恶寒甚。发其汗已，其脉如蛇。一云其脉浛浛。

[08] 暴腹胀大者，为欲解。脉如故，反伏弦者〔7〕，痓。

Annotations

[1] *Jing Xiang Qiang Ji*: Rigidity of the head and neck.

[2] *Mu Chi*: Eye redness (congestion).

[3] *Du Tou Dong Yao*: Shaking of the head and facial twitching.

[4] *Cu Kou Jin*: Paroxysmal lockjaw, upward and outward deviation of the mouth corner, elevated eyebrows, and a forced smile due to spasm of the masseter muscle.

[5] *Bei Fan Zhang*: Opisthotonus, a state of severe hyperextension and spasticity of the axial muscles along the neck and back.

[6] *Jing Bing*: A disease name in Chinese medicine. It is caused by external contraction of wind and characterized by neck rigidity, lockjaw and opisthotonos. It is similar to tetanus in modern medicine.

[7] *Bao Fu Zhang Da Zhe, Wei Yu Jie. Mai Ru Gu, Fa Fu Xian Zhe*: A soft, smooth pulse like the abdomen of a snake indicates the tetany is about to resolve. If the pulse remains as before or becomes hidden and wiry, this means an aggravated condition with pathogenic factors entering the interior; in other words, tetany may persist.

Interpretations

Clinical manifestations of tetany include fever, a cold sensation in the lower limbs, neck/back rigidity, aversion to cold, a hot sensation of the head, red face and eyes, facial twitching, sudden lockjaw and opisthotonos. External contraction of cold-dampness after sweating may exacerbate aversion to cold and cause the exterior to be more deficient. After sweating, the pulse of the patient feels soft and smooth like the enlarged abdomen of a snake. This is a sign that tetany is about to resolve. However, if the pulse remains as before or becomes hidden and wiry, the tetany may persist.

*****

[09] 夫痉脉，按之紧如弦〔1〕，直上下行〔2〕。一作筑筑而弦，《脉经》云："痉家其脉伏坚直上下。"

Annotations

[1] *Jin Ru Xian*: A tight, wiry and forceful pulse. A tight pulse is tense and forceful. A wiry pulse is straight and string-like. The *Yi Zong Jin Jian* (Golden Mirror of the Medical Tradition) states, "Patients with tetany present with spasm or rigidity symptoms and a tight, wiry pulse".

[2] *Zhi Shang Xia Xing*: The straight and wiry pulsation is felt in all the three regions (*Cun, Guan and Chi*). Here the word *Shang* refers to the *Cun* position, and the word *Xia* refers to the *Chi* position.

Interpretations

In tetany patients, the pulse is tight and wiry in all the three regions (*Cun*, *Guan* and *Chi*) when heavily pressed. The *Mai Jing* (Pulse Classic) states, "The pulse of tetany patients is deep, hidden and forceful in all the three regions".

*****

[10] 痉病有灸疮〔1〕，难治。

Annotations

[1] *Jiu Chuang*: Sores or ulcers due to skin burns from moxibustion. Spasm or convulsions resulting from moxibustion sores is more difficult to cure. The *Yi Xue Gang Mu* (Compendium of Medicine) states, "Spasticity due to moxibustion sores is tetanus".

Interpretations

Tetany coupled with moxibustion sores is difficult to cure.

*****

[11] 太阳病，其证备，身体强[1]，几几然，脉反沉迟[2]，此为痉，栝蒌桂枝汤[3]主之。栝蒌桂枝汤方：栝蒌根二两桂枝三两芍药三两甘草二两生姜三两大枣十二枚 右六味，以水九升，煮取三升。分温三服，取微汗。汗不出，食顷，啜热粥发之。

Annotations

[1] *Tai Yang Bing, Qi Zheng Bei, Shen Ti Qiang*: "*Tai Yang Bing, Qi Zheng Bei*" refer to fever, sweating or aversion to wind in exterior deficiency syndrome. "*Shen Ti Qiang*" refers to neck rigidity and opisthotonos.

[2] *Mai Fan Chen Chi*: Generally, the pulse in tetany is wiry and tight. Damage to body fluids may cause a deep, slow pulse; however, the pulse is still, at the same time, wiry and tight.

[3] *Gua Lou Gui Zhi Tang* (Trichosanthis and Cinnamon Twig Decoction): *Gou Lou Gen* (Radix Trichosanthis) + *Gui Zhi Tang* (Cinnamon Twig Decoction), a modified formula to relax muscles, remove pathogenic factors, regenerate fluids and nourish the tendons/sinews.

Interpretations

In patients with Taiyang syndrome, symptoms of exterior deficiency syndrome (fever, sweating and aversion to wind) combined with notable neck/back rigidity as well as a deep, slow pulse indicate a soft tetany, which should be treated with *Gua Lou Gui Zhi Tang* (Trichosanthis and Cinnamon Twig Decoction).

Gua Lou Gui Zhi Tang

[Ingredients]

栝蒌根	*guā lóu gēn*	2 *liǎng*	Radix Trichosanthis
桂枝	*guì zhī*	3 *liǎng*	Ramulus Cinnamomi
芍药	*sháo yào*	3 *liǎng*	Radix Paeoniae
甘草	*gān cǎo*	2 *liǎng*	Radix et Rhizoma Glycyrrhizae
生姜	*shēng jiāng*	3 *liǎng*	Rhizoma Zingiberis Recens
大枣	*dà zǎo*	12 pieces	Fructus Jujubae

Decoct the above ingredients in nine *shēng* of water to get three *shēng*. Drink the decoction when it is warm in three times (doses) to induce mild sweating. If the patients do not sweat, eat hot porridge to promote sweating.

*****

[12] 太阳病，无汗而小便反少〔1〕，气上冲胸〔2〕，口噤不得语，欲作刚痉，葛根汤〔3〕主之。

葛根汤方：葛根四两，麻黄三两去节，桂枝二两去皮，芍药二两，甘草二两炙，生姜三两，大枣十二枚，右七味。咀，以水一升，先煮麻黄、葛根。减二升，去沫。内诸药，煮取三升，去滓。温服一升。覆取微似汗，不须啜粥。余如桂枝汤法将息及禁忌。

Annotations

[1] *Xiao Bian Fan Shao:* Scanty urine or urine retention due to contracture of the lower abdomen.

[2] *Qi Shang Chong Xiong:* Qi rushing up to the chest.

[3] *Ge Gen Tang* (Pueraria Decoction): A formula to induce sweating, release the exterior, regenerate fluids and relax tendons/sinews.

Interpretations

In patients with Taiyang syndrome, symptoms of exterior excess syndrome (fever, aversion to cold and absence of sweating), scanty urine, qi rushing up to the chest, and lockjaw are warning signs of a hard tetany, which should be treated with *Ge Gen Tang* (Pueraria Decoction).

Ge Gen Tang

[Ingredients]

葛根	*gé gēn*	4 *liǎng*	Radix Puerariae Lobatae
麻黄	*má huáng*	3 *liǎng*	Herba Ephedrae
桂枝	*guì zhī*	2 *liǎng*	Ramulus Cinnamomi
芍药	*sháo yào*	2 *liǎng*	Radix Paeoniae
炙甘草	*zhì gān cǎo*	2 *liǎng*	Radix et Rhizoma Glycyrrhizae Praeparata
生姜	*shēng jiāng*	3 *liǎng*	Rhizoma Zingiberis Recens
大枣	*dà zǎo*	12 pieces	Fructus Jujubae

Chop up the above ingredients. Decoct *Ma Huang* and *Ge Gen* in one *Dou* of water to get eight *shēng*. Then remove the foam and add the rest of the ingredients to decoct and get three *shēng*. Remove the dregs and take one *shēng* of the decoction when it is warm for each dose. Then cover the patient with bedclothes to induce mild sweating. The cautionary notes and contraindications are the same as *Gui Zhi Tang*. If the patient sweats and recovers after one dose, he/she does not need to take the remaining two doses. If the patient does not sweat, take another dose. If it still doesn't work, take another dose. The three doses need to be taken within 6 hours. For severe cases, the patient needs to take the decoction both day and night for a 24-hour observation. During the treatment, the patient needs to stay away from raw, cold, greasy or spicy food such as meat, alcohol, cheese, union and garlic.

*****

[13] 痉〔1〕为病一本痉字上有刚字。胸满〔2〕，口噤，卧不着席〔3〕，脚挛急，必齿齘〔4〕，可与大承气汤〔5〕。

大承气汤方：大黄四两酒洗，厚朴半斤炙去皮，枳实五枚炙，芒硝三合，右四味，以水一斗，先煮二物，取五升，去滓，内大黄，煮取二升，去滓。内芒硝，更上火微一二弗。分温再服，得下止服。

Annotations

[1] *Jing*: Tetany. In the *Yu Han Jing* (Jade Case Classic) and *Mai Jing* (the Pulse Classic), *Jing* is recorded as *Gang Jing* (hard tetany).

[2] *Xiong Man*: Chest tightness. According to the *Jin Gui Yao Lüè Fang Lun Kao Zheng* (Textual Research on Prescriptions in the 'Essentials from the Golden Cabinet'), the word *Man* here means "tightness" instead of "fullness", which is often coupled with a distending sensation.

[3] *Wo Bu Zhuo Xi*: Severe opisthotonos.

[4] *Xie Chi*: Teeth grinding.

[5] *Da Cheng Qi Tang* (Major Purgative Decoction): A formula to unblock *Fu*-organs, clear heat, promote bowel movements and preserve yin fluids. However, this formula is symptom-oriented for tetany. According to the *Yi Men Fa Lǜ* (Precepts for Physicians), this is a "narrow escape" method.

Interpretations

Da Cheng Qi Tang (Major Purgative Decoction) can be prescribed for patients with tetany present with chest tightness (difficulty breathing), clenched jaw, teeth grinding, severe opisthotonos, and spasticity of the four limbs.

Da Cheng Qi Tang

[Ingredients]

大黄	*dà huáng*	4 *liǎng*	Radix et Rhizoma Rhei (soaked in wine)
厚朴	*hòu pò*	0.5 *jīn*	Cortex Magnoliae Officinalis
枳实	*zhǐ shí*	5	Fructus Aurantii Immaturus Praeparata
芒硝	*máng xiāo*	3 *gě*	Natrii Sulfas

Decoct *Hou Po* and *Zhi Shi* in one *Dou* of water to get five *shēng*. Remove the dregs and add *Da Huang* to decoct and get two *shēng*. Then add *Mang Xiao* and decoct until boiling (once or twice). Take the decoction when it is warm in two times (doses). Stop taking the formula as soon as the constipation is alleviated.

*****

[14] 太阳病，关节疼痛而烦〔1〕，脉沉而细〔2〕一作缓者，此名湿痹〔3〕。《玉函》云：中湿。湿痹之候，小便不利，大便反快〔4〕，但当利其小便〔5〕。

Annotations

[1] *Guan Jie Teng Tong Er Fan*: Severe joint pain.

[2] *Mai Chen Er Xi*: A deep, thready pulse. The *Yu Han Jing* (Jade Case Classic) and *Mai Jing* (the Pulse Classic) record that "the pulse is deep and mildly slow". Generally, the pulse is superficial in an exterior Taiyang syndrome; however, external contraction of dampness (characterized by heaviness, turbidity and stickiness) causes the pulse to be deep, thready or mildly slow.

[3] *Shi Bi*: As previously mentioned, patients present with severe joint pain due to retention of dampness in the exterior, it does not mean damp-impediment. Actually, both the *Yu Han Jing* (Jade Case Classic) and *Mai Jing* (the Pulse Classic) record, "*Ci Ming Zhong Shi* (it is known as retention of dampness)".

[4] *Shi Bi Zhi Hou, Xiao Bian Bu Li, Da Bian Fan Kuai*: Major symptoms of damp impediment (internal retention of dampness) are inhibited urination and free passing of stools.

[5] *Dan Dang Li Qi Xiao Bian*: The treatment strategy for inhibited urination is to promote urination, which helps to resolve dampness, unblock yang qi and restore qi transformation. Li Dongyuan (1180–1251), a well-known physician states, "It's essential to promote urination to resolve dampness".

Interpretations

In patients with exterior Taiyang syndrome, symptoms of fever and aversion to cold, coupled with severe joint pain, a deep, thready or deep, mildly slow pulse indicate retention of dampness. However, damp impediment (internal retention of dampness) is characterized by inhibited urination and free passing of stools. The treatment strategy for damp impediment is to promote urination.

*****

[15] 湿家〔1〕之为病，一身尽疼一云疼烦，发热，身色如熏黄〔2〕也。

Annotations

[1] *Shi Jia*: Patients who are affected by dampness.

[2] *Xun Huang*: A smoky, yellow skin color. The *Jin Gui Yao Lüè Xin Dian* (Personal Standards for the 'Essentials from the Golden Cabinet') records, "Heat intertwined with dampness may cause a smoky, yellow skin color. A dark, yellow color results from damp-qi stagnation".

Interpretations

Patients who are affected by damp-heat accumulation present with severe body ache, fever and a smoky, yellow skin color.

*****

[16] 湿家，其人但头汗出，背强，欲得被覆向火[1]。若下之早则哕[2]，或胸满，小便不利一云利，舌上如胎[3]者，以丹田[4]有热，胸上有寒，渴欲得饮而不能饮，则口燥烦也。

Annotations

[1] *Yu De Bei Fu Xiang Huo*: The aversion to cold is so severe that patients desire to be covered with bedclothes or close to the fire to stay warm.

[2] *Yue*: Hiccups or vomiting.

[3] *She Shang Ru Tai*: A dark tongue coating that resembles coal dust.

[4] *Dan Tian*: The name of an acupuncture point located in the abdomen below the umbilicus. It may refer to Qihai (Ren 6), Shimen (Ren 5), Guanyuan (Ren 4) and Zhongji (Ren 3). Here it refers to the lower abdomen.

Interpretations

Patients who are affected by dampness may present with sweats on the head alone, back rigidity and severe aversion to cold (with a desire to be covered with bedclothes or close to the fire to stay warm). If doctors mistake dampness (based on the sweats on the head) for interior heat and use purgation method, patients may develop hiccups/vomiting, abdominal fullness/distension, inhibited urination and a dark tongue coating that resembles coal dust. This is because there is heat in the lower abdomen but cold-dampness in the chest. In addition, patients may also experience an inability to drink despite a desire for water and subsequently, an extremely dry mouth.

*****

[17] 湿家下之[1]，额上汗出，微喘[2]，小便利一云不利[3]者死。若下利不止[4]者，亦死。

Annotations

[1] *Shi Jia Zhi Xia*: Wrong use of purgation method for dampness. The *Jin Gui Yao Lüè Xin Dian* (Personal Standards for the 'Essentials from the Golden Cabinet') records, "The treatment strategy for dampness in the exterior is to induce sweating, whereas the strategy for dampness in the interior is to promote urination. Purgation method is only used for damp-heat accumulation".

[2] *E Shang Han Chu, Wei Chuan*: Sweating on the forehead and mild panting due to damage to interior yang by purgation method.

[3] *Xiao Bian Li, Yi Yun Bu Li*: Urinary incontinence or inhibited urination.

[4] *Xia Li Bu Zhi*: Fecal incontinence, a critical sign of yin-yang separation.

Interpretations

For patients who are affected by dampness, sweating on the forehead, panting, urinary incontinence/inhibited urination due to inappropriate use of purgation method are life-threatening signs. Fecal incontinence is also a critical sign.

*****

[18] 风湿相搏〔1〕，一身尽疼痛，法当汗出而解，值天阴雨不止，医云：此可发汗。汗之，病不愈者，何也？盖发其汗，汗大出者，但风气〔2〕去，湿气〔3〕在，是故不愈也。若治风湿者，发其汗，但微微似欲出汗者，风湿俱去也。

Annotations

[1] *Feng Shi Xiang Bo*: Combined pathogenic wind and cold. According to the *Shang Han Lun Wen Zi Kao* (Textual Research on Descriptions in 'Treatise on Cold Damage'), the word *Xiang* here means "combined" instead of "mutual". The word *Bo* means attack. As a result,

Xiang Bo means wind and dampness in combination instead of mutual contending".

[2] *Feng Qi:* Pathogenic wind.

[3] *Shi Qi*: Pathogenic dampness.

Interpretations

Patients who are affected by wind and dampness in combination may present with body ache. Usually, the pain can be alleviated by inducing sweating. However, during a run of wet weather (external humidity affects the removal of dampness within the body), patients fail to recovery after sweating. Why is this?

The Master answered: Profuse sweating helps to remove wind out of the body; however, dampness retains within the body. This is why the patients fail to recovery. To remove wind and resolve dampness, it's advisable to induce mild but persistent sweating.

*****

[19] 湿家病身疼发热，面黄而喘〔1〕。头痛鼻塞而烦，其脉大〔2〕，自能饮食，腹中和无病。病在头中寒湿，故鼻塞。内药鼻中〔3〕则愈。

Annotations

[1] *Shi Jia Bing, Shen Tong Fa Re, Mian Huang Er Chuan*: Dampness may cause body ache, fever, a yellow complexion and panting. These descriptions are not consistent with "*Bing Zai Tou Zhong Han Shi* (cold-dampness in the head)" and "*Nei Yao Bi Zhong Ze Yu* (the recovery can be achieved by placing the medicine into the nostrils)". These eleven words are not mentioned in the text of *Mai Jing* (the Pulse Classic).

[2] *Mai Da:* A wide, large pulse that indicates heat.

[3] *Nei Yao Bi Zhong*: An external therapy, i.e., nasal administration. The *Qian Jin Yao Fang Bi Bing* (Nasal Problems, Important Formulas Worth a Thousand Gold Pieces) records a formula for nasal congestion

with thin, clear discharge: *Tong Cao* (Important Formulas Worth a Thousand Gold Pieces), *Xin Yi* (Flos Magnoliae), *Xi Xin* (Radix et Rhizoma Asari), *Gan Sui* (Radix Kansui), *Gui Xin* (Ramulus Cinnamomi), *Chuan Xiong* (Rhizoma Chuanxiong) and *Fu Zi* (Radix Aconiti Lateralis Praeparata). Grind these ingredients into a fine powder. Mix with honey and then place the wrapped honeyed pills into the nostrils.

Interpretations

Patients who are affected by dampness may experience body ache, fever, a sallow complexion and panting. Alternatively, they may also present with headache, severe nasal congestion, a large pulse, normal appetite, and absence of abdominal discomfort. This is cold-dampness in the head characterized by nasal congestion (with runny nose). This condition can be treated with an external therapy—placing medicine into the nostrils.

*****

[20] 湿家身烦疼，可与麻黄加术汤〔1〕，发其汗为宜，慎不可以火攻〔2〕之。

麻黄加术汤方：麻黄三两去节，桂枝二两去皮,甘草一两炙，杏仁七十个去皮尖，白术四两，右五味，以水九升，先煮麻黄，减二升，去上沫，内诸药，煮取二升半，去滓。温服八合。

覆取微似汗。

Annotations

[1] *Ma Huang Jia Zhu Tang*: *Ma Huang Tang* (Ephedra Decoction) + *Bai Zhu* (Rhizoma Atractylodis Macrocephalae). The *Ma Huang Tang* has a strong effect on inducing sweating (to remove wind-cold). With the addition of *Bai Zhu*, the modified formula mildly induces sweating, removes cold and resolves dampness. *Bai Zhu* acts to stop sweating and resolve dampness. According to the *Yi Men Fa Lǜ* (Precepts for Physicians), "*Bai Zhu* helps to counterbalance the strong effect of *Ma*

Huang in inducing sweating, whereas *Ma Huang* helps *Bai Zhu* to resolve dampness".

[2] *Huo Gong:* An ancient sweat-inducing method using warming needle, fumigation and hot compression. This method promotes sweating and circulates qi and blood. It is no longer used today because it may damage the bodily fluids.

Interpretations

For patients who are affected by cold-dampness may experience severe body ache (coupled with fever, aversion to cold and absence of sweating), *Ma Huang Jia Zhu Tang* (Ephedra Decoction plus white atractylodes) can be used to induce mild sweating. Cautionary note: It's not advisable to induce excessive sweating.

Ma Huang Jia Zhu Tang

[Ingredients]

麻黄	*má huáng*	3 *liǎng*	Herba Ephedrae
桂枝	*guì zhī*	2 *liǎng*	Ramulus Cinnamomi
炙甘草	*zhì gān cǎo*	1 *liǎng*	Radix et Rhizoma Glycyrrhizae Praeparata
杏仁	*xìng rén*	70 pieces	Semen Armeniacae Amarum
白术	*bái zhú*	4 *liǎng*	Rhizoma Atractylodis Macrocephalae

Decoct *Ma Huang* first in nine *shēng* of water and get seven *shēng*. Remove the dregs and add the rest four ingredients to decoct and get two and a half *shēng*. Remove the dregs and take eight *gě* (per dose) of the decoction when it is warm. Then cover the patient with bedclothes to induce mild sweating.

*****

[21] 病者一身尽疼，发热，日晡[1]所剧者，名风湿[2]。此病伤于汗出当风，或久伤取冷所致也。可与麻黄杏仁薏苡甘草汤[3]。

麻黄杏仁薏苡甘草汤方：麻黄去节，半两，汤泡，甘草一两炙，薏苡仁半两，杏仁十个，去皮尖，炒右锉麻豆大，每服四钱匕，水盏半，煮八分，去滓。温服。有微汗，避风。

Annotations

[1] *Ri Bu*: 3-5 PM.

[2] *Feng Shi*: Wind-dampness characterized by fever and body ache.

[3] *Ma Huang Xing Ren Yi Yi Gan Cao Tang* (Ephedrae, Armeniacae, Coicis and Glycyrrhizae Decoction): A formula to release the exterior, remove wind, resolve dampness and clear heat.

Interpretations

Body ache and fever that aggravates in the late afternoon are symptoms of wind-dampness. Contributing factors include exposure to wind-cold during sweating or eating raw/cold food for a long period of time. This condition can be treated with *Ma Huang Xing Ren Yi Yi Gan Cao Tang* (Ephedrae, Armeniacae, Coicis and Glycyrrhizae Decoction).

Ma Huang Xing Ren Yi Yi Gan Cao Tang

[Ingredients]

麻黄	*má huáng*	0.5 *liǎng*	Herba Ephedrae (nodes removed and water-soaked)
炙甘草	*zhì gān cǎo*	1 *liǎng*	Radix et Rhizoma Glycyrrhizae Praeparata
薏苡仁	*yì yǐ rén*	0.5 *liǎng*	Semen Coicis
杏仁	*xìng rén*	10 pieces	Semen Armeniacae Amarum (Skin and tips removed and fried)

Grind the above ingredients into the size of hemp seeds. For each dose, add four coin-spoonfuls (approximately 8g) of the ingredients to one and a half cups of water to get eight *fen*. Remove the dregs and take the decoction when it is warm. It's important for the patient to avoid exposure to wind-cold after mild sweating from taking the decoction.

*****

[22] 风湿，脉浮〔1〕、身重〔2〕、汗出恶风〔3〕者，防己黄芪汤〔4〕主之。

防己黄芪汤方：防己一两，甘草半两炒，白术七钱半，黄芪一两一分，去芦右剉麻豆大，每抄五钱匕，生姜四片，大枣一枚，水盏半，煎八分，去滓。温服。良久再服。喘者加麻黄半两，胃中不和者加芍药三分。气上冲者加桂枝三分，下有陈寒者加细辛三分。服后当如虫行皮中〔5〕，从腰下如冰，后坐被上，又以一被绕腰以下，温令微汗，差。

Annotations

[1] *Mai Fu*: A superficial pulse indicating pathogenic factors affecting the exterior.

[2] *Shen Zhong*: A heavy sensation (no pain) of the body, probably coupled with edema, indicating wind-dampness affecting the exterior.

[3] *Han Chu E Feng*: Aversion to wind after sweating (no fever) indicating qi deficiency.

[4] *Fang Ji Huang Qi Tang* (Stephania Root and Astragalus Decoction): A formula to supplement qi and resolve dampness.

[5] *Ru Chong Xing Pi Zhong*: A sensation that resembles small insects crawling on/under the skin, indicating a gradual recovery of health conditions.

Interpretations

A superficial pulse, a heavy sensation of the body (edema may also be present), and aversion to wind after sweating due to wind-dampness affecting the exterior can be treated with *Fang Ji Huang Qi Tang* (Stephania Root and Astragalus Decoction).

Fang Ji Huang Qi Tang

[Ingredients]

防己	*fáng jǐ*	1 *liǎng*	Radix Stephaniae Tetrandrae
甘草	*gān cǎo*	0.5 *liǎng*	Radix et Rhizoma Glycyrrhizae (stir-fried)
白术	*bái zhú*	7.5 *qián*	Rhizoma Atractylodis Macrocephalae
黄芪	*huáng qí*	10 (top removed)	Radix Astragali

Grind the above ingredients into the size of hemp seeds. For each dose, add five coin-spoonfuls (approximately 10g) of the ingredients, four slices of fresh ginger and one jujube fruit to one and a half cups of water to get eight *fen*. Remove the dregs and take the decoction when it is warm. Take the second dose after a couple of hours.

Modifications

✓ For panting, add *Ma Huang* (Herba Ephedrae) (0.5 *liǎng*).

✓ For stomach discomfort, add *Shao Yao* (Radix Paeoniae) (3 *fen*).

✓ For adverse ascending of pathogenic qi, add *Gui Zhi* (Ramulus Cinnamomi) (3 *fen*).

✓ For a cold sensation from the waist down, add *Xi Xin* (Radix et Rhizoma Asari) (3 *fen*).

After taking the decoction, patients may experience a sensation of small insects crawling on/under the skin. Patients with an extremely cold sensation from the waist down need to sit on a bed cover and cover with another bedcover around the waist to induce mild sweating. In this way, patients may recover.

*****

[23] 伤寒八九日，风湿相搏〔1〕，身体疼烦，不能自转侧。不呕不渴〔2〕，脉浮虚而〔3〕者，桂枝附子汤〔4〕主之。若大便坚，小便自利〔5〕者，去桂加白术汤〔6〕主之。

桂枝附子汤方：桂枝四两去皮，生姜三两切,附子三枚，炮去皮，破片，甘草三两炙，大枣十二枚擘右五味，以水六升，煮取二升，去滓。分温三服。

白术附子汤方：白术二两附子一枚半，炮，去皮甘草一两炙生姜一两半切大枣六枚右五味，以水三升，煮取一升，去滓。分温三服。一服觉身痹〔7〕，半日许再服，三服都尽，其人如冒状〔8〕，勿怪，即是术，附并走皮中，逐水气，未得除故耳。

Annotations

[1] *Shang Han Ba Jiu Ri, Feng Shi Xiang Bo:* After cold affects the body for eight or nine days (fever, aversion to wind and sweating), patients are additionally exposure to wind-dampness.

[2] *Bu Ou Bu Ke*: Neither vomiting (indicating that pathogenic factors still remaining in the exterior) nor thirst (indicating that dampness has not transformed into heat).

[3] *Mai Fu Xu Er*: A superficial and deficient pulse, indicating wind-dampness remaining in the exterior, coupled with yang deficiency.

[4] *Gui Zhi Fu Zi Tang* (Cinnamon Twig and Aconite Decoction): A formula to remove wind, resolve dampness, warms meridians and dissipate cold.

[5] *Da Bian Jian, Xiao Bian Zi Li*: Normal bowel and bladder movements, indicating pathogenic factors remaining in the exterior.

[6] *Qu Gui Jia Bai Zhu Tang* (aka *Bai Zhu Fu Zi Tang*) (Atractylodes Macrocephala and Aconite Decoction): A formula to resolve dampness and dissipate cold.

[7] *Shen Bi*: Skin numbness.

[8] *Ru Mao Zhuang*: Dizziness and blurred vision.

Interpretations

After pathogenic cold affects the body for eight or nine days (fever, aversion to wind and sweating), patients are additionally exposed to wind-dampness, manifesting as severe body ache, inability to turn sides, absence of vomiting or thirst, and a superficial, deficient and hesitant pulse. This condition can be treated with *Gui Zhi Fu Zi Tang* (Cinnamon Twig and Aconite Decoction). If patients have normal bowel and bladder movements, remove *Gui Zhi* (Cinnamon Twig) and add *Bai Zhu* (Rhizoma Atractylodis Macrocephalae) to the formula.

Gui Zhi Fu Zi Tang

[Ingredients]

桂枝	*guì zhī*	4 *liǎng*	Ramulus Cinnamomi (bark removed)
生姜	*shēng jiāng*	3 *liǎng*	Rhizoma Zingiberis Recens (slices)
附子	*fù zǐ*	3 pieces	Radix Aconiti Lateralis Praeparata (8 slices)
炙甘草	*zhì gān cǎo*	2 *liǎng*	Radix et Rhizoma Glycyrrhizae Praeparata
大枣	*dà zǎo*	12 pieces	Fructus Jujubae

Decoct the above ingredients in six *shēng* of water to get two *shēng*. Remove the dregs and divide the decoction into three doses. Take the decoction when it is warm.

Bai Zhu Fu Zi Tang

[Ingredients]

白术	*bái zhú*	2 *liǎng*	Rhizoma Atractylodis Macrocephalae
生姜	*shēng jiāng*	1 *liǎng*	Rhizoma Zingiberis Recens (slice)
附子	*fù zǐ*	1.5 pieces	Radix Aconiti Lateralis Praeparata (8 slices)
炙甘草	*zhì gān cǎo*	1 *liǎng*	Radix et Rhizoma Glycyrrhizae Praeparata
大枣	*dà zǎo*	6 pieces	Fructus Jujubae

Decoct the above ingredients in three *shēng* of water to get one *shēng*. Remove the dregs and divide the decoction into three doses. Take the decoction when it is warm. After the first dose, patients may feel skin numbness. Take another dose after approximately 6 hours. After the three doses, patients may experience dizziness and blurred vision, which are normal reactions when *Bai Zhu* (Rhizoma Atractylodis Macrocephalae) and *Fu Zi* (Radix Aconiti Lateralis Praeparata) move under the skin to remove cold and resolve dampness.

*****

[24] 风湿相搏，骨节疼烦，掣痛不得屈伸，近之则痛剧，汗出、短气、小便不利，恶风不欲去衣，或身微肿者。甘草附子汤[1]主之。

甘草附子汤方：甘草二两炙，附子二枚，炮，去皮，白术二两，桂枝四两去皮　右四味，以水六升，煮取三升，去滓。温服一升，日三服。初服得微汗则解，能食。汗出复烦者，服五合。恐一升多者，服六七合为妙。

Annotations

[1] *Gan Cao Fu Zi Tang* (Licorice and Aconite Decoction): A basic formula for *Bi*-impediment syndrome due to wind, cold and dampness. Actions: Warms yang, removes wind and resolves dampness.

Interpretations

Wind-dampness affecting the exterior may cause severe joint pain, impaired flexion and extension, and tenderness. Other symptoms include sweating, shortness of breath, inhibited urination, severe aversion to wind (reluctance to remove clothing in severe cases) and mild edema. This condition can be treated with *Gan Cao Fu Zi Tang* (Licorice and Aconite Decoction).

Gan Cao Fu Zi Tang

[Ingredients]

炙甘草	*zhì gān cǎo*	2 *liǎng*	Radix et Rhizoma Glycyrrhizae Praeparata
附子	*fù zǐ*	2 pieces	Radix Aconiti Lateralis Praeparata (skin removed)
白术	*bái zhú*	2 *liǎng*	Rhizoma Atractylodis Macrocephalae
桂枝	*guì zhī*	4 *liǎng*	Ramulus Cinnamomi (bark removed)

Decoct the above ingredients in six *shēng* of water to get three *shēng*. Remove the dregs and divide the decoction into three doses. Take the decoction when it is warm. Mild sweating after taking the formula helps to alleviate symptoms and increase the appetite. In case the severe pain persists after sweating, take another five *gě* of the decoction. If you fear one *shēng* is too much for one dose, take six or seven *gě*.

*****

[25] 太阳中暍[1]，发热恶寒，身重而疼痛，其脉弦细芤迟[2]。小便已，洒洒然毛耸[3]，手足逆冷。小有劳，身即热，口前开板齿燥[4]。若发其汗，则其恶寒甚；加温针[5]，则发热甚；数下之，则淋甚[6]。

Annotations

[1] *Zhong Ye:* Heat stroke characterized by fever, excessive thirst, sweating and a deficient pulse.

[2] *Mai Xian Xi Kong Chi*: A wiry, thready, hollow (like a scallion-stalk) and slow pulse. Heat consuming yang qi causes a wiry, thready pulse. Sweating consuming yin fluids causes a hollow, slow pulse.

[3] *Sa Sa Ran Mao Song*: Shivering that resembles a sensation of pouring water over the body. *Mao Song* means the body hair standing on end.

[4] *Kou Qian Kan Ban Chi Zao*: Breathing with an open mouth, and dryness of the front teeth.

[5] *Wen Zhen*: A combination of acupuncture and moxibustion, known as warming needle therapy.

[6] *Ze Lin*: Dribbling urine and painful urination.

Interpretations

Summer heat affecting the exterior may cause fever, chills and a wiry, thready or hollow (like scallion stalk), slow pulse. Since summer heat is liable to associate itself with dampness, patients may also experience body ache with a heavy sensation. After urination, patients may experience shivering with body hair standing on end and cold hands/feet. Mild physical exertion may trigger fever, breathing with an open mouth and dryness of the front teeth. Sweat-inducing method may aggravate the condition. Warming needle therapy may aggravate the fever. Repeated heat-clearing method may cause scanty, dribbling urine and painful urination.

*****

[26] 太阳中热[1]者，暍是也。汗出、恶寒、身热而渴。白虎加人参汤[2]主之。

白虎加人参汤方：知母六两，石膏一斤碎，甘草二两，粳米六合，人参三两，右五味，以水一斗，煮米熟汤成，去滓，温服一升，日三服。

Annotations

[1] *Zhong Re:* aka Zhong Ye, heat stroke.

[2] *Bai Hu Jia Ren Shen Tang* (White Tiger Decoction Plus Ginseng): A formula to clear summer heat and supplement qi and yin.

Interpretations

Summer heat affecting the exterior may cause sweating, aversion to cold (heat consuming qi), fever and thirst (heat consuming bodily fluids). This condition can be treated with *Bai Hu Jia Ren Shen Tang* (White Tiger Decoction Plus Ginseng).

Bai Hu Jia Ren Shen Tang

[Ingredients]

知母	*zhī mŭ*	6 *liăng*	Rhizoma Anemarrhenae
石膏	*shí gāo*	1 *jīn*	Gypsum Fibrosum
甘草	*gān căo*	2 *liăng*	Radix et Rhizoma Glycyrrhizae
粳米	*jīng mĭ*	6 *gĕ*	Oryza Sativa L.
人参	*rén shēn*	3 *liăng*	Radix et Rhizoma Ginseng

Decoct the above ingredients in one *Dou* of water until the rice is cooked. Remove the dregs and take 1 *shēng* for each dose, 3 doses in total.

*****

[27] 太阳中暍，身热疼重，而脉微弱[1]，此以夏月伤冷水，水行皮中所致也。一物瓜蒂汤[2]主之。

一物瓜蒂汤方：瓜蒂二七，个右锉，以水一升，煮取五合，去滓，顿服[3]。

Annotations

[1] *Mai Wei Ruo:* A mildly thready, deep and weak pulse due to summer heat consuming qi and yin.

[2] *Yi Wu Gua Di Tang* (Melon Stalk Decoction): Formulas that use melon stalk are recorded four times in the books by Zhang Zhongjing. Three formulas (a small dose of powder) are used to induce sweating. Here a large dose of melon stalk was used for summer-heat stroke. The mechanism needs further study, because melon stalk is toxic.

[3] *Dun Fu*: Drink up at a draught.

Interpretations

Summer heat affecting the exterior may cause fever, body ache with a heavy sensation, and a mildly thready and weak pulse. This is caused by over-drinking of cold water and retention of water-dampness in the exterior. This condition can be treated with *Yi Wu Gua Di Tang* (Melon Stalk Decoction).

Cut 27 melon stalks and decoct with water to get five *gě*. Remove the dregs and drink up at a draught.

百合狐惑阴阳毒病证治第三
Chapter 3 *Bai He*, *Hu Huo* and Yin-Yang Toxin—Patterns and Treatment

Overview

This chapter discusses three conditions with unusual names—Bai He (Lily disease), Hu Huo (Behcet's syndrome) and yin-yang toxin. The *Jin Gui Yao Lüè Qian Zhu* (Simple Annotation on the 'Essentials from the Golden Cabinet') states, "*Bai He* (Lily disease), *Hu Huo* (Behcet's syndrome) and yin-yang toxin are all extraordinary conditions". The three conditions are discussed together because they are all associated with externally contracted febrile diseases and share common signs and symptoms. Patients with Lily disease or Behcet's syndrome may present with difficulty sleeping and poor appetite. Patients with Behcet's syndrome and yin-yang toxin may present with sore throat.

*****

[01] 论曰：百合病〔1〕者，百脉一宗，悉致其病〔2〕也。意欲食，复不能食，常默默〔3〕，欲卧不能卧，欲行不能行。饮食或有美时，或有不用闻食臭时。如寒无寒，如热无热。口苦，小便赤。诸药不能治，得药则剧吐利〔4〕，如有神灵者。身形如和〔5〕，其脉微数〔6〕。

每溺时头痛者，六十日乃愈；若溺时头不痛淅然〔7〕者，四十日愈；若溺快然〔8〕，但头眩者，二十日愈。其证或未病而预见，或病四五日而出，或病二十日或一月微见者，各随证治之。

Annotations

[1] *Bai He Bing*: Lily disease. It often occurs as a result of internal heat due to yin deficiency after febrile diseases. This condition is characterized by poor appetite, an inability to sleep or walk, a bitter mouth, dark-yellow urine, and a mildly rapid pulse. It is named the lily disease because *Bai He* (Bulbus Lilii) is primarily used to treat this condition. The *Wen Re Jing Wei* (Warp and Woof of Warm-Heat Diseases) states, "Lily diseases are associated with seasonal pandemic...such as epidemic warm heat". In modern medicine, it is similar to post-infectious (febrile) disease syndrome.

[2] *Bai Mai Yi Zong, Xi Zhi Qi Bing*: Despite a variety of symptoms involving all meridians, they share the same root cause.

[3] *Mo Mo:* Reserved and reluctance to talk.

[4] *Ju Tu Li*: Aggravated condition.

[5] *Shen Xing Ru He*: Having normal body shape.

[6] *Mai Wei Shuo*: A mildly thready and rapid pulse (internal heat due to yin deficiency).

[7] *Xi Ran*: *Tou Xi Xi Ran* recorded in the *Jin Gui Yao Lüè* (Supplement to and Corrections on Simple Annotation on the 'Essentials from the Golden Cabinet'), meaning dizziness and tinnitus.

[8] *Ni Kuai Ran*: Uninhibited urination (the color of urine is no longer reddish).

Interpretations

The Medical Classic states, "For patients with lily disease, symptoms may be associated with any meridians. However, they all share a same root cause. Patients may have a desire to eat but does not want to swallow food, and they are often reserved and reluctance to talk. They want to sleep but get restlessness when they lie down. They want to move around but cannot walk far. They sometimes enjoy the delicious food but sometimes cannot even bear the smell of food. They sometimes feel cold and sometimes hot, and yet they have neither cold nor heat. In addition, they may have a bitter taste in the mouth and reddish urine. They do not respond to any medicine. Instead, the symptoms aggravated after taking medicine, as if they were possessed by a spirit. Despite all the symptoms, they appear completely normal in body shape; however, their pulse is mildly thready and rapid".

(This condition has a favorable prognosis and generally resolves within 1 or 2 months. The duration is related to the retention of pathogenic factors and severity of yin deficiency-related heat). Patients with reddish urine coupled with headache need sixty days to recover. Patients with reddish urine coupled with dizziness and tinnitus need forty days to recover. Patients with uninhibited urination (no reddish urine) coupled with dizziness only need twenty days to recover.

Symptoms such as headache or dizziness may occur before the occurrence of lily disease. Some patients may experience these symptoms four to five days after the occurrence, and some may experience mild symptoms twenty days or around one month after the occurrence. It's advisable to treat patients according to individual signs and symptoms.

*****

[02] 百合病，发汗后〔1〕者，百合知母汤〔2〕主之。

百合知母汤方：百合七枚擘， 知母三两切,右先以水洗百合，渍一宿，当白沫出，去其水，更以泉水[3]二升，煎取一升，去滓；别以泉水二升，煎知母，取一升，去滓。后合和，煎取一升五合。分温再服。

Annotations

[1] *Fa Han Hou*: Inappropriate use of sweating method.

[2] *Bai He Zhi Mu Tang* (Lily Bulb and Anemarrhenae Decoction): A formula to clear the heart, calm the mind, regenerate fluids and alleviate thirst.

[3] *Quan Shui*: Uncontaminated well water or spring water. Actions: Clears the lung, nourishes the stomach and regenerates fluids.

Interpretations

After the inappropriate use of sweating method, patients with lily disease may present with restlessness and thirst due to aggravated deficiency heat. These symptoms can be treated with *Bai He Zhi Mu Tang* (Lily Bulb and Anemarrhenae Decoction).

Bai He Zhi Mu Tang

[Ingredients]

百合	*bǎi hé*	7 pieces	Bulbus Lilii (break)
知母	*zhī mǔ*	6 *liǎng*	Rhizoma Anemarrhenae (cut)

Wash *Bai He* with clean water, and then soak in clean water overnight. Discard the water when white foam is present. Decoct *Bai He* in two *shēng* of spring water to get one *shēng* and remove the dregs. Decoct *Zhi Mu* with another two *shēng* of spring water to get one *shēng* and remove the dregs. Blend the two decoctions and re-decoct to get one *shēng* and five *gě*. Divide the decoction into two doses and drink when it is warm.

*****

[03] 百合病下之后〔1〕者，滑石代赭汤〔2〕主之。

滑石代赭汤方：百合七枚擘,滑石三两碎，绵裹,代赭石如弹丸大一枚，碎，绵裹[3]。右先以水洗百合，渍一宿，当白沫出，去其水。更以泉水二升，煎取一升，去滓；别以泉水二升煎滑石、代赭，取一升，去滓；后合和重煎，取一升五合。分温服。

Annotations

[1] *Xia Zhi Hou*: After the inappropriate use of downward draining (purgative) method. The purgative method may consume body fluids, aggravate deficiency heat and disturb the descending of stomach qi, resulting in scanty urination, vomiting and hiccups.

[2] *Hua Shi Dai Zhe Tang* (Talcum and Haematitum Decoction): A formula to clear the heart, calm the mind, promote urination and regulate stomach qi.

[3] *Mian Guo*: One of the Chinese herbal decoction methods: certain herbs are wrapped in cotton cloth before decoction.

Interpretations

After the inappropriate use of downward draining (purgative) method, patients may experience scanty urination, vomiting and hiccups due to damage to body fluids and aggravated deficiency heat. This can be treated with *Hua Shi Dai Zhe Tang* (Talcum and Haematitum Decoction).

Hua Shi Dai Zhe Tang

[Ingredients]

百合	*bǎi hé*	7 pieces	Bulbus Lilii (break)
滑石	*huá shí*	3 *liǎng*	Talcum (crushed and wrapped in cotton)
代赭石	*dài zhě shí*	1 piece (pellet-sized)	Haematitum (crushed and wrapped in cotton)

Wash *Bai He* with clean water, and then soak in clean water overnight. Discard the water when white foam is present. Decoct *Bai He* in two *shēng* of spring water to get one *shēng* and remove the dregs. Decoct *Hua Shi and Dai Zhe Shi* separately with another two *shēng* of spring water to get one *shēng* and remove the dregs.

Blend the two decoctions and re-decoct to get one *shēng* and five *gě*. Divide the decoction into two doses and drink when it is warm.

*****

[04] 百合病，吐之后〔1〕者，百合鸡子汤〔2〕主之。

百合鸡子汤方：百合七枚擘，鸡子黄[3]一枚，右先以水洗百合，渍一宿，当白沫出，去其水。更以泉水二升，煎取一升，去滓。内鸡子黄，搅匀，煎五分。温服。

Annotations

[1] *Tu Zhi Hou*: After the inappropriate use of vomit-inducing method, patients may experience restlessness, insomnia and stomach upset due to damage to stomach yin and ascending of deficiency fire.

[2] *Bai He Ji Zi Tang* (Lily Bulb and Egg Yolk Decoction): A formula to clear the heart, calm the mind, nourish yin and alleviate restlessness.

[3] *Ji Zi Huang:* Egg yolk. Actions: Nourishes yin, alleviates restlessness and calms the mind.

Interpretations

After the inappropriate use of vomit-inducing method, patients may experience restlessness, insomnia and stomach upset due to damage to stomach yin and ascending of deficiency fire. This can be treated with *Bai He Ji Zi* (Lily Bulb and Egg Yolk Decoction).

Bai He Ji Zi Tang

[Ingredients]

百合	*bǎi hé*	7 pieces	Bulbus Lilii (break)
鸡子黄	*jī zǐ huáng*	1	Egg yolk

Wash *Bai He* with clean water, and then soak in clean water overnight. Discard the water when white foam is present. Decoct *Bai He* in two *shēng* of spring water to get one *shēng* and remove the dregs. Add the egg yolk to the decoction and blend evenly. Then re-decoct to get five *fēn*. Drink the decoction in one dose when it is warm.

*****

[05] 百合病，不经吐、下，发汗，病形如初〔1〕者。百合地黄汤〔2〕主之。

百合地黄汤方：百合七枚擘，生地黄汁一升，右以水洗百合，渍一宿，当白沫出，去其水。更以泉水二升，煎取一升，去滓。内地黄汁，煎取一升五合。分温再服。中病〔3〕勿更服，大便当如漆〔4〕。

Annotations

[1] *Bing Xing Ru Chu*: Patients present with the signs and symptoms indicative of lily disease.

[2] *Bai He Di Huang Tang* (Lily Bulb and Rehmannia Decoction): A major formula for lily disease. Actions: Clears the heart, calms the mind, nourishes yin and clears heat.

[3] *Zhong Bing:* Alleviation or absence of symptoms.

[4] *Da Bian Dang Ru Qi*: It literally means the stool is as black as lacquer. However, according to the *Jin Gui Yao Lüè Fang Lun Kao Zheng* (Textual Research on Formulas in 'Essentials from the Golden Cabinet'), here it means loose stools.

Interpretations

For signs and symptoms of lily disease before the use of vomit-inducing, downward draining and sweat-inducing methods, *Bai He Di Huang Tang* (Lily Bulb and Rehmannia Decoction) can be employed.

Bai He Di Huang Tang

[Ingredients]

百合	*bǎi hé*	7 pieces	Bulbus Lilii (break)
生地	*shēng dì*	1 *Shēng*	Radix Rehmanniae (fresh juice)

Wash *Bai He* with clean water, and then soak in clean water overnight. Discard the water when white foam is present. Decoct *Bai He* in two *shēng* of spring water to get one *shēng* and remove the dregs. Add the rehmammiae juice to the decoction and get one *shēng* and five *gě*. Divide the decoction into two doses and drink when it is warm. If patients get better with alleviated or absent symptoms, stop taking the decoction; otherwise, they may have loose stools.

*****

[06] 百合病一月不解，变成渴者，百合洗方[1]主之。

百合洗方：右以百合一升，以水一斗，渍之一宿。以洗身。洗已，食煮饼[2]，勿以盐豉[3]也。

Annotations

[1] *Bai He Xi Fang*: An externally-used formula for lily disease. Over time, patients with lily disease may experience thirsty from internal heat due to yin deficiency. In addition to orally administered medicine, external therapy needs to be combined to facilitate the efficacy of clearing heat and moistening dryness.

[2] *Zhu Bing*: Cake made from wheat flour and water, i.e., noodles. Actions: Supplements qi and regenerates fluids.

[3] *Yan Chi:* Salty fermented beans. It's contraindicated for patients with thirsty due to yin deficiency.

Interpretations

For patients with lily disease, if their symptoms fail to resolve within one month after treatment but start to experience thirsty, in addition to orally administered medicine, they need to wash the body with *Bai He Xi Fang*.

Method: Soak 1 *Shēng* of lily into one *Dou* of water overnight. Use the liquid to bathe the body. After this, eat the cake made from wheat flour and water, but avoid salty, fermented beans.

*****

[07] 百合病，渴不差[1]者，栝蒌牡蛎散[2]主之。

栝蒌牡蛎散方：栝蒌根,牡蛎,熬等分,右为细末。饮服方寸匕[3]，日三服。

Annotations

[1] *Ke Bu Cha*: Unresolved thirsty after internal and external therapies. This is caused by hyperactive fire (due to yin deficiency) consuming bodily fluids.

[2] *Gua Lou Mu Li San* (Trichosanthes and Oyster Shell Powder): A formula to regeneraet bodily fluids and alleviate thirst.

[3] *Fang Cun Bi:* A tool to measure herbal medicine. The word *Bi* means a spoon, referring to a square-inch-spoonful capacity, which is approximately 2 grams of mineral powder and 1gram of herbal powder.

Interpretations

Persistent thirst in patients with chronic lily disease should be treated with *Gua Lou Mu Li San* (Trichosanthes and Oyster Shell Powder).

Gua Lou Mu Li San

[Ingredients]

栝蒌根	*guā lóu gēn*	Radix Trichosanthis
牡蛎	*mŭ lì*	Concha Ostreae

Grind equal amount of the above two ingredients into a fine powder, take a square-inch-spoonful (approximately 2g) with hot water for each dose, three doses a day.

*****

[08] 百合病变发热〔1〕者一作发寒热，百合滑石散〔2〕主之。

百合滑石散方：百合一两炙，滑石三两，右为散。饮服方寸匕，日三服。当微利〔3〕者，止服，热则除。

Annotations

[1] *Bian Fa Re*: Generally patients with lily disease do not have fever. However, persistent lily disease may cause internal heat and result in low-grade fever, inhibited urination or dribbling, painful urination.

[2] *Bai He Hua Shi San* (Lily Bulb and Talcum Powder): A formula to nourish yin, clear heat and promote urination.

[3] *Wei Li:* Mild improvement of inhibited urination.

Interpretations

Low-grade fever (some texts recorded chills and fever) in patients with chronic lily disease should be treated with *Bai He Hua Shi San* (Lily Bulb and Talcum Powder).

Bai He Hua Shi San

[Ingredients]

百合	*bǎi hé*	1 *liǎng*	Bulbus Lilii (fried)
滑石	*huá shí*	3 *liǎng*	Talcum

Grind the above two ingredients into a fine powder, take a square-inch-spoonful (approximately 2g) with hot water for each dose, three doses a day. Stop immediately when the inhibited urination improved, because it indicates that the interior heat has been eliminated.

*****

[09] 百合病见于阴者，以阳法救之〔1〕；见于阳者，以阴法救之〔2〕。见阳攻阴，复发其汗，此为逆；见阴攻阳，乃复下之，此亦为逆。

Annotations

[1] *Jian Yu Yin Zhe, Yi Yang Fa Jiu Zhi*: Cold syndrome in lily disease should be treated with yang-warming methods. However, there is no cold syndrome in lily disease, because most patients present with internal heat due to yin deficiency.

[2] *Jian Yu Yang Zhe, Yi Yin Fa Jiu Zhi:* Heat syndrome in lily disease should be treated with yin-nourishing methods. According to the *Jin Gui Yi Shi* (Interpretations of Essentials from the Golden Cabinet), "Lily disease is more of a deficiency syndrome in Chinese medicine. As a result, it needs to be managed with reinforcing healthy qi. The yin-nourishing method refers to the use of formulas like *Bai He Di Huang Tang* (Lily Bulb and Rehmannia Decoction).

Interpretations

Cold syndrome in lily disease should be treated with yang-warming methods. Heat syndrome in lily disease should be treated with yin-nourishing methods. As for manifestations due to an exterior syndrome, it is wrong to treat interior syndrome first and then resolve the exterior syndrome by sweating-inducing methods. As for manifestations due to an interior syndrome, it is wrong to treat the exterior syndrome first and then deal with the interior syndrome with purgation methods.

*****

[10] 狐惑〔1〕之为病，状如伤寒，默默欲眠〔2〕，目不得闭，卧起不安。蚀于喉为惑，蚀于阴为狐〔3〕。不欲饮食，恶闻食臭。其面目乍赤、乍黑、乍白〔4〕。蚀于上部〔5〕则声喝〔6〕一作嗄〔7〕。甘草泻心汤〔8〕主之。

甘草泻心汤方：甘草四两；黄芩，人参，干姜各三两；黄连一两；大枣十二枚；半夏半升；右七味，水一斗，煮取六升，去滓再煎。温服一升，日三服。

Annotations

[1] *Hu Huo*: A condition in Chinese medicine resulting from severe damp heat. It is characterized by throat ulcers, genital ulcers and eye inflammation. This condition is named *Hu Huo* in Chinese because its ulcerative symptoms make people suspicious and confused. Today it's known as Behçet's syndrome, which is classically characterized as a triad of symptoms that include recurring crops of mouth ulcers (aphthous ulcers, canker sores), genital ulcers, and inflammation of a specialized area around the pupil of the eye.

[2] *Zhuang Ru Shang Han, Mo Mo Yu Mian:* The "*Zhuang Ru Shang Han*" means that the systemic symptoms of *Hu Huo* are similar to those of cold damage. The "*Mo Mo Yu Mian*" means no desire to talk and feel sleepy. This is similar to "drowsiness" in Shaoyin disease instead of "fever and chills" in Taiyang disease.

[3] *Shi Yu Hou Wei Huo, Shi Yu Yin Wei Hu:* The two sentences are intertextual in describing localized symptoms of *Hu Huo*—the ulceration can be seen in the throat or genital areas. The first word "*Shi*" means erosion or ulceration. The *Jin Gui Yao Lüè Fang Lun Kao Zheng* (Textual

Research on Prescriptions in Essentials from the Golden Cabinet) states, "It is absurd to separate *Hu* and *Huo* into two different conditions; the two words *Hu Huo* simply mean suspicious and confused".

[4] *Mian Mu Zha Chi, Zha Hei, Zha Bai*: The first two words *Mian Mu* mean face and eyes; however, they focus on the eyes. The eyes can be red with black or white (pus-filled) sockets.

[5] *Shi Yu Shang Bu*: Erosion of the throat.

[6] *Sheng Ye*: Low, husky voice.

[7] *Sha*: Hoarseness.

[8] *Gan Cao Xie Xin Tang* (Licorice Heart-Draining Decoction): A formula to clear heat, resolve dampness, and remove toxins.

Interpretations

Patients with *Hu Huo* (Behçet's syndrome) may present with cold damage (Shaoyin disease) symptoms—no desire to talk, feeling sleepy but too restless to close the eyes or fall asleep, ulcerations inside the throat or in genital areas, a poor appetite with aversion to food smell, and red eyes with black or white (pus-filled) eye sockets. Throat ulcers may cause a low, husky voice or hoarseness. This condition can be treated with *Gan Cao Xie Xin Tang* (Licorice Heart-Draining Decoction).

Gan Cao Xie Xin Tang

[Ingredients]

甘草	*gān cǎo*	4 *liǎng*	Radix et Rhizoma Glycyrrhizae
黄芩	*huáng qín*	3 *liǎng*	Radix Scutellariae
人参	*rén shēn*	3 *liǎng*	Radix et Rhizoma Ginseng
干姜	*gān jiāng*	3 *liǎng*	Rhizoma Zingiberis
黄连	*huáng lián*	1 *liǎng*	Rhizoma Coptidis
大枣	*dà zǎo*	12 pieces	Fructus Jujubae
半夏	*bàn xià*	0.5 *shēng*	Rhizoma Pinelliae

Decoct the above seven ingredients in 1 *Dou* of water to get 6 *shēng* and remove the dregs. Then re-decoct to get 3 *shēng*. Drink 1 *shēng* in one dose when it is warm, 3 doses a day.

*****

[11] 蚀于下部〔1〕则咽干〔2〕。苦参汤〔3〕洗之。

Annotations

[1] *Shi Yu Xia Bu*: The "*Xia Bu*" here refers to genital areas.

[2] *Yan Gan*: The throat becomes dry. It is doubtful that this is a mistake of "*Yin Gan*", which means the genital areas become dry. In the case of throat ulcers, a dry throat may also be present.

[3] *Ku Shen Tang* (Sophorae Flavescentis Decoction): An external washing formula for genital sores. The *Jin Gui Yu Han Yao Lüè Ji Yi* (Summaries on the Jade Case Essentials of the Golden Cabinet) states, "Decoct 1 *shēng* of *Ku Shen* in 1 *Dou* of water to get 7 *shēng*. Remove the dregs and wash the genital area 3 times a day". Actions of *Ku Shen* (Radix Sophorae Flavescentis): Clears heat, resolves dampness, kills insects and stops itching. It's advisable to fumigate and wash the genital areas with *Ku Shen* decoction and at the same time, take *Gan Cao Xie Xin Tang* to achieve a better effect.

Interpretations

Genital ulcers coupled with a dry throat should be fumigated and washed with *Ku Shen Tang* (Sophorae Flavescentis Decoction).

*****

[12] 蚀于肛者，雄黄〔1〕熏之。

雄黄　右一味为末，筒瓦二枚合之〔2〕，烧向肛熏之〔3〕。《脉经》云：病人或从呼吸上蚀其咽，或从下焦〔4〕蚀其肛阴，蚀上为惑，蚀下为狐。狐惑病者，猪苓散〔5〕主之。

Annotations

[1] *Xiong Huang* (Realgar): A toxic, arsenic sulfide mineral often used externally to remove toxins and dry dampness.

[2] *Jian Wa Er Mei He Zhi*: Place two concave tiles together to form a tube.

[3] *Shao Xiang Gan Xun Zhi:* The *Jin Gui Shi An* (Annotations to Essentials from the Golden Cabinet) states, "Use two tiles to form a tube and burn the realgar to fumigate the anus".

[4] *Xia Jiao*: the lower abdomen.

[5] *Zhu Ling San* (Polyporus Powder): please see annotation 13 in Chapter 17 Retching, Vomiting, Hiccups and Diarrhea.

Interpretations

Anal or perianal ulcers should be fumigated with *Xiong Huang Fang* (Realgar).

Grind the realgar into a fine powder, place two tiles to form a tube, and burn the realgar to fumigate the anal area. According to the *Mai Jing* (The Pulse Classic), some patients experience throat ulcers, known as *Huo*; and some patients experience genital ulcers, known as *Hu*. These patients can take *Zhu Ling San* (Polyporus Powder) orally.

*****

[13] 病者脉数〔1〕，无热，微烦〔2〕，默默但欲卧，汗出。初得之三四日，目赤如鸠眼〔3〕；七八日，目四眦一本此有黄字黑〔4〕。若能食者，脓已成也〔5〕。赤豆当归散〔6〕主之。

赤豆当归散方：赤小豆三升，浸，令芽出，曝干〔7〕 当归 右二味，杵为散，浆水〔8〕服方寸匕，日三服。

Annotations

[1] *Mai Shuo:* Rapid (increased) pulse rate. It is often seen in heat syndrome or deficiency syndrome.

[2] *Wu Re*, *Wei Fan*: Absence of fever or chills; presence of mild fever (deficiency heat).

[3] *Mu Chi Ru Jiu Yan:* The eyes are as red as those of a turtledove. It is known as iritis.

[4] *Si Zi Hei*: Black eye sockets.

[5] *Ruo Neng Shi Zhe, Nong Yi Cheng*: Along with the alleviation of systemic symptoms, patients start to have a better appetite and pus formation in the anterior chamber of the eye (i.e., hypopyon).

[6] *Chi Dou Dang Gui San* (Rice Bean and Chinese Angelica Powder): A formula to drain pus, remove toxins, circulate blood and resolve stasis. It can also be used for bleeding of the lower body (please see annotation 16 in Chapter 16, Fright, Palpitations, Hematemesis, Nosebleed and Bleeding of the Lower Body).

[7] *Jin, Ling Ya Chu, Pu Gan*: Soak the rice bean in water until the presence of bean sprouts. Then take it out and dry in the sun.

[8] *Jiang Shui:* Also known as *Suan Jiang* (sour syrup). Preparation method: soak the cooked millet in cold water for 5 or 6 days. It is sour in taste and white in color. Actions: Removes toxins.

Interpretations

Patients with *Hu Huo* may present with a rapid pulse but no chills or fever in an exterior syndrome; however, they may have a mild fever, no desire to talk, feeling sleepy, and sweating. Patients may develop red eyes like those of a turtledove three or four days after the initial onset. After seven or eight days, they may further progress to black (or brown yellow) eye sockets. At this time, the systemic systems start to alleviate, patients begin to have a better appetite. They may experience pus formation in the anterior chamber of the eye (actually they are already blind). This condition can be treated with *Chi Xiao Dou Dang Gui San* (Rice Bean and Chinese Angelica Powder).

Chi Xiao Dou Dang Gui San

[Ingredients]

赤小豆	*chì xiǎo dòu*	3 *shēng*	Rice bean
当归	*dāng guī*		Radix Angelicae Sinensis

Soak 3 *shēng* of rice bean in water until the presence of bean sprouts. Dry *Dang Gui* and grind the two ingredients into a fine powder. Then take a square-inch-spoonful (approximately 2g) with the prepared sour syrup for one dose, 3 doses a day.

*****

[14] 阳毒〔1〕之为病，面赤斑斑如锦文〔2〕，咽喉痛，唾脓血〔3〕。五日可治，七日不可治〔4〕。升麻鳖甲汤〔5〕主之。

阴毒〔6〕之为病，面目青〔7〕，身痛如被杖〔8〕，咽喉痛〔9〕，五日可治，七日不可治。升麻鳖甲汤去雄黄、蜀椒〔10〕主之。

升麻鳖甲汤方：升麻〕二两　当归一两　蜀椒炒去汗〔11〕，一两　甘草二两　鳖甲手指大〔12〕一片炙　雄黄半两研　右六味，以水四升，煮取一升，顿服之。老小再服，取汗《肘后》〔13〕、《千金方》〔14〕：阳毒用升麻汤，无鳖甲，有桂；阴毒用甘草汤，无雄黄。

Annotations

[1] *Yang Du:* Yang toxin that involves the heat in the qi phase. Yin yang toxin is an epidemic febrile disease. It is clinically characterized by a sore throat and eruption of macules on the face. It often has an acute onset and an unfavorable prognosis. Yang toxin affects the qi phase and is clinically characterized by the presence of macules on the face, a sore throat and spitting of purulent blood. This condition is similar to scarlet fever.

[2] *Mian Chi Ban Ban Ru Jin Wen:* The presence of brocade-like macules on the face.

[3] *Tuo Nong Xue*: Spitting of pus and blood due to exuberant toxic heat.

[4] *Wu Ri Ke Zhi, Qi Ri Bu Ke Zhi:* Yang toxin is curable within five days, but incurable after seven days. However, five or seven are not fixed numbers. They just signify the crucial importance of early treatment.

[5] *Sheng Ma Bie Jia Tang* (Cimicifuga and Turtle Shell Decoction): A formula to clear heat, remove toxins, nourish yin and resolve stasis. This formula is later used for scarlet fever.

[6] *Yin Du:* Yin toxin that involves heat in the blood phase. It is a critical condition characterized by a bluish facial complexion, a sore throat and generalized pain.

[7] *Mian Mu Qing:* Dark, bluish macules on the face due to toxic heat entering the blood phase.

[8] *Shen Tong Ru Bei Zhang:* Pain as if beaten by a stick.

[9] *Yan Hou Tong*: A red, swollen and sore throat due to exuberant toxic heat, coupled with spitting of pus and blood.

[10] *Sheng Ma Bie Jia Tang Qu Xiong Huang, Shu Jiao*: Since Yin toxins enter the blood phase and cause stasis heat in the interior, *Shu Jiao* (Pericarpium Zanthoxyli) and *Xiong Huang* (Realgar) are (pungent in flavor and dispersing in property) only effective in the qi phase.

[11] *Chao Qu Han*: Heat and fry the ingredients to remove their oil.

[12] *Shou Zhi Da*: Big finger. It was recorded as "big hand" in the *Wai Tai Mi Yao* (Arcane Essentials from the Imperial Library).

[13] *Zhou Hou*: *Zhou Hou Bei Ji Fang* (Emergency Formulas to Keep Up One's Sleeve) by Ge Hong.

[14] *Qian Jin Fang*: *Qian Jin Yao Fang* (Important Formulas Worth a Thousand Gold Pieces) by Sun Simiao.

Interpretations

Yin yang toxin includes yang toxin and yin toxin. Yang toxin causes brocade-like bright macules on the face, a red, swollen, sore throat, and spitting of pus and blood. Early treatment is crucial to this condition. It is curable within five days and might become incurable after seven days. Yang toxin can be treated with *Sheng Ma Bie Jia Tang* (Cimicifuga and Turtle Shell Decoction).

Yin toxin causes dark, bluish macules on the face, generalized pain as if beaten by a stick and a red, swollen, sore throat (coupled with spitting of pus and blood). Likewise, early treatment is crucial. It is curable within 5 days and might become incurable after seven days. Yin toxin can be treated with *Sheng Ma Bie Jia Tang* (Cimicifuga and Turtle Shell Decoction) by removing *Shu Jiao* (Pericarpium Zanthoxyli) and *Xiong Huang* (Realgar).

Sheng Ma Bie Jia Tang

[Ingredients]

升麻	*shēng má*	2 *liǎng*	Rhizoma Cimicifugae
当归	*dāng guī*	1 *liǎng*	Radix Angelicae Sinensis
蜀椒	*huā jiāo*	1 *liǎng*	Pericarpium Zanthoxyli (oil removed)
甘草	*gān cǎo*	2 *liǎng*	Radix et Rhizoma Glycyrrhizae
鳖甲	*biē jiǎ*	Finger-sized piece	Carapax Trionycis
雄黄	*xióng huáng*	0.5 *liǎng*	Realgar (powder)

Decoct the above six ingredients in 4 *shēng* of water to get 1 *shēng* and drink up at a draught. The elderly and children should take the decoction in two doses. Patients often sweat after taking this formula. According to the *Zhou Hou Bei Ji Fang* (Emergency Formulas to Keep Up One's Sleeve) and *Qian Jin Yao Fang* (Important Formulas Worth a Thousand Gold Pieces), Yang toxin is treated with *Sheng Ma Bie Jia Tang* by replacing *Bie Jia* (turtle shell) with *Gui Zhi* (Ramulus Cinnamomi); and yin toxin is treated with *Gan Cao Tang* (Licorice Decoction) by removing *Xiong Huang* (Realgar).

疟病脉证并治第四
Chapter 4 Malaria—Pulses, Patterns and Treatment

Overview

This chapter specifically focuses on malaria (*Nüè Ji*). The *Shuo Wen Jie Zi* (Explaining Graphs and Analyzing Characters) states, "Nüè is a disease characterized by alternating episodes of chills and fever (intermittent)". Based on the *Nei Jing Su Wen Nüè Lun* (Discussions on Malaria, Basic Questions, Yellow Emperor's Inner Classic), this chapter categorizes malaria into three sub-patterns, namely, heat malaria (*dan nüè*), warm malaria (*wen nüè*) and cold malaria (*pin nüè*). It also contains a detailed discussion of the mother-of-malaria, coupled with formulas for malarial diseases.

*****

[01] 师曰：疟脉自弦〔1〕，弦数者多热；弦迟者多寒〔2〕。弦小紧者，下之差〔3〕；弦迟者，可温之〔4〕；弦紧者，可发汗针灸也〔5〕；浮大者，可吐之〔6〕；弦数者，风发也〔7〕，以饮食消息止之〔8〕。

Annotations

[1] *Nüè Mai Xi Xuan:* A wiry pulse is indicative of Shaoyang disease located in between the exterior and interior. Shaoyang disease is also characterized by alternating chills and fever. A wiry pulse is long, straight and string-like. However, patients with malaria may not present with a wiry pulse.

[2] *Xuan Shuo Zhe Duo Re, Xuan Chi Zhe Duo Han*: A wiry, rapid pulse indicates heat, whereas a wiry, slow pulse indicates cold. This suggests that malaria is mainly characterized by alternating fever and chills, and its syndrome differentiation is based on predominance of fever or chills.

[3] *Xian Xiao Jin Zhe, Xia Zhi Cha*: A wiry, small and tight (i.e., deep, small and tight) pulse indicates pathogenic factors affecting the lower part of the body (intestines), which should be treated with purgation.

[4] *Xuan Chi Zhe, Ke Wen Zhi:* A wiry, slow pulse indicates interior cold, which should be treated with warming methods.

[5] *Xuan Jin Zhe, Ke Fa Han Zhen Jiu Ye:* A wiry and tight pulse indicates exterior cold, which should be treated with acupuncture to induce sweating. According to the *Mai Jing* (the Pulse Classic), "a wiry and tight pulse can be understood as a tight and rapid pulse".

[6] *Fu Da Zhe, Ke Tu Zhi:* A superficial and large pulse indicates pathogenic factors affecting the upper part of the body (stomach), which should be treated with vomiting methods.

[7] *Xuan Shuo Zhe, Feng Fa Ye:* A wiry and rapid pulse indicates exuberant heat. "*Feng Fa Ye*" describes a sudden onset.

[8] *Yi Yin Shi Xiao Xi Zhi Zhi*: The "*Yin Shi*" here refers to take medicine; and "*Xiao Xi*" means to modify the ingredients in a formula. Unlike inducing sweating by acupuncture, this means to alleviate fever or chills through modifications of formulas.

Interpretations

The master said, "Patients with malaria often present with a wiry pulse (indicating a disease located in between the exterior and interior and characterized by alternating chills and fever): a wiry and rapid pulse indicates heat, whereas a wiry and slow pulse indicates cold (sweating, vomiting, purgation, warming and clearing methods can be adopted according to the disease severity and location). A wiry, small and tight pulse indicates problems of the intestines, which should be treated with purgation; a wiry and slow pulse indicates interior cold, which should be treated with yang warming methods; a wiry and tight pulse indicates exterior cold, which should be treated with sweating method by acupuncture; a superficial and large pulse indicates problems of the stomach, which should be treated with vomiting methods; and a wiry and rapid pulse indicates a sudden onset of exuberant heat, which should be treated with (heat-clearing) formulas.

*****

[02] 病疟以月一日发，当以十五日愈〔1〕。设不差，当月尽解〔2〕。如其不差，当如何？师曰：此结为症瘕〔3〕，名曰疟母〔4〕。急治之〔5〕，宜鳖甲煎丸〔6〕。

鳖甲煎丸方：鳖甲十二分〔7〕炙乌扇三分烧黄芩三分柴胡六分鼠妇三分熬干姜三分大黄三分　芍药五分桂枝三分葶苈一分熬石韦三分去毛厚朴三分牡丹五分去心瞿麦二分　紫葳三分半夏一分人参一分䗪虫五分熬阿胶三分炙蜂窠四分熬赤硝十二分蜣螂六分熬桃仁二分 右二十三味，为末，取煅灶下灰〔8〕一斗，清酒一斛〔9〕五斗，浸灰，候酒尽一半，着鳖甲于中，煮令泛烂如胶漆，绞取汁，内诸药，煎为丸，如梧子大。空心服七丸，日三服。《千金方》用鳖甲十二片，又有海藻三分，大戟一分，䗪虫五分，无鼠妇、赤硝二味，以鳖甲煎和诸药为丸。

Annotations

[1] *Bing Nüè Yi Yue Yi Ri Fa, Dang Yi Shi Wu Ri Yu:* Malaria usually lasts 15 days and resolves when anti-pathogenic qi prevails over pathogenic factors.

[2] *She Bu Cha, Dang Yue Jin Jie:* If fever and chills do not resolve after 15 days, they should be completely resolved by the end of the month.

[3] *Zheng Jia:* Abdominal masses: solid, painful (with a fixed location) and immobile masses are called "*Zheng*", whereas painful (no fixed location) and movable masses are known as "*Jia*".

[4] *Nüè Mu:* Mother of malaria, i.e., splenomegaly. It occurs when recurrent fever and chills consumes anti-pathogenic qi and, over time, stagnant phlegm and blood retain below the left subcostal region.

[5] *Ji Zhi Zhi:* Fever and chills in malaria require early and urgent treatment; otherwise, it takes longer period of time once the splenomegaly is present.

[6] *Bie Jia Jian Wan* (Turtle Shell Decocted Pill): A formula to supplement healthy qi, remove pathogenic factors, soften hardness and resolve masses.

[7] *Shi Er Fen:* 12 *fēn*, the dosage is 11 *fēn* in Xu's version.

[8] *Zao Xia Hui:* Also known as *Zao Xin Tu* or *Fu Long Gan*, it means ashes from a cooking stove. Actions: Warms the spleen and stomach, dries dampness, stops bleeding and relieves vomiting.

[9] *Qing Jiu Yi Hu*: The "*Qing Jiu*" means rice wine. *Hu* is a unit of capacity: 1 *hu*=10 *dou*.

Interpretations

Malaria that occurs on the first day of the month should resolve spontaneously on the fifteenth day. If not, the chills and fever alleviate by the end of the month. What happens if it still lingers by then? The master says, "This may form abdominal masses (*Zheng Jia*) known as the mother of malaria. That's why malaria requires early and urgent treatment. Once the mother of malaria forms, it takes longer period of time to recover. *Bie Jia Jian Wan* (Turtle Shell Decocted Pill) is recommended for this stage".

Bie Jia Jian Wan

[Ingredients]

鳖甲	*biē jiǎ*	12 *fēn*	Carapax Trionycis (mix-fried)
射干	*shè gān*	3 *fēn*	Rhizoma Belamcandae (burnt)
黄芩	*huáng qín*	3 *fēn*	Radix Scutellariae
柴胡	*chái hú*	6 *fēn*	Radix Bupleuri
鼠妇	*shǔ fù*	3 *fēn*	Porcellio (boiled)
干姜	*gān jiāng*	3 *fēn*	Rhizoma Zingiberis

Bie Jia Jian Wan

[Ingredients]

大黄	*dà huáng*	3 *fēn*	Radix et Rhizoma Rhei
芍药	*sháo yào*	5 *fēn*	Radix Paeoniae
桂枝	*guì zhī*	3 *fēn*	Ramulus Cinnamomi
葶苈子	*tíng lì zǐ*	1 *fēn*	Semen Lepidii (boiled)
石韦	*shí wéi*	3 *fēn*	Folium Pyrrosiae (hair removed)
厚朴	*hòu pò*	3 *fēn*	Cortex Magnoliae Officinalis
牡丹皮	*mǔ dān pí*	5 *fēn*	Cortex Moutan (core removed)
瞿麦	*qú mài*	2 *fēn*	Herba Dianthi
紫葳	*zǐ wēi*	3 *fēn*	Flos Campsis
半夏	*bàn xià*	1 *fēn*	Rhizoma Pinelliae
人参	*rén shēn*	1 *fēn*	Radix et Rhizoma Ginseng
蛰虫	*zhé chóng*	5 *fēn*	Eupolyphaga seu Steleophaga (boiled)
阿胶	*ē jiāo*	3 *fēn*	Colla Corii Asini (mix-fried)
蜂房	*fēng fáng*	4 *fēn*	Nidus Vespae (mix-fried)
赤硝	*chì xiāo*	12 *fēn*	Nitrum Rubrum
蜣螂	*qiāng lang*	6 *fēn*	Catharsius (boiled)
桃仁	*táo rén*	2 *fēn*	Semen Persicae

Grind the above twenty-three ingredients into a powder. Soak 1 *dou* of ashes from a cooking stove in 15 *dou* of rice wine until half of the wine left, and then add *Bie Jia* to decoct until it becomes mushy like glue or lacquer. Wring to get its juice and decoct with the aforementioned powder to make pellets the size of firmiana seeds. Take seven pellets on an empty stomach for each dose, 3 doses a day.

[Note] The *Qian Jin Yao Fang* (Important Formulas Worth a Thousand Gold Pieces) records another formula for *Bie Jia Jian Wan*: 12 turtle shell pieces, 3 *fen* of *Hai Zao* (sargassum), 1 *fen* of *Da Ji* (Radix Knoxiae) and 5 *fen* of *Zhe Chong* (ground beetle).

*****

[03] 师曰：阴气孤绝，阳气独发〔1〕，则热而少气烦冤〔2〕，手足热而欲呕〔3〕，名曰瘅疟〔4〕。若但热不寒者，邪气内藏于心，外舍分肉之间，令人消铄脱肉〔5〕。

Annotations

[1] *Yin Qi Gu Jue, Yang Qi Du Fa:* A quotation from the *Huang Di Nei Jing Su Wen Nüè Lun* (Discussions on Malaria, Basic Questions, Yellow Emperor's Inner Classic), means that when yin qi is blocked, yang qi effuses alone. Instead of "being expired", the "*Gu Jue*" here means blockage between yin qi and yang qi.

[2] *Shao Qi Fan Yuan:* The "*Shao Qi*" means shortness of breath due to exuberant heat. The "*Fan Yuan*" means vexation and restlessness.

[3] *Shou Zu Re Er Yu Ou:* Heat in both the exterior and interior. The "*Shou Zu Re*" means heat in the extremities due to heat affecting the exterior. The "*Yu Ou*" means recurrent, persistent vomiting due to heat affecting the interior (stomach)".

[4] *Dan Nüè:* Pure-heat malaria characterized by fever alone without chills.

[5] *Xiao Shuo Tuo Rou:* Wasting of muscles or emaciation.

Interpretations

The master said, "When yin qi is blocked, yang qi effuses alone. This may result in fever, shortness of breath, vexation, restlessness, hot sensations in the extremities, and persistent vomiting. This is known as pure-heat malaria (absence of chills), a condition that causes wasting of muscles because pathogenic heat affects the stomach internally and the surface of the body externally".

*****

[04] 温疟〔1〕者，其脉如平〔2〕，身无寒但热〔3〕，骨节疼烦，时呕〔4〕。白虎加桂枝汤〔5〕主之。

白虎加桂枝汤方：

知母六两甘草二两炙石膏一斤粳米二合桂去皮三两　右锉，每五钱，水一盏半，煎至八分，去滓。温服，汗出愈。

Annotations

[1] *Wen Nüè:* Warm malaria characterized by fever followed by chills. Heat malaria manifests as heat in both the exterior and interior. Warm malaria manifests as exterior cold and interior heat.

[2] *Qi Mai Ru Ping:* Regarding the pulse in patients with malaria, there are two interpretations through the ages: the pulse is wiry or the pulse is not wiry. The *Jin Gui Yao Lüè Jin Shi* (Modern Interpretation of the 'Essentials from the Golden Cabinet') states, "A wiry pulse is characteristic of malaria. When the pulse is described as "normal" (for a malaria patient), it simply means it is not wiry, but not the same as seen in a healthy person". Clinical observations have shown that malaria patients with fever always present with a rapid pulse—either surging and rapid or wiry and rapid.

[3] *Shen Wu Han Dan Re:* More fever than chills or fever followed by chills.

[4] *Gu Jie Teng Fan, Shi Ou*: The "*Gu Jie Teng Fan*" means severe joint pain, indicating exterior cold. The "*Shi Ou*" means occasional vomiting, indicating interior heat. Heat malaria (severe interior heat) causes persistent vomiting, whereas warm malaria (mild interior heat) causes occasional vomiting. The *Mai Jing* (the Pulse Classic) defines warm malaria as "malaria that occurs in the morning and resolves in the evening or malaria that occurs in the evening and resolves by the morning".

[5] *Bai Hu Jia Gui Zhi Tang* (White Tiger Decoction plus Cinnamon Twig): The *Bai Hu Tang* (White Tiger Decoction) clears interior heat. *Gui Zhi* (Ramulus Cinnamomi) resolves exterior cold.

Interpretations

Patients with warm malaria present with the same pulse as other types of malaria. They experience mild chills but severe fever, coupled with noticeable joint pain and occasional vomiting. Warm malaria should be treated with *Bai Hu Jia Gui Zhi Tang* (White Tiger Decoction Plus Cinnamon Twig).

Bai Hu Jia Gui Zhi Tang

[Ingredients]

知母	*zhī mǔ*	6 *liǎng*	Rhizoma Anemarrhenae
甘草	*gān cǎo*	2 *liǎng*	Radix et Rhizoma Glycyrrhizae (mix-fried)
石膏	*shí gāo*	1 *jīn*	Gypsum Fibrosum
粳米	*jīng mǐ*	2 *ge*	Oryza Sativa L.
桂枝	*guì zhī*	3 *liǎng*	Ramulus Cinnamomi (bark removed)

Grind the above five ingredients into a powder. For each dose, decoct 5 *qián* of the powder in one and a half cups of water to get 80% of the liquid. Remove the dregs and take the decoction when it is warm. Sweating contributes to a quick recovery.

*****

[05] 疟多寒者〔1〕，名曰牡疟〔2〕。蜀漆散〔3〕主之。

蜀漆散方：蜀漆烧，去腥〔4〕云母烧二日龙骨等分右三味，杵为散。未发前以浆水〔5〕服半钱。温疟加蜀漆半分，临发时服一钱匕一方云母作云实。

Annotations

[1] *Nüè Duo Han*: Pronounced shivering.

[2] *Mu Nüè:* Malaria characterized by chills followed by fever.

[3] *Shu Qi San* (Dichroa Leaf Powder): The earliest specific formula for cold malaria as well as warm malaria; however, it has to be taken (2 hours) before the onset of chills and fever. Actions: Resolves phlegm and alleviates malaria.

[4] *Qu Xing:* Remove the fishy smell.

[5] *Jiang Shui*: Vinegar-mixed millet water. It acts to stop vomiting. Please see annotation 10 in Chapter 20, Pregnancy—Diseases, Pulses and Syndromes, "For vomiting, use vinegar-mixed millet water".

Interpretations

Malaria characterized by severe chills (or chills followed by fever) is known as cold malaria. It should be treated with *Shu Qi San* (Dichroa Leaf Powder).

Shi Qi San

[Ingredients]

蜀漆	*shŭ qī*	Folium Dichroae (wash to remove the fishy smell)
云母	*yún mŭ*	Muscovite (burnt for two full days)
龙骨	*lóng gŭ*	Os Draconis

Grind equal parts of the above three ingredients into a fine powder and take 0.5 *qián* of the powder with vinegar-contained millet water before the onset of fever and chills. Add additional 0.5 *fēn* of *Shu Qi* (Folium Dichroae) for warm malaria and take 1 *qián* spoon of the mixed liquid with vinegar-contained millet water before the onset of chills and fever.

One formula uses *Yun Shi* (Mysore thorn seeds) (actions: clears heat and resolves dampness) instead of *Yun Mu* (Muscovite).

Attached formula from the *Wai Tai Mi Yao* (Arcane Essentials from the Imperial Library)

*****

牡蛎汤：治牝疟。

牡蛎四两熬 麻黄四两去节 甘草二两 蜀漆三两

右四味，以水八升，先煮蜀漆、麻黄，去上沫，得六升，内诸药，煮取二升。温服一升。若吐，则勿更服。

Formula # 1 *Mu Li Tang* (Oyster Shell Decoction) for cold malaria

牡蛎	*mǔ lì*	4 *liǎng*	Concha Ostreae (boiled)
麻黄	*má huáng*	4 *liǎng*	Herba Ephedrae (nodes removed)
甘草	*gān cǎo*	2 *liǎng*	Radix et Rhizoma Glycyrrhizae
蜀漆	*shǔ qī*	3 *liǎng*	Folium Dichroae

First decoct *Shu Qi* (Folium Dichroae) and *Ma Huang* (Herba Ephedrae) in 8 *shēng* of water. Remove the foamy scum off the top and get 6 *shēng*. Add the rest of the ingredients to decoct and get 2 *shēng*. Take 1 *shēng* for each dose when the decoction is warm. If vomiting occurs, do not take the decoction any more.

Annotation

The *Mu Li Tang* (Oyster Shell Decoction) is a variation of *Shu Qi San* (Dichroa Leaf Powder) by removing *Yun Mu* (Muscovite) and *Long Gu* (Os Draconis) and adding *Mu Li* (Concha Ostreae), *Ma Huang* (Herba Ephedrae) and *Gan Cao* (Radix et Rhizoma Glycyrrhizae). This formula enhances the effect of releasing the exterior by inducing sweating.

*****

柴胡去半夏加栝蒌汤：治疟病发渴者，亦治劳疟。

柴胡八两人参黄芩甘草各三两栝蒌根四两生姜二两大枣十二枚

右七味，以水一斗二升，煮取六升，去滓，再煎，取三升。温服一升，日二服。

Formula # 2 *Chai Hu Qu Ban Xia Jia Gua Lou Tang* (Bupleurum Decoction minus Pinellia plus Trichosanthes Root) for malaria-related thirst and chronic malaria

柴胡	chái hú	8 *liǎng*	Radix Bupleuri
黄芩	*huáng qín*	3 *liǎng*	Radix Scutellariae
人参	*rén shēn*	3 *liǎng*	Radix et Rhizoma Ginseng
甘草	*gān cǎo*	3 *liǎng*	Radix et Rhizoma Glycyrrhizae
栝蒌根	*guā lóu gēn*	4 *liǎng*	Radix Trichosanthis
生姜	*shēng jiāng*	2 *liǎng*	Rhizoma Zingiberis Recens
大枣	*dà zǎo*	12 pieces	Fructus Jujubae

Decoct the above seven ingredients in 12 *shēng* of water to get six *shēng*. Remove the dregs and re-decoct to get 3 *shēng*. Take 1 *shēng* for each dose when it is warm, 2 doses a day.

Annotation

The *Chai Hu Qu Ban Xia Jia Gua Lou Tang* (Bupleurum Decoction minus Pinellia plus Trichosanthes Root) is a variation of *Xiao Chai Hu Tang* (Minor Bupleurum Decoction). This formula enhances the effect of releasing the exterior by inducing sweating. According to the *Shang Han Lun* (Treatise on Cold Damage), the *Xiao Chai Hu Tang* is indicated for "alternating chills and fever, fullness in the chest and subcostal region, no desire to talk, a poor appetite, restlessness and vomiting". As exuberant heat consumes fluids and causes thirst, *Ban Xia* (Rhizoma Pinelliae, pungent in flavor and warm in property) is removed and *Gua Lou* (Radix Trichosanthis, bitter in flavor and cool in property) is added to the formula. This formula harmonizes and releases Shaoyang, removes pathogenic heat, reinforces deficiency, nourishes yin and engenders fluids. Consequently, it can also be used for chronic malaria.

*****

柴胡桂姜汤：治疟寒多，微有热，或但寒不热。服一剂如神。

柴胡半斤桂枝三两去皮干姜二两栝蒌根四两黄芩三两牡蛎三两熬甘草二两炙

右七味，以水一斗二升，煮取六升，去滓。再煎，取三升。温服一升，日三服。初服微烦，复服汗出，便愈。

Formula # 3 *Chai Hu Gui Jiang Tang* (Bupleurum, Cinnamon Twig and Dried Ginger Decoction) for severe chills, mild fever or chills alone.

柴胡	*chái hú*	0.5 *jīn*	Radix Bupleuri
桂枝	*guì zhī*	3 *liǎng*	Ramulus Cinnamomi (bark removed)
干姜	*gàn jiāng*	2 *liǎng*	Rhizoma Zingiberis
栝蒌根	*guā lóu gēn*	4 *liǎng*	Radix Trichosanthis
黄芩	*huáng qín*	3 *liǎng*	Radix Scutellariae
牡蛎	*mǔ lì*	3 *liǎng*	Concha Ostreae (boiled)
甘草	*gān cǎo*	2 *liǎng*	Radix et Rhizoma Glycyrrhizae (mix-fried)

Decoct the above seven ingredients in 12 *liǎng* of water to get six *shēng*. Remove the dregs and re-decoct to get 3 *shēng*. Take 1 *shēng* for each dose when it is warm, 3 doses a day. Patients may experience mild vexation after the first dose and sweating after the second dose. After this, they obtain a full recovery.

Annotation

The *Chai Hu Gui Jiang Tang* (Bupleurum, Cinnamon Twig and Dried Ginger Decoction) is a variation of *Xiao Chai Hu Tang* (Minor Bupleurum Decoction). According to the *Shang Han Lun* (Treatise on Cold Damage), *Chai Hu* (Radix Bupleuri) harmonizes and releases Shaoyang, *Gui Zhi* (Ramulus Cinnamomi) and *Gan Jiang* (Rhizoma Zingiberis) warms yang and removes cold. This formula harmonizes and releases Shaoyang and balances yin and yang.

中风历节病脉证并治第五
Chapter 5 Wind Stroke and Joint Diseases—Pulses, Patterns, and Treatment

Overview

This chapter discusses wind stroke and joint diseases. Wind stroke is characterized by a sudden onset of hemiplegia and deviation of the mouth and eyes. In severe cases, faint and unconsciousness may be present. Joint diseases often manifest as migratory joint pain and swelling. The two conditions are discussed together because they are both associated with pathogenic wind (featured by constant moving and rapid changes) and share similar signs and symptoms such as motor impairment.

*****

[01] 夫风〔1〕之为病，当半身不遂〔2〕。或但臂不遂者，此为痹〔3〕。脉微而数〔4〕，中风使然。

Annotations

[1] *Feng:* Wind stroke.

[2] *Ban Shen Bu Sui:* Inability to initiate voluntary movement.

[3] *Bi:* Impediment caused by pathogenic wind, cold and dampness. There are three types of impediment. Wandering impediment (due to more wind than cold or damp) is characterized by migratory joint pain. Cold impediment is characterized by joint pain that worsens upon exposure to cold. Fixed impediment (due to more damp than wind or cold) is characterized by joint pain in a fixed position. In modern medicine,

Bi-impediment syndrome includes rheumatic arthritis, rheumatoid arthritis, gouty arthritis, osteoarthritis, etc.

[4] *Mai Wei Er Ruo*: The pulse is faint and rapid. A faint pulse indicates deficiency of qi and blood. A rapid pulse indicates excessive pathogenic factors. This explains wind stroke occurs as a result of deficiency of qi and blood coupled with contraction of wind.

Interpretations

Wind stroke causes inability to initiate voluntary movement on one side of the body. Motor impairment of one arm or leg is called Bi-impediment syndrome. A faint, rapid pulse is often seen in wind stroke caused by deficiency of qi and blood coupled with external contraction of wind.

*****

[02] 寸口脉〔1〕浮而紧，紧则为寒，浮则为虚〔2〕。寒虚相搏，邪在皮肤〔3〕。浮者血虚，络脉〔4〕空虚。贼邪不泻〔5〕。或左或右。邪气〔6〕反缓，正气〔7〕即急，正气引邪，㖞僻〔8〕不遂。

邪在于络，肌肤不仁；邪在于经，即重不胜；邪入于府〔9〕，即不识人；邪入于藏〔10〕，舌即难言，口吐涎。

Annotations

[1] *Cun Kou Mai:* Pulsation in the *Cunkou* (radial artery) region. Here it refers to conditions of the upper *jiao*.

[2] *Jin Ze Wei Han, Fu Ze Wei Xu:* Etiological factors of deviation of the mouth corner—exposure to cold (external) and deficiency of qi and blood (internal).

[3] *Pi Fu:* Here it refers to skin on the face.

[4] *Luo Mai:* Superficial branches of meridians.

[5] *Zei Xie Bu Xie*: Retention of pathogenic cold due to deficiency of anti-pathogenic qi.

[6] *Xie Qi*: It refers to the affected side of the face.

[7] *Zheng Qi*: It refers to the (unaffected) healthy side of the face.

[8] *Wo Pi*: Deviation of the mouth corner.
[9] *Fu*: Fu organs. Here it specifically refers to the brain.
[10] *Zang*: Zang organs.

Interpretations

A superficial, tight pulse in the Cunkou region is indicative of abnormal changes in the facial skin due to deficiency of qi and blood coupled with external contraction of cold. Because the blood qi in superficial collaterals becomes deficient, pathogenic wind cold retains and affects the left or right-sided face. The skin on the affected side becomes flaccid, whereas the skin on the healthy side becomes relatively tightened. As a result, deviation of the eyes and mouth occurs.

Wind affecting the collaterals causes skin insensitivity (sensory disturbance). Wind affecting the meridians causes body heaviness (motor impairment). Wind affecting the brain causes mental unconsciousness (conscious disturbance). Wind entering the zang-organs causes drooling and tongue stuffiness with an inability to speak.

*****

[03] 侯氏黑散〔1〕：治大风〔2〕四肢烦重〔3〕，心中恶寒不足者。《外台》〔4〕治风癫〔5〕。

菊花四十分白术十分细辛三分茯苓三分牡蛎三分桔梗八分防风十分人参三分矾石三分黄芩五分当归三分干姜三分芎䓖三分桂枝三分 右十四味，杵为散。酒服方寸匕，日一服。初服二十日，温酒调服。禁一切鱼肉、大蒜。常宜冷食，六十日止，即药积在腹中不下也。热食即下矣，冷食自能助药力。

Annotations

[1] *Hou Shi Hei San:* Hou's Black Powder. Unlike the other formulas often placed after the signs and symptoms in this text, this one is placed

before clinical manifestations. So many commentators suspect that it is not a formula by Zhang Zhongjing. It's named black powder because *Zao Fan* (Alumen), one of the ingredients, appears black. This is the earliest formula for wind stroke. Of the ingredients, *Ju Hua* (Flos Chrysanthemi) acts as the monarch; and *Fang Feng* (Radix Saposhnikoviae) and *Bai Zhu* (Rhizoma Atractylodis Macrocephalae) act as the ministers. Actions: Removes wind, clears fire, resolves phlegm and stasis, and reinforces deficiency.

[2] *Da Feng*: A sudden onset of wind stroke.

[3] *Fan Zhong:* Severe heaviness.

[4] *Wai Tai*: the *Wai Tai Mi Yao* (Arcane Essentials from the Imperial Library) by Wang Tao.

[5] *Feng Dian*: Episodic mental disorder. It is similar to epilepsy.

Interpretations

The *Hou Shi Hei San* (Hou's Black Powder) is used for sudden wind stroke with limb heaviness, a cold sensation in the chest, and fatigue. According to the *Wai Tai Mi Yao* (Arcane Essentials from the Imperial Library), this formula is indicated for episodic epilepsy.

Hou Shi Hei San

[Ingredients]

菊花	*jú huā*	40 *fēn*	Flos Chrysanthemi
白术	*bái zhú*	10 *fēn*	Rhizoma Atractylodis Macrocephalae
细辛	*xì xīn*	3 *fēn*	Radix et Rhizoma Asari
茯苓	*fú líng*	3 *fēn*	Poria
牡蛎	*mŭ lì*	3 *fēn*	Concha Ostreae
桔梗	*jié gěng*	8 *fēn*	Radix Platycodonis
防风	*fáng fēng*	10 *fēn*	Radix Saposhnikoviae
人参	*rén shēn*	3 *fēn*	Radix et Rhizoma Ginseng

Hou Shi Hei San

[Ingredients]

矾石	*fán shí*	3 *fēn*	Alumen
黄芩	*huáng qín*	3 *fēn*	Radix Scutellariae
当归	*dāng guī*	3 *fēn*	Radix Angelicae Sinensis
干姜	*gān jiāng*	3 *fēn*	Rhizoma Zingiberis
川芎	*chuān xiōng*	3 *fēn*	Rhizoma Chuanxiong
桂枝	*guì zhī*	3 *fēn*	Ramulus Cinnamomi

Grind the above ingredients into a fine powder. Take 1 square-inch-spoon with wine for each dose, 1 dose a day. Take it with warm wine for the first 20 days and avoid fish, meat and garlic.

It's advisable to eat cold-property food. Take the medicine for 60 days to allow its medicinal potency. Hot-property food may attenuate the medicinal efficacy, whereas the cold-property food may enhance the medicinal efficacy.

*****

[04] 寸口脉迟而缓〔1〕，迟则为寒，缓则为虚〔2〕；营缓则为亡血，卫缓则为中风〔3〕。邪气中经〔4〕，则身痒而瘾疹〔5〕；心气不足〔6〕，邪气入中〔7〕，则胸满而短气。

Annotations

[1] *Cun Kou Mai Chi Er Huan*: A slow and delayed pulse. Here it refers to the disease location (the whole body) and pathogenesis (slow circulation of blood).

[2] *Chi Ze Wei Han, Huan Ze Wei Xu:* The two sentences are intertextual—a slow pulse indicates cold and a delayed pulse indicates deficiency, which further explains the root cause of the disease—deficiency cold.

[3] *Ying Huan Ze Wang Xue, Wei Huan Ze Zhong Feng:* Both *Ying*-nutrients qi and *Wei*-defensive qi are transformed from water and grains. The *Ying*-nutrients dominates blood and circulates within the blood vessels, whereas *Wei*-defense dominates qi and circulates outside the blood vessels. Deficiency cold of the Ying-nutrients and Wei-defense may cause loss of blood or wind stroke.

[4] *Xie Qi Zhong Jing:* Pathogenic factors affecting the exterior.

[5] *Yin Zhen:* Skin conditions caused by wind, i.e., urticaria or hives.

[6] *Xin Qi Bu Zu:* Deficiency of (heart) blood qi.

[7] *Xie Qi Ru Zhong:* Pathogenic wind affecting the interior.

Interpretations

A slow and delayed (slack) pulse is caused by deficiency cold. Deficiency cold of the *Ying*-nutrients and *Wei*-defense can be seen in loss of blood or wind stroke. Pathogenic wind affecting the exterior may cause urticaria. Pathogenic wind entering the interior due to blood qi deficiency may cause chest tightness and shortness of breath.

*****

[05] 风引汤〔1〕：除热瘫痫〔2〕。

大黄干姜龙骨各四两 桂枝三两 甘草牡蛎各二两 寒水石滑石赤石脂白石脂紫石英石膏各六两 右十二味，杵，粗筛，以韦囊〔3〕盛之。取三指撮，井花水〔4〕三升，煮三沸。温服一升。治大人风引，少小惊痫瘈疭〔5〕，日数十发，医所不疗，除热方。巢氏〔6〕云：脚气〔7〕宜风引汤。

Annotations

[1] *Feng Yin Tang* (Wind-Extinguishing Decoction): A formula for exuberant heat stirring wind and causing epilepsy. Consisting of six medicinal minerals, *Long Gu* (Os Draconis), *Mu Li* (Concha Ostreae), *Da Huang* (Radix et Rhizoma Rhei), etc., this formula submerges yang, clears heat and extinguishes wind. Enlightened by this formula, Zhang Xichun, a contemporary physician developed *Jian Ling Tang* (Down Sweeping

Decoction) to use heavy-weight medicinals to treat hypertension or cerebral hemorrhage.

[2] *Chu Re Tan Xian:* Alleviates heat-induced paralysis and epilepsy.

[3] *Wei Nang:* A leather bag to hold medicinals.

[4] *Jing Hua Shui:* Clear spring water drawn from a well early in the morning.

[5] *Zhi Zong:* Convulsions.

[6] *Chao Shi:* the *Zhu Bing Yuan Hou Lun* (Treatise on the Origins and Manifestations of Various Diseases) by Chao Yuanfang.

[7] *Jiao Qi:* Beriberi characterized by leg weakness, numbness, soreness or swelling.

Interpretations

The *Feng Yin Tang* (Wind-Extinguishing Decoction) acts to clear heat and alleviates fright. It is indicated for heat-induced paralysis and fright-induced epilepsy.

Feng Yin Tang

[Ingredients]

大黄	*dà huáng*	4 *liǎng*	Radix et Rhizoma Rhei
干姜	*gān jiāng*	4 *liǎng*	Rhizoma Zingiberis
龙骨	*lóng gǔ*	4 *liǎng*	Os Draconis
桂枝	*guì zhī*	3 *liǎng*	Ramulus Cinnamomi
甘草	*gān cǎo*	2 *liǎng*	Radix et Rhizoma Glycyrrhizae
牡蛎	*mǔ lì*	2 *liǎng*	Concha Ostreae
寒水石	*hán shuǐ shí*	6 *liǎng*	Glauberitum
滑石	*huá shí*	6 *liǎng*	Talcum
赤石脂	*chì shí zhī*	6 *liǎng*	Halloysitum Rubrum
白石脂	*bái shí zhī*	6 *liǎng*	Kaolinitum
紫石英	*zǐ shí yīng*	6 *liǎng*	Fluoritum
石膏	*shí gāo*	6 *liǎng*	Gypsum Fibrosum

Mash the above twelve ingredients, sieve and store in a leather bag. Take a three-finger pinch of the powder and decoct with 3 *shēng* of well water drawn in the early morning three times. Take 1 *shēng* for each dose when it is warm. It is indicated for wind-related paralysis and epilepsy in adults. For fright-induced epilepsy or convulsions that recur dozens of times a day in children, this formula is helpful to clear heat. The *Zhu Bing Yuan Hou Lun* (Treatise on the Origins and Manifestations of Various Diseases) by Chao Yuanfang states, "Weak feet can be treated with *Feng Yin Tang* (Wind-Extinguishing Decoction)".

*****

[06] 防己地黄汤[1]治病如狂状[2]、妄行、独语不休，无寒热，其脉浮[3]。

防己一分桂枝三分防风三分甘草二分　右四味，以酒一杯，渍之一宿，绞取汁；生地黄二斤，　咀，蒸之如斗米饭久，以铜器盛其汁，更绞地黄汁，和。分再服。

Annotations

[1] *Fang Ji Di Huang Tang* (Stephania Root and Rehmannia Decoction): A formula for blood deficiency stirring wind and causing mania. Actions: Nourishes blood and removes wind. It can also be used for dizziness in the elderly. The *Di Huang Yin Zi* (Rehmannia Drink) recorded in the *Huang Di Nei Jing Su Wen* (Basic Questions, Yellow Emperor's Inner Classic) is actually a variation of this formula indicated for inability to speak or hemiplegia after stroke.

[2] *Ru Kuang Zhuang*: the word "*Kuang*" means mental disorder (mania).

[3] *Qi Mai Fu*: A superficial pulse.

Interpretations

The *Fang Ji Di Huang Tang* (Stephania Root and Rehmannia Decoction) is used to treat patients with mania-like symptoms including reckless behaviors, constantly talking gibberish, and an absence of fever or chills. The pulse is superficial.

Fang Ji Di Huang Tang

[Ingredients]

防己	*fáng jǐ*	1 *fēn*	Radix Stephaniae Tetrandrae
桂枝	*guì zhī*	3 *fēn*	Ramulus Cinnamomi
防风	*fáng fēng*	3 *fēn*	Radix Saposhnikoviae
甘草	*gān cǎo*	2 *fēn*	Radix et Rhizoma Glycyrrhizae

Soak the four ingredients in a cup of wine overnight and then wring out the juice. Cut 2 *jīn* of *Sheng Di Huang* (Radix Rehmanniae) into small pieces, steam them for approximately the length of time that it takes to cook a *dòu* of rice, and then wring out the juice. Mix the two juices and take in two equal doses.

*****

[07] 头风摩散方：〔1〕

大附子一枚炮盐等分右二味为散，沐了，以方寸匕，已摩疢上〔2〕，令药力行。

Annotations

[1] *Tou Feng Mo San Fang*: Head Wind Rubbing Powder, an externally used formula for head wind—episodic dizziness and headache. Actions: Removes wind, dissipates cold, and alleviates pain.

[2] *Yi Mo Chen Shang:* Apply the powder to the painful area.

Tou Feng Mo San Fang

[Ingredients]

附子	*fù zǐ*	1 large piece	Radix Aconiti Lateralis Praeparata
盐	*yán*		Salt

Ground the two equal portions of *Da Fu Zi* (Radix Aconiti Lateralis Praeparata) and salt into a powder. Wash the hair and immediately apply 1 square-inch-spoon of the powder to the painful area to achieve the medicinal efficacy.

*****

[08] 寸口脉沉而弱〔1〕，沉即主骨，弱即主筋〔2〕。沉即为肾，弱即为肝〔3〕。汗出入水中，如水伤心〔4〕。历节黄汗出，故曰历节。

Annotations

[1] *Cun Kou Mai Chen Er Ruo*: A deep, weak pulse. A deep pulse indicates interior and a weak pulse indicates deficiency. This suggests that the root cause of joint disorders is interior deficiency.

[2] *Chen Ji Zhu Gu, Ruo Ji Zhu Jin:* The two sentences are intertextual in describing the disease location—bones and sinews.

[3] *Chen Ji Wei Shen, Ruo Ji Wei Gan:* The two sentences are intertextual in describing the internal etiological factor of the joint disorder—deficiency of the liver and kidney.

[4] *Ru Shui Shang Xin:* Water dampness damages the blood vessels (which is dominated by the heart). This explains the external etiological factor of the joint disorder—exposure to cold dampness.

Interpretations

Interior deficiency is one of the major etiological factors of joint disorders. It may cause a deep, weak pulse. The internal causative factor is deficiency of the liver and kidney. The external causative factor is exposure to water upon sweating. As a result, water dampness affects the blood vessels and causes joint pain, swelling and yellow pus exudation, known as joint disease (due to dampness transforming into heat).

*****

[09] 趺阳脉[1]浮而滑，滑则谷气实[2]，浮则汗自出。

[10] 少阴脉[3]浮而弱，弱则血不足，浮则为风，风血相搏，即疼痛如掣。

Annotations

[1] *Fu Yang Mai*: The pulsation felt at the dorsal artery of the foot, at the acupuncture point Chongyang (ST 42). Ancient physicians believe feeling this pulsation can tell the abundance or insufficiency of stomach qi.

[2] *Gu Qi Shi:* Replenish stomach qi.

[3] *Shaoyin Mai:* The pulsation felt at Taixi (KI 3), located at the posterior aspect of the medial malleolus. Feeling this pulsation can tell the abundance or insufficiency of kidney qi.

Interpretations

A superficial, slippery pulse at the dorsal artery of the foot indicates replenish stomach qi. Individuals may experience spontaneous sweating and aversion to heat (instead of cold). A superficial, weak pulse at Taixi (KI 3) indicates insufficiency of yin blood (internally) and exposure to wind (externally). This may result in pulling pain in the joints.

*****

[11] 盛人脉涩小[1]，短气，自汗出，历节疼，不可屈伸，此皆饮酒汗出当风[2]所致。

Annotations

[1] *Sheng Ren Mai Se Xiao:* A hesitant, small pulse in obese people. The "*Sheng Ren*" means obese people. In Chinese medicine, obesity is caused by phlegm dampness. A hesitant, small pulse indicates interior yang deficiency. This sentence suggests that the internal causative factor of joint disorder is yang deficiency coupled with dampness retention.

[2] *Yin Jiu Han Chu Dang Feng*: Exposure to wind upon sweating after drinking wine. This explains the external causative factor of joint disorder—exposure to wind dampness.

Interpretations

A hesitant, small pulse (due to interior yang deficiency) in obese people, coupled with shortness of breath, spontaneous sweating, and joint pain with impaired flexion and extension are often caused by exposure to wind upon sweating after drinking wine. (The joint disorder caused by dampness retention due to yang deficiency, coupled with exposure to wind dampness.)

*****

[12] 诸肢节疼痛，身体魁瘰〔1〕，脚肿如脱，头眩、短气、温温欲吐〔2〕。桂枝芍药知母汤〔3〕主之。

桂枝芍药知母汤方：

桂枝四两芍药三两甘草二两麻黄二两生姜五两白术五两知母四两防风四两附子二两炮 右九味，以水七升，煮取二升。温服七合，日三服。

Annotations

[1] *Shen Ti Kui Luo:* The first two words "*Shen Ti*" here refers to joints. The latter two words "*Kui Luo*" means joint swelling.

[2] *Wen Wen Yu Tu:* Stomach stuffiness and discomfort.

[3] *Gui Zhi Shao Yao Zhi Mu Tang* (Cinnamon Twig, Peony, and Anemarrhena Decoction): A formula to remove wind, resolve dampness, warm the meridians, dissipate cold, nourish yin and clear heat.

Interpretations

The *Gui Zhi Shao Yao Zhi Mu Tang* (Cinnamon Twig, Peony and Anemarrhena Decoction) is indicated for pain and swelling of multiple joints. The joint swelling on the foot is so severe that individuals may feel it being separated from the body. Associated symptoms include dizziness, shortness of breath, stomach discomfort, nausea and vomiting.

Gui Zhi Shao Yao Zhi Mu Tang

[Ingredients]

桂枝	*guì zhī*	4 *liǎng*	Ramulus Cinnamomi
芍药	*sháo yào*	3 *liǎng*	Radix Paeoniae
甘草	*gān cǎo*	2 *liǎng*	Radix et Rhizoma Glycyrrhizae
麻黄	*má huáng*	2 *liǎng*	Herba Ephedrae
生姜	*shēng jiāng*	5 *liǎng*	Rhizoma Zingiberis Recens
白术	*bái zhú*	5 *liǎng*	Rhizoma Atractylodis Macrocephalae
知母	*zhī mǔ*	4 *liǎng*	Rhizoma Anemarrhenae
防风	*fáng fēng*	4 *liǎng*	Radix Saposhnikoviae
附子	*fù zǐ*	2 *liǎng*	Radix Aconiti Lateralis Praeparata

Decoct the above nine ingredients in 7 *shēng* of water to get 2 *shēng*. Take 3 *gě* when it is warm for each dose, 3 doses a day.

*****

[13] 味酸则伤筋，筋伤则缓，名曰泄；咸则伤骨，骨伤则痿，名曰枯〔1〕。枯泄相搏，名曰断泄。荣气不通，卫不独行，荣卫俱微〔2〕，三焦无所御，四属断绝〔3〕。身体羸瘦，独足肿大，黄汗出，胫冷〔4〕。假令发热，便为历节〔5〕也。

Annotations

[1] *Wei Suan Ze Shang Jin, Shang Jin Ze Huan, Ming Yue Xie; Xian Ze Shang Gu, Gu Shang Ze Wei, Ming Yue Ku:* Sour-tasting food

damages the sinew. When sinews are damaged, they slacken. This is called flaccidity. Salt-tasting food damages the bone. When bones are damaged, they weaken. This is called withering away. Actually the sour and salt tastes here refer to all five tastes. This sentence suggests that improper diet may cause sinews to become flaccid and bones withered away.

[2] *Rong Qi Bu Tong, Wei Bu Du Xing, Rong Wei Ju Wei:* As the circulation of Ying-nutrients and Wei-defense are obstructed, qi, blood, *Ying*-nutrients and *Wei*-defense become deficient.

[3] *San Jiao Wu Suo Yu, Si Shu Duan Juan:* The "*San Jiao*" here refers to the entire body, including the lung in the upper jiao, spleen and stomach in the middle jiao and kidney in the lower jiao. The whole sentence means, "The body lacks sufficient supply of qi and blood, and the four limbs are malnourished".

[4] *Shen Ti Lei Shou, Du Zu Zhong Da, Huang Han Chu, Jing Leng*: Weight loss, joint swelling of the lower limb with exudation of yellow pus, and a cold sensation of the lower leg. Instead of joint disorder, this condition is actually tuberculous bones and joints.

[5] *Jia Ling Fa Re, Bian Wei Li Jie*: A hot sensation upon palpating the swollen joint indicates a joint disorder.

Interpretations

Sour-tasting food damages the sinew. When sinews are damaged, they slacken. This is called flaccidity. Salt-tasting food damages the bone. When bones are damaged, they weaken. This is called withering away. Flaccidity of sinews combined with withering of bones is called "erosive flaccidity". When the circulation of *Ying*-nutrients and *Wei*-defense is obstructed, the body lacks sufficient supply of qi and blood, and the four limbs are malnourished. As a result, patients may present with weight loss, joint swelling of the lower limb coupled with exudation of yellow pus, and a cold sensation of the lower leg. The presence of a hot sensation upon palpation indicates a joint disorder.

*****

[14] 病历节[1]，不可屈伸，疼痛。乌头汤[2]主之。

麻黄芍药黄芪各三两甘草炙川乌五枚，㕮咀，以蜜二升，煎取一升，即出乌头。右五味。㕮咀四味，以水三升，煮取一升，去滓。内蜜煎中，更煎之。服七合。不知，尽服之。

Annotations

[1] *Bing Li Jie:* Joint pain.

[2] *Wu Tou Tang* (Aconite Main Root Decoction): A formula to warm the meridians, dissipate cold, resolve dampness and alleviate pain.

Interpretations

Impaired joint flexion and extension and joint pain that aggravates upon physical exertion should be treated with *Wu Tou Tang* (Aconite Main Root Decoction).

Wu Tou Tang

[Ingredients]

麻黄	*má huáng*	3 *liǎng*	Herba Ephedrae
芍药	*sháo yào*	3 *liǎng*	Radix Paeoniae
黄芪	*huáng qí*	3 *liǎng*	Radix Astragali
甘草	*gān cǎo*	2 *liǎng*	Radix et Rhizoma Glycyrrhizae
川乌	*chuān wū*	5 *pieces*	Radix Aconiti

Decoct five pieces of *Chuan Wu* (Radix Aconiti) with 2 *shēng* of honey to get 1 *shēng* and take out the *Wu Tou* (Aconite main root). Cut off the other four ingredients into pieces and decoct in 3 *shēng* of water to get 1 *shēng*. Remove the dregs and re-decoct with the previous honey solution. Take 7 *gě* first. If there is no noticeable effect, take the rest of the decoction in one dose.

*****

[15] 矾石汤〔1〕：治脚气冲心〔2〕。

矾石二两右一味，以浆水〔3〕一斗五升，煎三五沸，浸脚良。

Annotations

[1] *Fan Shi Tang* (Alum Decoction): An externally used formula for beriberi coupled with palpitations and vomiting.

[2] *Jiao Qi Chong Xin:* Beriberi with complications of palpitations, panting, vomiting, etc.

[3] *Jiang Shui*: See the same item in Chapter 3.

Interpretations

The *Fan Shi Tang* (Alum Decoction) can be used to treat beriberi with complications of palpitations and vomiting.

Method: Decoct 2 *liǎng* of *Fan Shi* (Alumen) in 15 *shēng* of millet water until it begins to boil. When it cools down, re-decoct to boil for 3-5 times. Soak the feet in the boiled liquid.

*****

[16]《古今录验》〔1〕续命汤〔2〕：治中风痱〔3〕。身体不能自收，口不能言，冒昧〔4〕不知痛处。或拘急不得转侧。姚云：与大续命同，兼治妇人产后失血者及老人小儿。

麻黄桂枝当归人参石膏干姜甘草各三两芎䓖一两杏仁四十枚右九味，以水一斗，煮取四升。温服一升。当小汗，薄覆脊，凭几坐，汗出则愈。不汗，更服。无所禁，勿当风。并治但伏不得卧，咳逆上气、面目浮肿。

Annotations

[1] *Gu Jin Lu Yan*: Ancient and Modern Records of Proven Formulas compiled by Zhen Liyan in the Tang Dynasty (618-907). This text has been lost.

[2] *Xu Ming Tang* (Life Prolonging Decoction): A formula for wind stroke. Actions: Tonifies qi and blood, removes wind and expels pathogenic factors. Since it contains qi-supplementing and blood-nourishing ingredients such as *Ren Shen* (Radix et Rhizoma Ginseng), *Dang Gui* (Radix Angelicae Sinensis) and *Chuan Xiong* (Rhizoma Chuanxiong), this formula can be used for bleeding after childbirth. Since it also contains lung qi-dispersing ingredients such as *Ma Huang* (Herba Ephedrae), *Shi Gao* (Gypsum Fibrosum) and *Xing Ren* (Semen Armeniacae Amarum), this formula can be used for coughing or asthma in the elderly or children.

[3] *Fei*: Disuse muscle atrophy after wind stroke.

[4] *Mao Mei*: Blurred vision.

Interpretations

The *Xu Ming Tang* (Life Prolonging Decoction) recorded in the *Gu Jin Lu Yan* (Ancient and Modern Records of Proven Formulas) can be used for wind stroke of the meridians with an inability to initiate body movement or grasp objects with the hand, tongue stiffness, blurred vision, skin insensitivity to pain, and in some cases, difficulty turning sides. Yao said, like *Da Xu Ming Tang* (Major Life Prolonging Decoction), this formula can also be used for bleeding after childbirth or coughing/asthma in the elderly or children.

Xu Ming Tang

[Ingredients]

麻黄	*má huáng*	3 *liǎng*	Herba Ephedrae
桂枝	*guì zhī*	3 *liǎng*	Ramulus Cinnamomi
当归	*dāng guī*	3 *liǎng*	Radix Angelicae Sinensis
人参	*rén shēn*	3 *liǎng*	Radix et Rhizoma Ginseng
石膏	*shí gāo*	3 *liǎng*	Gypsum Fibrosum
干姜	*gān jiāng*	3 *liǎng*	Rhizoma Zingiberis

甘草	*gān cǎo*	3 *liǎng*	Radix et Rhizoma Glycyrrhizae
川芎	*chuān xiōng*	1 *liǎng*	Rhizoma Chuanxiong
杏仁	*xìng rén*	40 kernels	Semen Armeniacae Amarum

Decoct the above nine ingredients in 1 *dòu* of water to get 4 *shēng*. Take 1 *shēng* when it is warm for each dose. Slight sweating helps to get a better effect. It's advisable to keep the back warm and sit leaning over a table. If there is no sweating, take another dose. It's important to avoid exposure to wind after sweating.

This formula can also be used to treat an inability to lie flat, coughing with rapid breathing and facial puffiness.

*****

[17]《千金》三黄汤[1]，治中风手足拘急，百节疼痛，烦热心乱，恶寒，经日不欲饮食。

麻黄五分独活四分细辛二分黄芪二分黄芩三分右五味，以水六升，煮取二升。分温三服，一服小汗，二服大汗。心热加大黄二分；腹满加枳实一枚；气逆加人参三分；悸，加牡蛎三分；渴，加栝蒌根三分；先有寒，加附子一枚。

Annotations

[1] *Qian Jin San Huang Tang* (Three Yellow Decoction) recorded in the *Qian Jin Yao Fang* (Important Formulas Worth a Thousand Gold Pieces): A formula to remove wind, supplemens qi and clear heat.

Interpretations

The *San Huang Tang* (Three Yellow Decoction) can be used for wind stroke with contracture of the limbs, joint pain, vexation, aversion to cold and a poor appetite.

Qian Jin San Huang Tang

[Ingredients]

麻黄	*má huáng*	5 *fēn*	Herba Ephedrae
独活	*dú huó*	4 *fēn*	Radix Angelicae Pubescentis
细辛	*xì xīn*	2 *fēn*	Radix et Rhizoma Asari
黄芪	*huáng qí*	2 *fēn*	Radix Astragali
黄芩	*huáng qín*	3 *fēn*	Radix Scutellariae

Decoct the five ingredients in 6 *shēng* of water to get 2 *shēng*. Take when it is warm in three doses. Patients may experience mild sweating after the first dose and profuse sweating after the second and third doses.

Modifications

For stomach heat, add 2 *fēn* of *Da Huang* (Radix et Rhizoma Rhei) to promote bowel movements and clear heat;

For abdominal distension, add 1 piece of *Zhi Shi* (Fructus Aurantii Immaturus) to circulate qi;

For ascending of stomach qi (belching), add 3 *fēn* of *Ren Shen* (Radix et Rhizoma Ginseng) to tonify and down-regulate qi;

For palpitations, add 3 *fēn* of *Mu Li* (Concha Ostreae) to tranquilize the mind;

For thirst, add 3 *fēn* of *Gua Lou Gen* (Radix Trichosanthis) to engender fluids;

For pre-existing deficiency cold, add 1 piece of *Fu Zi* (Radix Aconiti Lateralis Praeparata) to warm the middle jiao and dissipate cold.

*****

[18]《近效方》[1] 术附子汤[2]，治风虚头重，眩苦极[3]。不知食味，暖肌补中，益精气。

白术二两附子一枚半，炮，去皮甘草一两炙右三味，锉。每五钱匕，姜五片，枣一枚，水盏半，煎七分，去滓。温服。

Annotations

[1] *Jin Xiao Fang* (Formulas for Instant Effect) compiled by Li Jianyi in the Tang Dynasty (618-907). This text has been lost.

[2] *Zhu Fu Tang* (Atractylodes Macrocephala and Aconite Decoction): A formula to warm the kidney, supplement essence, strengthen the spleen and regulate the middle jiao.

[3] *Feng Xu Tou Zhong, Xuan Ku Ji*: Severe dizziness and heaviness in the head.

Interpretations

The *Zhu Fu Tang* (Atractylodes Macrocephala and Aconite Decoction) can be used for severe dizziness, heaviness in the head, and loss of appetite. This formula acts to warm the kidney, reinforce the middle jiao and supplement essential qi.

Zhu Fu Tang

[Ingredients]

白术	*bái zhú*	*2 liǎng*	Rhizoma Atractylodis Macrocephalae
附子	*fù zǐ*	1.5 pieces	Radix Aconiti Lateralis Praeparata (bark removed and baked)
甘草	*gān cǎo*	*1 liǎng*	Radix et Rhizoma Glycyrrhizae

Grind the above three ingredients into a fine powder. Decoct 5 *qian*-spoons of the powder, 5 ginger slices and 1 piece of Chinese date in one and half cups of water to get 7 *fēn*. Remove the dregs and take when it is warm.

*****

[19] 崔氏八味丸[1]，治脚气上入，少腹不仁[2]。

干地黄八两 山茱萸 署蓣各四两 泽泻 茯苓 牡丹皮各三两 桂枝 附子炮，各一两 右八味，末之，炼蜜和丸，梧子大。酒下十五丸，日再服。

Annotations

[1] *Cui Shi Ba Wei Wan* (Cui's Eight Ingredient Pill): Originally known as *Ba Wei Shen Qi Wan* (Eight Ingredient Kidney Qi Pill) (see Chapter 6, 12 and 13), it is indicated for chronic deficiency, phlegm-fluid retention, or wasting-thirsting disorder (diabetes). It's called Cui's Eight Ingredient Pill because Cui applied this formula to beriberi. It is recorded as *Zhang Zhongjing Ba Wei Wan* (Zhang Zhongjing's Eight Ingredient Pill). Actions: Supplements kidney qi and warms/transforms cold and dampness. As a well-recognized kidney-tonifying formula, it is later known as *Jin Kui Shen Qi Wan* (Golden Cabinet's Kidney Qi Pill) or *Fu Gui Ba Wei Wan* (Aconite and Cinnamomi Eight Ingredient Pill).

[2] *Shao Fu Bu Ren:* Beriberi is a systemic condition. It begins with leg weakness and impaired sensory perception (needle-pricking sensation or sensation that resembles that of small insects crawling on/under the skin), and may develop into skin insensitivity. In severe cases, palpitations, shortness of breath and vomiting may be present. These symptoms result from the failure of kidney qi to transform cold and dampness.

Interpretations

The *Cui Shi Ba Wei Wan* (Cui's Eight Ingredient Pill) can be used for beriberi, coupled with skin insensitivity of the bilateral lower abdomen.

Cui Shi Ba Wei Wan

[Ingredients]

干地黄	*gān dì huáng*	8 *liǎng*	Radix Rehmanniae
山茱萸	*shān zhū yú*	4 *liǎng*	Fructus Corni
山药	*shān yào*	4 *liǎng*	Rhizoma Dioscoreae
泽泻	*zé xiè*	3 *liǎng*	Rhizoma Alismatis
茯苓	*fú líng*	3 *liǎng*	Poria
牡丹皮	*mǔ dān pí*	3 *liǎng*	Cortex Moutan
桂枝	*guì zhī*	1 *liǎng*	Ramulus Cinnamomi
附子	*fù zǐ*	1 *liǎng*	Radix Aconiti Lateralis Praeparata

Grind the above eight ingredients into a fine powder and blend with the heated honey to make pellets the size of firmiana seeds. Take 15 pellets with wine for each dose, 2 doses a day.

*****

[20]《千金》越婢加术汤〔1〕：治肉极〔2〕，热则身体津脱，腠理开，汗大泄，厉风气，下焦脚弱〔3〕。

麻黄六两石膏半斤生姜三两甘草二两白术四两大枣十五枚　右六味，以水六升，先煮麻黄，去上沫，内诸药，煮取三升。分温三服。恶风，加附子一枚炮。

Annotations

[1] *Qian Jin Yue Bi Jia Zhu Tang* (Maidservant from Yue Decoction plus Atractylodes): A formula to remove wind, clear heat, strengthen the spleen, and benefit qi.

[2] *Zhi Rou Ji:* Extreme of the muscle, one of the six extremes (the other five are extremes of qi, blood, sinew, bone, and essence). Extreme of the muscle means severe muscle fatigue and weakness.

[3] *Li Feng Qi, Xiao Jiao Jiao Ruo*: Leg weakness due to severe pathogenic wind.

Interpretations

The *Yue Bi Jiao Zhu Tang* (Maidservant from Yue Decoction plus Atractylodes) recorded in the *Qian Jin Yao Fang* (Important Formulas Worth a Thousand Gold Pieces) can be used to treat muscle fatigue and weakness due to severe loss of body fluids from profuse sweating (caused by exuberant interior heat), coupled with an exposure to wind upon sweating.

Yue Bi Jiao Zhu Tang

[Ingredients]

麻黄	má huáng	6 *liǎng*	Herba Ephedrae
石膏	*shí gāo*	8 *liǎng*	Fructus Corni
生姜	*shēng jiāng*	3 *liǎng*	Rhizoma Zingiberis Recens
甘草	*gān cǎo*	2 *liǎng*	Radix et Rhizoma Glycyrrhizae
白术	*bái zhú*	4 *liǎng*	Rhizoma Atractylodis Macrocephalae
大枣	*dà zǎo*	15 pieces	Fructus Jujube

Decoct *Ma Huang* (Herba Ephedrae) first in 6 *shēng* of water, remove the foam and add the rest of the ingredients to decoct and get 3 *shēng*. Take the decoction when it is warm in 3 doses. For aversion to wind, add 1 piece of *Fu Zi* (Radix Aconiti Lateralis Praeparata).

血痹虚劳病脉证并治第六
Chapter 6 Blood Impediment and Deficiency Exhaustion—Pulses, Patterns and Treatment

Overview

This chapter discusses blood impediment and deficiency exhaustion. Blood impediment results from blocked yang qi and obstructed blood flow. This is often caused by deficiency of qi and blood coupled with an exposure to wind. Deficiency exhaustion is a collective term for congenitally deficient or chronic debilitating, progressive conditions due to consumptions of qi and blood of the five-zang organs. With a slow onset and long duration, it begins with deficiency, over time, progresses into consumption and further into exhaustion. The *Lin Zheng Zhi Nan Yi An* (Case Records as a Guide to Clinical Practice) states, "As for the sequence of deficiency, consumption and exhaustion, chronic, persistent deficiency is called consumption, and persistent, extreme consumption is called exhaustion".

The two conditions are discussed together because they share the similar pathological process. The *Jin Kui Xuan Jie* (Explanation of Unresolved Issues in the 'Essentials from the Golden Cabinet') records, "Blood impediment definitely involves deficiency exhaustion. Blood impediment in people who appear strong but have weak sinews or bones is often caused by sweating upon fatigue. Deficiency exhaustion definitely progresses into blood impediment, causing blood stasis, rough skin and dark circles under the eyes".

*****

[01] 问曰：血痹病〔1〕从何得之？师曰：夫尊荣人，骨弱肌肤盛〔2〕，重因疲劳汗出，卧不时动摇，加被微风〔3〕，遂得之。但以脉自微涩在寸口，关上小紧〔4〕，宜针引阳气，令脉和紧去则愈〔5〕。

Annotations

[1] *Xue Bi Bing*: Blood impediment disorder characterized by limb numbness due to deficiency of qi and blood coupled with an exposure to exogenous pathogenic factors.

[2] *Zun Rong Ren, Gu Ruo Ji Fu Sheng:* Entitled people who live a comfortable life and do little physical labor may appear strong but actually have weak bones or sinews.

[3] *Zhong Yin Pi Lao Han Chu, Wo Bu Shi Dong Yao, Jia Bei Wei Feng*: The "*Pi Lao* (fatigue)" here refers to sexual intercourse. The "*Wo Bu Shi Dong Yao*" refers to the body moving during sexual intercourse. The "*Jia Bai Wei Feng*" means exposure to mild wind.

[4] *Mai Zi Wei Se Zai Cun Kou, Guan Shang Xiao Jin*: A faint, hesitant pulse at the Cunkou area, small and tight at the *Guan* position. A faint pulse indicates yang qi insufficiency. A hesitant pulse indicates blood stagnation. A small and tight pulse at the *Guan* position indicates mild external wind cold.

[5] *Zhen Yin Yang Qi, Ling Ma He Jin Qu Ze Yu*: As blood impediment is caused by blockage of yang qi and obstruction of blood flow, it should be treated by activating yang qi with acupuncture. When yang qi moves, the blood circulates, the pulse becomes normal and the patients will recover.

Interpretations

Question: How does one get blood impediment?

Answer: Entitled people who live a comfortable life and do little physical labor appear strong; however, their bones and sinews are weak. In addition, sexual indulgence causes sweating during their sleep. If exposed to wind cold at this time, they will develop blood impediment with a faint, hesitant pulse at the *Cunkou* area and small, tight pulse at the *Guan* position. Since wind cold only affects the superficial region, this condition can be treated by activating yang qi with acupuncture. When yang qi moves, the pulse will become normal and the patients will recover.

*****

[02] 血痹阴阳俱微，寸口关上微，尺中小紧〔1〕，外证身体不仁，如风痹状〔2〕，黄耆桂枝五物汤〔3〕主之。

黄耆桂枝五物汤方：黄耆三两芍药三两桂枝三两生姜六两大枣十二枚右五味，以水六升，煮取二升。温服七合，日三服一方有人参。

Annotations

[1] *Yin Yang Ju Wei, Cun Kou Guan Shang Wei, Chi Zhong Xiao Jin*: Since the *Cunkou* area is considered yang and *Guan* position yin, the "*Yin Yang Ju Wei*" means a faint pulse at both the *Cunkou* area and *Guan* position. The "*Chi Zhong Xiao Jin*" means a small, tight pulse felt at the *Chi* position, indicating a deeper disease location.

[2] *Shen Ti Bu Ren, Ru Feng Bi Zhuang:* Generalized numbness that resembles wind impediment, which is characterized by numbness and pain. Blood impediment causes numbness alone.

[3] *Huang Qi Gui Zhi Wu Wu Tang* (Astragalus and Cinnamon Twig Five Ingredient Decoction): A modified *Gui Zhi Tang* (Cinnamon Twig Decoction) by removing *Gan Cao* (Radix et Rhizoma Glycyrrhizae), doubling the dose of *Sheng Jiang* (Rhizoma Zingiberis Recens) and adding *Huang Qi* (Radix Astragali). It is a major formula for blood impediment. Actions: Unblocks yang and alleviates impediment. Inspired by this formula, the *Bu Yang Huan Wu Tang* (Yang-Supplementing and Five-Returning Decoction) for wind stroke contains a big dose of *Huang Qi* (Radix Astragali).

Interpretations

The *Huang Qi Gui Zhi Wu Wu Tang* (Astragalus and Cinnamon Five Ingredient Decoction) can be used for blood impediment with a faint pulse at the *Cunkou* area and *Guan* position and a small, tight pulse felt at the *Chi* position (blocked yang qi, obstructed blood flow, coupled with exposure to severe wind cold) and generalized numbness that resembles wind impediment.

Huang Qi Gui Zhi Wu Wu Tang

[Ingredients]

黄芪	*huáng qí*	3 *liǎng*	Radix Astragali
芍药	*sháo yào*	3 *liǎng*	Radix Paeoniae
桂枝	*guì zhī*	3 *liǎng*	Ramulus Cinnamomi
生姜	*shēng jiāng*	6 *liǎng*	Rhizoma Zingiberis Recens
大枣	*dà zǎo*	12 pieces	Fructus Jujubae

Decoct the above five ingredients in 6 *shēng* of water to get 2 *shēng*. Take 7 *gě* when it is warm for each dose, 3 doses a day. An alternative version of this formula contains *Ren Shen* (Radix Ginseng) for people with deficiency of qi and blood.

*****

[03] 夫男子平人〔1〕，脉大为劳〔2〕，极虚亦为劳〔3〕。

Annotations

[1] *Nan Zi Ping Ren*: The "*Nan Zi*" means men. Here it refers to all men (both men and women). The "*Ping Ren*" means a group of people appear normal but actually have insufficiency of qi and blood of the five-zang organs.

[2] *Mai Da Wei Lao:* Deficiency exhaustion with a large, weak pulse.

[3] *Ji Xu Yi Wei Lao*: Deficiency exhaustion with a deficient, soft and weak pulse.

Interpretations

Deficiency exhaustion is often seen in men and women who appear normal on the outside but actually have insufficiency of qi and blood of the five-zang organs. They may present with two categories of manifestations: deficiency exhaustion with a big pulse (deficiency of both yin and yang and floating of deficiency yang) and deficiency exhaustion with a soft and weak pulse (deficiency of yin and yang and failure of essential qi).

*****

[04] 男子面色薄〔1〕者，主渴及亡血〔2〕，卒喘悸〔3〕，脉浮者〔4〕，里虚也。

Annotations

[1] *Mian Se Bao*: A thin, pale and lusterless complexion.

[2] *Zhu Ke Ji Wang Xue:* The "*Ke*" here refers to wasting and thirsting disorder. The "*Wang Xue*" means lack of blood, anemia. This sentence suggests a history of wasting and thirsting disorder or anemia.

[3] *Cu Chuan Ji*: Paroxysmal panting and palpitations.

[4] *Mai Fu*: A big, superficial and weak pulse.

Interpretations

A thin, pale and lusterless complexion, a known history of wasting and thirsting disorder or anemia, paroxysmal panting and palpitations and a big, superficial and weak pulse indicate deficiency exhaustion due to qi deficiency of the five-zang organs.

*****

[05] 男子脉虚沉弦[1]，无寒热，短气里急，小便不利[2]，面色白，时目瞑[3]，兼衄[4]，少腹满，此为劳使之然[5]。

Annotations

[1] *Mai Xu Chen Xian*: A deep, wiry and weak pulse, indicating deficiency exhaustion.

[2] *Duan Qi Li Ji, Xiao Bian Bu Li:* Shortness of breath, a swift pulse due to interior deficiency and inhibited urination. These symptoms are caused by yang qi deficiency.

[3] *Mian Se Bai, Shi Mu Ming, Jian Nǜ*: A thin, pale complexion, frequent blurred vision and nosebleed. These symptoms are caused by yin blood deficiency.

[4] *Shao Fu Man*: Bilateral lower abdominal fullness and distension caused by inhibited urination (due to yang qi deficiency).

[5] *Ci Wei Lao Shi Zhi Ran*: All these symptoms are caused by deficiency of yin, yang, qi and blood.

Interpretations

In patients with deficiency exhaustion, the pulse is deep, wiry and weak. Although the chills and fever are absent, they experience rapid breathing, contracture of the lower abdomen, inhibited urination, a thin, white complexion, and frequent blurred vision, sometimes coupled with nosebleed and bilateral lower abdominal fullness and distension. These are all signs and symptoms indicative of deficiency exhaustion due to deficiency of yin, yang, qi and blood.

*****

[06] 劳之为病，其脉浮大[1]，手足烦[2]，春夏剧，秋冬瘥，阴寒精自出[3]，酸削[4]不能行。

Annotations

[1] *Mai Fu Da*: A superficial, big and weak pulse.

[2] *Shou Zu Fan:* Feverish sensations in the palms and soles.

[3] *Yin Han Jing Zi Chu:* Impotence (coldness in external genitalia) and seminal emissions.

[4] *Suan Xiao*: Soreness and pain.

Interpretations

Deficiency exhaustion manifests a superficial, big and weak pulse and feverish sensations in the palms and soles. The symptom aggravates in spring and summer but alleviates in autumn and winter. Impotence and seminal emissions due to coldness in the external genitalia may also be present. Some patients may experience difficulty walking due to sore, painful limbs.

*****

[07] 男子脉浮弱而涩〔1〕，为无子〔2〕，精气清冷〔3〕一作冷。

Annotations

[1] *Mai Fu Ruo Er Se*: A superficial, rapid and hesitant pulse.

[2] *Wu Zi:* Sterility.

[3] *Jing Qi Qing Leng:* Thin, clear and scanty semen.

Interpretations

A superficial, weak and hesitant pulse in men often indicate sterility due to thin, clear and scanty semen.

*****

[08] 夫失精家〔1〕少腹弦急，阴头寒〔2〕，目眩一作目眶痛。发落〔3〕。脉极虚芤迟，为清谷、亡血、失精〔4〕。脉得诸芤动微紧，男子失精，女子梦交〔5〕，桂枝龙骨牡蛎汤〔6〕主之。

桂枝加龙骨牡蛎汤方：《小品》〔7〕云：虚羸浮热汗出〔8〕者，除桂，加白薇，附子各三分，故曰二加龙骨汤〔9〕。

桂枝芍药生姜各三两甘草二两大枣十二枚龙骨牡蛎　右七味，以水七升，煮取三升。分温三服。

Annotations

[1] *Shi Jing Jia*: Patients with chronic seminal emissions or spermatorrhea.

[2] *Shao Fu Xuan Ji, Yin Tou Han:* Contracture of the lower abdomen and impotence due to yang qi deficiency.

[3] *Mu Xuan Yi Zuo Mu Kuang Tong, Fa Luo*: Blurred vision and hair loss are caused by deficiency of yin blood. The "*Mu Kuang Tong*" means pain in the eye socket due to stagnant heat in the liver meridian.

[4] *Mai Ji Xu Kong Chi, Wei Qing Gu, Wang Xue, Shi Jing:* An extremely deficient (superficial, big and weak), hollow and slow (superficial, big and scallion-stalk) pulse can be seen in diarrhea with stools containing undigested food, loss of blood or seminal emissions (different conditions manifesting the same pulse).

[5] *Mai De Zhu Kong Dong Wei Jin, Nan Zi Shi Jing, Nǚ Zi Meng Jiao*: A scallion-stalk and stirring (superficial of deficiency yang) pulse or faint and tight (yang qi deficiency) pulse can be seen in men with nocturnal emissions or women with sexual intercourse in dream (same conditions manifesting different pulses).

[6] *Gui Zhi Long Gu Mu Li Tang* (Cinnamon Twig Decoction plus Dragon Bone and Oyster Shell): A formula to harmonize yin and yang.

[7] *Xiao Pin*: It refers to the *Xiao Pin Fang* (A Humble Judgment on the Classical Formulas) compiled by Chen Yanzhi in the Northern and Southern Dynasties (420-589). This text has been lost.

[8] *Xu Lei Fu Re Han Chu*: In addition to nocturnal emissions, patients also present with deficiency heat, sweating, weight loss and fatigue.

[9] *Er Jia Long Gu Tang* (Dragon Bone Decoction with Two Additions): A modified version of *Gui Zhi Long Gu Mu Li Tang* (Cinnamon Twig Decoction plus Dragon Bone and Oyster Shell) by removing *Gui Zhi* (Ramulus Cinnamomi) and adding *Bai Wei* (Radix et Rhizoma Cynanchi Atrati) and *Fu Zi* (Radix Aconiti Lateralis Praeparata). Actions: Warms yang, astringes the essence and clears heat.

Interpretations

Patients with chronic seminal emissions may experience contracture of the lower abdomen, coldness in external genitalia, impotence, dizziness, blurred vision (or pain in the eye socket) and hair loss. An extremely deficient or scallion-stalk, slow pulse can also be seen in diarrhea with stools containing undigested food, loss of blood or loss of essence. A scallion-stalk, stirring or faint and tight pulse can be seen in men with nocturnal emission or women with sexual intercourse in dream. These signs and symptoms can be treated with *Gui Zhi Long Gu Mu Li Tang* (Cinnamon Twig Decoction plus Dragon Bone and Oyster Shell).

The *Xiao Pin Fang* (A Humble Judgment on the Classical Formulas) states, "For patients with seminal emissions, deficiency heat, sweating, weight loss and fatigue, remove *Gui Zhi* (Ramulus Cinnamomi) and add 3 *fēn* of *Bai Wei* (Radix et Rhizoma Cynanchi Atrati) and *Fu Zi* (Radix Aconiti Lateralis Praeparata) respectively. This is called *Er Jia Long Gu Tang* (Dragon Bone Decoction with Two Additions).

Gui Zhi Long Gu Mu Li Tang

[Ingredients]

桂枝	*guì zhī*	3 *liǎng*	Ramulus Cinnamomi
芍药	*sháo yào*	3 *liǎng*	Radix Paeoniae
生姜	*shēng jiāng*	3 *liǎng*	Rhizoma Zingiberis Recens
甘草	*gān cǎo*	2 *liǎng*	Radix et Rhizoma Glycyrrhizae
大枣	*dà zǎo*	12 pieces	Fructus Jujubae
龙骨	*lóng gǔ*	3 *liǎng*	Os Draconis
牡蛎	*mǔ lì*	3 *liǎng*	Concha Ostreae

Decoct the above seven ingredients in 7 *shēng* of water to get 3 *shēng*. Take when it is warm in 3 doses.

*****

[09] 天雄散〔1〕方：天雄三两，炮白术八两桂枝六两龙骨三两右四味，杵为散。酒服半钱匕，日三服。不知，稍增之〔2〕。

Annotations

[1] *Tian Xiong San* (Aconitum carmichaeli Debx Powder): A formula to tonify yang and astringe yin.

[2] *Shao Zeng Zhi:* Gradually increase the dosage.

Interpretations

The *Tian Xiong San* (Aconitum carmichaeli Debx Powder) is indicated for seminal emissions due to yang deficiency.

Tian Xiong San

[Ingredients]

天雄	*tiān xióng*	3 *liǎng*	Aconitum carmichaeli Debx (prepared)
白术	*bái zhú*	8 *liǎng*	Rhizoma Atractylodis Macrocephalae
桂枝	*guì zhī*	6 *liǎng*	Ramulus Cinnamomi
龙骨	*lóng gǔ*	3 *liǎng*	Os Draconis

Grind the above four ingredients into a fine powder. Take half a qian-spoon powder with wine for each dose, 3 doses a day. If patients do not respond, gradually increase the dosage.

*****

[10] 男子平人，脉虚弱细微者，善盗汗〔1〕也。

Annotations

[1] *Mai Xu Ruo Xi Wei Zhe, Shan Dao Han*: A weak pulse indicates yang deficiency. A thready and faint pulse indicates yin deficiency. Yang deficiency or internal heat due to yin deficiency can both cause night sweats.

Interpretations

Patients with deficiency exhaustion may appear normal on the outside; however, they often have a weak or faint, thready pulse and experience night sweats.

*****

[11] 人年五六十，其病脉大者〔1〕，痹侠背行〔2〕，苦肠鸣〔3〕，马刀侠瘿〔4〕者，皆为劳得之。

Annotations

[1] *Ren Nian Wu Liu Shi, Qi Bing Mai Da Zhe*: A superficial, big and weak pulse seen in people in their 50s or 60s with decline of essential qi.

[2] *Bi Xia Bei Hang*: Back/low back pain (bone spur or intervertebral disc herniation). This is *Bi*-impediment, not deficiency exhaustion.

[3] *Chang Ming*: Bowel sounds, loose stools and poor digestion.

[4] *Ma Dao Xia Ying*: Scrofula (tuberculous cervical lymphadenitis), one of the deficiency exhaustions.

Interpretations

In their 50s or 60s, people start to experience decline of essential qi. A superficial, big and weak pulse (superficial of deficiency yang) can be seen in the following conditions: *Bi*-impediment manifesting as back/low back pain or deficiency exhaustion manifesting as bowel sounds, chronic diarrhea, poor digestion or scrofula.

*****

[12] 脉沉小迟，名脱气[1]，其人疾行则喘喝，手足逆寒[2]，腹满，甚则溏泄，食不消化也[3]。

Annotations

[1] *Mai Chen Xiao Chi, Ming Tuo Qi*: A deep, small and slow pulse indicates yang deficiency and qi consumption, therefore known as collapse of qi.

[2] *Ji Xing Ze Chuan He, Shou Zu Ni Han:* Panting upon physical exertion. This is caused by kidney yang deficiency.

[3] *Fu Man, Shen Ze Tang Xie, Shi Bu Xiao Hua Ye:* Abdominal fullness, loose stools and poor digestion. These are caused by spleen yang deficiency (failure of respiratory and circulatory function).

Interpretations

A deep, small and slow pulse (due to collapse of yang qi) is known as collapse of qi. Patients with this condition present with panting upon physical exertion, cold limbs, and abdominal fullness and distension. In severe cases, loose stools containing undigested food may be present.

*****

[13] 脉弦而大，弦则为减，大则为芤[1]，减则为寒，芤则为虚，虚寒相搏，此名为革[2]，妇人则半产漏下[3]，男子则亡血失精[4]。

Annotations

[1] *Mai Xian Er Da, Xian Ze Wei Jian, Da Ze Wei Kong*: A wiry pulse indicates cold, a big pulse indicates deficiency. The "*Xian* (wiry)" here means wiry and weak. The "*Da* (big)" here means big and hollow.

[2] *Jian Ze Wei Han, Kong Ze Wei Xu, Xu Han Xiang Bo, Ci Ming Wei Ge:* A wiry, weak, big and hollow pulse is known as (*Ge*) drumskin

pulse. It is often caused by deficiency cold and seen in deficiency exhaustion with deficiency of essence and blood.

[3] *Ban Chan Lou Xia:* Miscarriage or bleeding during menstruation or after childbirth.

[4] *Wan Xue Shi Jing*: Loss of blood and seminal emissions.

Interpretations

A wiry, weak, big and hollow pulse is called a drumskin pulse. It is caused by deficiency cold (deficiency exhaustion with loss of essence and blood). It is often seen in bleeding after miscarriage, during menstruation or after childbirth in women; or loss of blood or seminal emissions in men.

*****

[14] 虚劳里急〔1〕，悸、衄〔2〕，腹中痛，梦失精，四肢酸疼，手足烦热〔3〕，咽干口燥，小建中汤〔4〕主之。

小建中汤方：

桂枝三两去皮甘草三两炙大枣十二枚芍药六两生姜二两胶饴一升 右六味，以水七升，煮取三升，去滓，内胶饴，更上微火消解。温服一升，日三服，呕家不可用建中汤〔5〕，以甜故也。

《千金》疗男女因积冷气滞，或大病后不复常，苦四肢沉重，骨肉痠疼，吸吸少气，行动喘乏，胸满气急〔6〕，腰背强痛，心中虚悸，咽干唇燥，面体少色〔7〕，或饮食无味，胁肋腹胀，头重不举，多卧少起，甚者积年，轻者百日，渐致瘦弱，五脏气竭〔8〕，则难可复常，六脉〔9〕俱不足，虚寒乏气，少腹拘急，羸瘠〔10〕百病，名曰黄芪建中汤〔11〕，又有人参二两。

Annotations

[1] *Li Ji*: Contracture of the abdomen due to interior deficiency of yin, yang, qi and blood.

[2] *Ji, Nü:* Heart deficiency causes palpitations; and liver deficiency causes nosebleed.

[3] *Shou Zu Fan Re:* Feverish sensations in the palms, soles and chest.

[4] *Xiao Jian Zhong Tang* (Minor Middle Jiao Fortifying Decoction): A modified version of *Gui Zhi Tang* (Cinnamon Twig Decoction) by doubling the dose of *Shao Yao* (Radix Paeoniae) and adding *Yi Tang* (Saccharum Granorum). Actions: Harmonizes yin and yang, and benefits the spleen and stomach.

[5] *Ou Jia Bu Ke Yong Jian Zhong Tang*: The *Xiao Jian Zhong Tang* (Minor Middle Jiao-Fortifying Decoction) is contraindicated for patients with vomiting because of its sweet flavor. Vomiting is associated with stomach heat and should be treated with medicinals that are bitter in taste and descending in property such as *Huang Lian* (Rhizoma Coptidis) or *Da Huang* (Radix et Rhizoma Rhei).

[6] *Xi Xi Shao Qi, Xing Dong Chuan Fa, Xiong Man Qi Ji*: Rapid breathing, panting upon physical exertion and chest fullness and distension (similar to emphysema or poor lung function).

[7] *Mian Ti Shao Se*: Lusterless body skin.

[8] *Wu Zang Qi Jie*: Functional failure of the zang-fu organs.

[9] *Liu Mai*: The positions of feeling the pulse, three regions (*Cun, Guan and Chi*) on each side.

[10] *Lei Ji*: Weight loss.

[11] *Huang Qi Jian Zhong Tang* (Astragalus Middle Jiao-Fortifying Decoction): a modified version of *Xiao Jian Zhong Tang* plus *Huang Qi* (Radix Astragali).

Interpretations

Abdominal contracture, palpitations, nosebleed, abdominal pain, nocturnal emissions, joint pain, feverish sensations in the palms, soles and chest, and a dry mouth and throat in patients with deficiency exhaustion can be treated with *Xiao Jian Zhong Tang* (Minor Middle Jiao-Fortifying Decoction).

Xiao Jian Zhong Tang

[Ingredients]

桂枝	*guì zhī*	3 *liǎng*	Ramulus Cinnamomi (bark removed)
甘草	*gān cǎo*	3 *liǎng*	Radix et Rhizoma Glycyrrhizae (fried)
大枣	*dà zǎo*	12 pieces	Fructus Jujubae
芍药	*sháo yào*	6 *liǎng*	Radix Paeoniae
生姜	*shēng jiāng*	2 *liǎng*	Rhizoma Zingiberis Recens
饴糖	*yí táng*	1 *shēng*	Saccharum Granorum

Decoct the first five ingredients in 7 *shēng* of water to get 3 *shēng*. Remove the dregs, add *Yi Tang* (Saccharum Granorum) and dissolve it with mild fire. Take 1 *shēng* when it is warm for each dose, 3 doses a day.

[Cautionary note] The *Xiao Jian Zhong Tang* (Minor Middle Jiao-Fortifying Decoction) is contraindicated for patients with vomiting because of its sweet flavor.

According to the *Qian Jin Yao Fang* (Important Formulas Worth a Thousand Gold Pieces for Emergency), *Huang Qi Jiang Zhong Tang* (Astragalus Middle Jiao-Fortifying Decoction) plus 2 *liǎng* of *Ren Shen* (Radix et Rhizoma Ginseng) can be used to treat disorders due to cold retention or qi stagnation or delayed recovery from major illnesses. Clinical manifestations include limb heaviness/fatigue, muscle/bone/joint pain, rapid breathing, panting upon physical exertion, back stiffness/pain, palpitations, dry mouth and lips, lusterless complexion and body skin, a poor appetite, distending pain in the right upper quadrant and subcostal region, heaviness in the head with a sense of difficulty lifting the head, a tendency to lie down with no desire to rise, gradual weight loss, functional failure of the zang-fu organs, and a deficient pulse felt at all the three regions on both hands.

*****

[15] 虚劳里急，诸不足[1]，黄芪建中汤[2]主之。于小建中汤内加黄芪一两半，余依上法。气短胸满者加生姜；腹满者去枣，加茯苓一两半。及疗肺虚损不足，补气加半夏三两。

Annotations

[1] *Zhu Bu Zu*: Deficiency of yin, yang, qi and blood of the five-zang organs. Since this formula contains *Huang Qi* (Radix Astragali), it is especially indicated for qi deficiency. In addition to deficiency exhaustion indicated by *Xiao Jian Zhong Tang* (Minor Middle Jiao-Fortifying Decoction), this formula is also indicated for spontaneous sweating, lack of qi and fatigue.

[2] *Huang Qi Jian Zhong Tang* (Astragalus Middle Jiao-Fortifying Decoction): a modified version of *Xiao Jian Zhong Tang* (Minor Middle Jiao-Fortifying Decoction) plus *Huang Qi* (Radix Astragali). Actions: Harmonizes yin and yang, supplements qi, and fortifies the spleen and stomach.

Interpretations

Abdominal contracture (due to deficiency exhaustion) and deficiency of yin, yang, qi and blood of the five-zang organs can be treated with *Huang Qi Jian Zhong Tang* (Astragalus Middle Jiao-Fortifying Decoction).

Add 1.5 *liǎng* of *Huang Qi* (Radix Astragali) to *Xiao Jian Zhong Tang* (Minor Middle Jiao-Fortifying Decoction) and follow the above preparation method. For shortness of breath and chest tightness, add *Sheng Jiang* (Rhizoma Zingiberis Recens); for abdominal fullness and distension, remove *Da Zao* (Fructus Jujubae) and add 1.5 *liǎng* of *Fu Ling* (Poria); and for lung qi deficiency, add 3 *liǎng* of *Ban Xia* (Rhizoma Pinelliae).

*****

[16] 虚劳腰痛，少腹拘急，小便不利〔1〕者，八味肾气丸〔2〕主之。方见脚气中。

Annotations

[1] *Xiao Bian Bu Li:* Inhibited urination or urinary dribbling due to kidney qi deficiency and impaired qi transformation of the urinary bladder.

[2] *Ba Wei Shen Qi Wan:* Also known as the *Cui Shi Ba Wei Wan* (Cui's Eight Ingredient Pill). Actions: Nourishes yin, warms yang and activates kidney qi.

Interpretations

Low back pain, lower abdominal contracture (pain) and inhibited urination in patients with deficiency exhaustion can be treated with the *Ba Wei Shen Qi Wan* (Eight Ingredient Kidney Qi Pill). The formula is also referred to as *Cui Shi Ba Wei Wan* (Cui's Eight Ingredient Pill) in chapter 5 or 22.

*****

[17] 虚劳诸不足，风气百疾〔1〕，薯蓣丸〔2〕主之。

薯蓣丸方：

薯蓣三十分当归桂枝曲干地黄豆黄卷各十分甘草二十八分人参七分芎䓖芍药白术麦门冬杏仁各六分柴胡桔梗茯苓各五分阿胶七分干姜三分白蔹］二分防风六分大枣百枚为膏 右二十一味，末之，炼蜜和丸，如弹子大。空腹酒服一丸，一百丸为剂。

Annotations

[1] *Xu Lao Zhu Bu Zu, Feng Qi Bai Ji:* Disorders caused by deficiency of yin, yang, qi and blood (due to deficiency exhaustion) coupled with

exposure to wind, such as dizziness, hemiplegia or wind-impediment (migratory pain and numbness).

[2] *Shu Yu Wan* (Dioscoreae Pill): A formula to supplement healthy qi and remove wind. *Shan Yao* (Rhizoma Dioscoreae), *Gan Cao* (Radix et Rhizoma Glycyrrhizae) and *Da Zao* (Fructus Jujubae) are the monarch medicinals to tonify the spleen. This formula also contains multiple medicinals to supplement qi and nourish blood and some medicinals to remove wind and regulate qi. This is a very influential spleen-tonifying formula. Actually, the combination of *Ren Shen* (Radix et Rhizoma Ginseng), *Bai Zhu* (Rhizoma Atractylodis Macrocephalae), *Fu Ling* (Poria) and *Gan Cao* (Radix et Rhizoma Glycyrrhizae) is later known as *Si Jun Zi Tang* (Four Gentlemen Decoction); the combination of *Dang Gui* (Radix Angelicae Sinensis), *Di Huang* (Radix Rehmanniae), *Chuan Xiong* (Rhizoma Chuanxiong) and *Bai Shao* (Radix Paeoniae Alba) is later known as *Si Wu Tang* (Four Ingredient Decoction); and the combination of the two formulas is later known as the *Ba Zhen Tang* (Eight Gem Decoction).

Interpretations

The *Shu Yu Wan* (Dioscoreae Pill) can be taken for a long period of time to treat numerous conditions (such as dizziness or hemiplegia) due to deficiency of yin, yang, qi and blood in deficiency exhaustion.

Shu Yu Wan

[Ingredients]

山药	*shān yào*	30 *fēn*	Rhizoma Dioscoreae
当归	*dāng guī*	10 *fēn*	Radix Angelicae Sinensis
桂枝	*guì zhī*	10 *fēn*	Ramulus Cinnamomi
神曲	*shén qū*	10 *fēn*	Massa Medicata Fermentata
干地黄	*gān dì huáng*	10 *fēn*	Radix Rehmanniae

豆黄卷	*dòu huáng juǎn*	10 *fēn*	Semen Sojae Germinatum
甘草	*gān cǎo*	28 *fēn*	Radix et Rhizoma Glycyrrhizae
人参	*rén shēn*	7 *fēn*	Radix et Rhizoma Ginseng
川芎	*chuān xiōng*	6 *fēn*	Rhizoma Chuanxiong
白术	*bái zhú*	6 *fēn*	Rhizoma Atractylodis Macrocephalae
芍药	*sháo yào*	6 *fēn*	Radix Paeoniae
麦冬	*mài dōng*	6 *fēn*	Radix Ophiopogonis
杏仁	*xìng rén*	6 *fēn*	Semen Armeniacae Amarum
柴胡	*chái hú*	5 *fēn*	Radix Bupleuri
茯苓	*fú líng*	5 *fēn*	Poria
阿胶	*ē jiāo*	5 *fēn*	Colla Corii Asini
干姜	*gān jiāng*	3 *fēn*	Rhizoma Zingiberis
白薇	*bái wēi*	2 *fēn*	Radix et Rhizoma Cynanchi Atrati
防风	*fáng fēng*	6 *fēn*	Radix Saposhnikoviae
大枣	*dà zǎo*	100 pieces	Fructus Jujubae

Grind the above twenty-one ingredients into a fine powder, and mix with the prepared honey to make pellets the size of slingshot balls. Take 1 pellet with wine for each dose on an empty stomach, 100 pellets make up a course of treatment.

*****

[18] 虚劳虚烦不得眠[1]，酸枣汤[2]主之。

酸枣汤方：

酸枣仁二升甘草一两知母二两茯苓二两芎䓖二两，《深师》[3]有生姜二两右五味，以水八升，煮酸枣仁，得六升，内诸药，煮取三升。分温三服。

Annotations

[1] *Xu Fan Bu De Mian*: An inability to sleep due to liver yin deficiency and subsequently, ascending of deficiency fire. Patients may also experience night sweats and feverish sensations in the palms, soles and chest. The "*Xu Fan*" means deficiency heat.

[2] *Suan Zao Tang* or *Suan Zao Ren Tang* (Sour Jujube Decoction): A major formula for insomnia. Actions: Nourishes the liver and calms the mind. Generally *Sheng Jiang* (Rhizoma Zingiberis Recens) is not included in the formula for clinical use.

[3] *Shen Shi*: The *Shen Shi Fang* (Shen Shi's Formula) compiled in the Northern and Southern Dynasties (420-589). This text has been lost.

Interpretations

Insomnia due to liver yin deficiency can be treated with the *Suan Zao Ren Tang* (Sour Jujube Decoction).

Suan Zao Ren Tang

[Ingredients]

酸枣仁	*suān zǎo rén*	2 *shēng*	Semen Ziziphi Spinosae
甘草	*gān cǎo*	1 *liǎng*	Radix et Rhizoma Glycyrrhizae (fried)
知母	*zhī mǔ*	2 *liǎng*	Rhizoma Anemarrhenae
茯苓	*fú líng*	2 *liǎng*	Poria
川芎	*chuān xiōng*	2 *liǎng*	Rhizoma Chuanxiong

Decoct *Suan Zao Ren* (Semen Ziziphi Spinosae) first in 8 *shēng* of water and get 6 *shēng*. Add the other ingredients to decoct and get 3 *shēng*. Take when it is warm in 3 doses.

According to Shen Shi, a physician in the Northern and Southern Dynasties (420-589), this formula also contains 2 *liǎng* of *Sheng Jiang* (Rhizoma Zingiberis Recens).

*****

[19] 五劳虚极羸瘦〔1〕，腹满不能饮食〔2〕，食伤、忧伤、饮伤、房室伤、饥伤、劳伤、经络营卫气伤，内有干血〔3〕。肌肤甲错，两目黯黑〔4〕。缓中补虚〔5〕，大黄䗪虫丸〔6〕主之。

大黄䗪虫丸方：大黄十分，蒸黄芩二两甘草三两桃仁一升杏仁一升芍药四两干地黄十两干漆一两虻虫一升水蛭百枚蛴螬一升䗪虫半升 右十二味，末之，炼蜜和丸，小豆大。酒饮服五丸，日三服。

Annotations

[1] *Wu Lao Xu Ji Lei Shou:* The "*Wu Lao*" means five exhaustions of the five-zang organs, such as exhaustion of the heart or lung. Patients in late stage deficiency of the five-zang organs may experience significant weight loss.

[2] *Fu Man Bu Neng Yin Shi*: A subjective sensation of abdominal fullness and distension (due to blood stasis) with no desire to eat food.

[3] *Shi Shang, You Shang, Yin Shang, Fang Shi Shang, Ji Shang, Lao Shang, Jing Luo Ying Wei Qi Shang, Nei You Gan Xue*: Multiple causative factors of deficiency exhaustion, including improper diet, seven emotions, alcohol drinking, sexual indulgence, irregular eating habits, or mental/physical overexertion. These factors may obstruct the flow of qi and blood of the zang-fu organs and result in blood stagnation.

[4] *Ji Fu Jia Cuo, Liang Mu An Hei:* Rough, scaly skin due to blood stagnation (blood failing to nourish the skin) and dark circles under the eyes.

[5] *Huan Zhong Bu Xu*: Resolve blood stasis and reinforces the deficiency (treatment strategy).

[6] *Da Huang Zhe Chong Wan* (Rhubarb and Eupolyphaga Pill): A formula to move blood, resolve stasis and reinforce the body.

Interpretations

In late stage deficiency of the five-zang organs, patients may present with emaciation, a subjective feeling of abdominal distension and fullness, and loss of appetite. These symptoms can be caused by multiple factors, including improper diet, emotions, alcohol drinking, sexual indulgence, irregular eating habits and physical/mental overexertion. All these factors may obstruct the flow of qi and blood in meridians, *Ying*-nutrients and *Wei*-defense, leading to internal retention of stagnant blood. As a result, rough, scaly skin and dark circles under the eyes are present. The *Da Huang Zhe Chong Wan* (Rhubarb and Eupolyphaga Pill) can be used to move blood, resolve stasis and reinforce the deficiency.

Da Huang Zhe Chong Wan

[Ingredients]

大黄	*dà huáng*	10 *fēn*	Radix et Rhizoma Rhei
黄芩	*huáng qín*	2 *liǎng*	Radix Scutellariae
甘草	*gān cǎo*	2 *liǎng*	Radix et Rhizoma Glycyrrhizae
桃仁	*táo rén*	1 *shēng*	Semen Persicae
杏仁	*xìng rén*	1 *shēng*	Semen Armeniacae Amarum
白芍	*bái sháo*	4 *liǎng*	Radix Paeoniae Alba
干地黄	*gān dì huáng*	10 *liǎng*	Radix Rehmanniae
干漆	*gān qī*	1 *liǎng*	Resina Toxicodendri
虻虫	*méng chóng*	1 *shēng*	Tabanus
水蛭	*shuǐ zhì*	100 pieces	Hirudo
蛴螬	*qí cáo*	1 *shēng*	Holotrichia
蛰虫	*zhé chóng*	0.5 *shēng*	Eupolyphaga seu Steleophaga

Grind the above twelve ingredients into a powder, mix with the prepared honey to make pellets the size of red beans. Take 5 pellets with wine for each dose, 3 doses a day.

*****

[20] 附《千金翼》〔1〕炙甘草汤一云复脉汤〔2〕，治虚劳不足，汗出而闷〔3〕，脉结悸〔4〕，行动如常，不出百日，危急者十一日死〔5〕。

甘草四两炙桂枝生姜各三两麦门冬半升麻仁半升人参阿胶各二两大枣三十枚生地黄一斤 右九味，以酒七升，水八升，先煮八味，取三升，去滓，内胶消尽。温服一升，日三服。

Annotations

[1] *Qian Jin Yi:* The *Qian Jin Yi Fang* (Supplement to 'Important Formulas Worth a Thousand Gold Pieces') by Sun Simiao in the Tang Dynasty (618-907).

[2] *Zhi Gan Cao Tang* (Honey-Fried Licorice Decoction): Also known as *Fu Mai Tang* (Pulse-Restoring Decoction), a formula to nourish heart yin and restore pulses. It has been praised by later physicians as the "pioneer formula for nourishing yin". Six yin-nourishing formulas are modified from this one, such as *Yi Jia Fu Mai Tang* (Pulse-Restoring Decoction plus Oyster Shell), *Er Jia Fu Mai Tang* (Pulse-Restoring Decoction plus Oyster Shell and Turtle Carapace) and *San Jiao Fu Mai Tang* (Pulse-Restoring Decoction plus Oyster Shell, Turtle Carapace and Tortoise plastron).

[3] *Xu Lao Bu Zu, Han Chu Er Men*: Sweating and chest tightness due to deficiency of yin, yang, qi and blood. In severe cases, profuse sweating and chest pain (similar to myocardial ischemia or angina pectoris) may be present.

[4] *Mai Jie Ju:* A slow, intermittent pulse and palpitations, indicating irregular heart rates (similar to arrhythmia or premature heart beats).

[5] *Bu Chu Bai Ri, Wei Ji Zhe Shi Yi Ri Si*: The "*Bai Ri* (100 days)" or "*Shi Yi Ri* (11 days)" here are not definite numbers, simply indicating critical conditions that require immediate attention.

Interpretations

The *Zhi Gan Cao Tang* (Honey-Fried Licorice Decoction) [also known as *Fu Mai Tang* (Pulse-Restoring Decoction)] can be used to treat sweating and chest tightness (chest pain), intermittent, irregular pulse rates and palpitations due to deficiency of yin, yang, qi and blood in deficiency exhaustion. Although these patients seem normal, their conditions are critical with an unfavorable prognosis: they may die suddenly within a dozen or hundred days.

Zhi Gan Cao Tang

[Ingredients]

甘草	*gān cǎo*	4 *liǎng*	Radix et Rhizoma Glycyrrhizae (honey-fried)
桂枝	*guì zhī*	3 *liǎng*	Ramulus Cinnamomi
生姜	*shēng jiāng*	3 *liǎng*	Rhizoma Zingiberis Recens
麦冬	*mài dōng*	0.5 *shēng*	Radix Ophiopogonis
火麻仁	*huǒ má rén*	0.5 *shēng*	Fructus Cannabis
人参	*rén shēn*	2 *liǎng*	Radix et Rhizoma Ginseng
阿胶	*ē jiāo*	2 *liǎng*	Colla Corii Asini
大枣	*dà zǎo*	30 pieces	Fructus Jujubae
生地黄	*shēng dì huáng*	1 *jīn*	Radix Rehmanniae Recens

Decoct the eight ingredients [except *E Jiao* (Colla Corii Asini)] in seven *shēng* of wine and 8 *shēng* of water to get three *shēng*. Remove the dregs and add *E Jiao* to dissolve it completely. Take 1 *shēng* when it is warm for each dose, 3 doses a day.

*****

[21]《肘后》獭肝散[1]，治冷劳[2]，又主鬼疰[3]，一门相染[4]。獭肝一具炙干末之。水服方寸匕，日三服。

Annotations

[1] *Zhou Hou Ta Gan San:* Otter Liver Powder recorded in the *Zhou Hou Bei Ji Fang* (Emergency Formulas to Keep Up One's Sleeve).

[2] *Leng Lao*: Cold deficiency exhaustion, similar to tuberculous diseases.

[3] *Gui Zhu*: Lung tuberculosis.

[4] *Yi Men Xiang Ran:* Contagious among family members

Interpretations

The *Ta Gan San* (Otter Liver Powder) from the *Zhou Hou Bei Ji Fang* (Emergency Formulas to Keep Up One's Sleeve) can be used to treat cold deficiency exhaustion and lung tuberculosis that is contagious among family members.

Method: Heat and fry one otter liver and grind into a fine powder. Take 1 square-inch-spoon powder (approximately 2 grams) with warm water for each dose, 3 doses a day.

肺痿肺痈咳嗽上气病脉证治第七
Chapter 7 Lung Decline, Lung Abscess, and Coughing with Panting—Pulses, Patterns and Treatment

Overview

This chapter includes lung declining, lung abscess and coughing with panting. Since the three conditions are all involved with the lung and share common symptoms (coughing with sputum and rapid breathing), they are discussed together.

*****

[01] 问曰：热在上焦者〔1〕，因咳为肺痿〔2〕。肺痿之病，何从得之？师曰：或从汗出，或从呕吐，或从消渴〔3〕，小便利数，或从便唯，又被快药〔4〕下利，重亡津液，故得之。

曰：寸口脉数〔5〕，其人咳，口中反有浊唾涎沫〔6〕者何？师曰：为肺痿之病。若口中辟辟燥〔7〕，咳即胸中隐隐痛，脉反滑数〔8〕，此为肺痈〔9〕，咳唾脓血。脉数虚者为肺痿，数实者为肺痈。

Annotations

[1] *Re Zai Shang Jiao*: Retained heat in the lung.

[2] *Fei Wei*: It literally means lung decline—a chronic, debilitating lung condition characterized by cough with turbid sputum and foamy saliva. It often results from yin deficiency. This condition is later referred to as chronic, fatigue-related cough, which is similar to "pulmonary tuberculosis" in modern medicine. According to the *Fu Ren Liang Fang*

(Fine Formulas for Women), symptoms of lung decline include "fever, chills, night sweats, and a chronic cough with blood-stained sputum".

[3] *Xiao Ke*: Wasting and thirsting disorder. For more information, please refer to chapter 13.

[4] *Kuai Yao:* It refers to harsh purgative medicinals such as *Da Huang* (Radix et Rhizoma Rhei).

[5] *Cun Kou Mai Shuo*: This shares the same meaning as *Re Zai Shang Jiao* (heat affecting the lung).

[6] *Zhuo Tuo Xian Mo*: The property of sputum. The *Zhuo Tuo* refers to thick sputum, whereas *Xian Mo* refers to thin, clear sputum.

[7] *Kou Zhong Pi Pi Zao*: Extremely dry mouth.

[8] *Mai Fan Hua Shuo*: Lung abscess may cause a slippery, rapid pulse. A slippery pulse indicates excess of yang qi, and a rapid pulse indicates heat. In summary, lung abscess is diagnosed as an excess heat syndrome.

[9] *Fei Yong*: A suppurative lung condition characterized by cough with purulent mucus or blood. It often results from exogenous wind heat and is similar to "suppurative pulmonary abscess" or "infection secondary to bronchial dilatation" in modern medicine.

Interpretations

Question: Retained heat in the lung may cause coughs and over time, result in lung decline. How does the decline of lung develop?

Answer: The decline of lung may result from excessive sweating, frequent vomiting, or increased urination due to wasting and thirsting disorder. Alternatively, it may occur as a result of severe damage to body fluids due to excessive diarrhea after taking purgative medicinals (such as *Da Huang*) for constipation.

Question: With retained heat in the lung, why do patients experience cough with thick or thin, clear sputum?

Answer: This indicates the lung decline. However, an extremely dry mouth, cough-induced chest pain, expectoration of purulent mucus or blood and a slippery, rapid pulse are manifestations indicative of lung abscess. Both conditions have retained heat in the lung; however, the lung decline causes a rapid, weak pulse (deficiency heat) and the lung abscess causes a rapid, forceful pulse (excess heat).

*****

[02] 问曰：病咳逆，脉之〔1〕何以知此为肺痈？当有脓血，吐之则死〔2〕。其脉何类〔3〕？师曰：寸口脉微而数，微则为风，数则为热〔4〕；微则汗出，数则恶寒〔5〕；风中于卫，呼气不入，热过于荣，吸而不出〔6〕。风伤皮毛，热伤血脉〔7〕，风舍于肺〔8〕，其人则咳，口干喘满，咽燥不渴〔9〕，时唾浊沫，时时振寒。热之所过，血为之凝滞〔10〕，畜结痈脓，吐如米粥〔11〕，始萌可救，脓成则死〔12〕。

Annotations

[1] *Mai Zhi*: Here it refers to all the four diagnostic methods—inspection, auscultation & olfaction, inquiry and palpation.

[2] *Dang You Tong Xue, Tu Zhi Ze Si*: Cough with pus and blood is the diagnostic basis for lung abscess. Here it means lung abscess has a poor prognosis, and therefore, requires an early treatment.

[3] *Qi Mai He Lei*: How does this condition develop? The word *Mai* (pulse) here refers to the pathologic process.

[4] *Cun Kou Mai Wei Er Shuo, Wei Ze Wei Feng, Shuo Ze Wei Re*: This explains lung abscess results from wind heat. The "*Wei Ze Wei Feng*" and "*Shuo Ze Wei Re*" are intertextual sentences.

[5] *Wei Ze Han Chu, Shuo Ze Wu Han*: Two intertextual sentences, indicating that early symptoms after exposure to wind cold are (fever), sweating and aversion to cold.

[6] *Feng Zhong Yu Wei, Hu Qi Bu Ru, Re Guo Yu Rong, Xi Er Bu Chu*: Four intertextual sentences, further elaborating that wind heat affecting the Ying-nutrients and Wei-defense may cause difficulty breathing.

[7] *Feng Shang Pi Mao, Re Shang Xue Mai*: Two intertextual sentences, indicating that wind heat entering the bloodstream (interior) via the skin and body hair (exterior).

[8] *Feng She Yu Fei:* Wind heat retains in the lung.

[9] *Yan Zao Bu Ke*: A dry throat but with no thirst.

[10] *Re Zhi Suo Guo, Xue Wei Zhi Ning Zhi*: Wind heat causes qi and blood to stagnate.

[11] *Xu Jie Yong Nong, Tu Ru Mi Zhou*: The formation of abscess causes thick sputum like glutinous rice porridge.

[12] *Shi Meng Ke Jiu, Nong Cheng Ze Si*: Lung abscess can be cured in an early stage; however, presence of thick sputum indicates an unfavorable prognosis.

Interpretations

Question: For cough with qi counterflow, how can we confirm the diagnosis of lung abscess through examinations?

Answer: A characteristic symptom is coughing with sputum that contains pus and blood. However, vomiting of pus and blood may indicate a poor prognosis.

Question: How does lung abscess develop?

Answer: Patients may first experience (fever), sweating, and aversion to cold upon exposure to wind heat. Wind heat entering the *Ying*-nutrients and *Wei*-defense may cause difficulty breathing. Wind heat entering from the exterior to the interior (retaining in the lung) may cause cough, a dry mouth, rapid breathing, chest obstruction, a dry throat, frequent presence of thick sputum, and occasional aversion to cold or chills. Wind heat causes the qi and blood to stagnate. Over time, stagnant qi and blood may develop into abscess. The formation of abscess may cause thick sputum like glutinous rice porridge. This condition can be cured in early stage; however, it can be very difficult to be cured in the later stage with sputum containing pus or blood.

*****

[03] 上气〔1〕面浮肿，肩息〔2〕，其脉浮大，不治，又加利尤甚〔3〕。

[04] 上气喘而躁[4]者，属肺胀[5]，欲作风水[6]，发汗则愈。

Annotations

[1] *Shang Qi*: Panting or rapid breathing.

[2] *Jian Xi:* Breathe with raising shoulders, indicating a severe shortness of breath.

[3] *Qi Mai Fu Da, Bu Zhi, You Jia Li You Shen*: A superficial, large and rootless pulse indicates failure of kidney to absorb qi (i.e., to maintain the depth of breathing). The presence of diarrhea indicates spleen yang deficiency. Deficiency of both the kidney and spleen is more difficult to be cured.

[4] *Chuan Er Zao:* Panting and rapid breathing.

[5] *Fei Zhang*: A lung condition characterized by cough with panting. It often results from wind cold blocking lung qi. It is similar to asthmatic bronchitis or bronchial asthma in modern medicine.

[6] *Feng Shui*: Wind water. For more information, please refer to chapter 14.

Interpretations

Rapid breathing, facial puffiness, breathing with raising shoulders and a superficial, large and rootless pulse (kidney failing to absorb qi) are difficult to be cured. The presence of diarrhea may aggravate the condition. Panting or rapid breathing due to (lung) qi fullness or distension with symptoms of wind water (fever, aversion to wind, and puffiness) seems more severe, but they can be treated by inducing sweating.

*****

[05] 肺痿吐涎沫而不咳[1]者，其人不渴，必遗尿，小便数，所以然者，以上虚不能制下故也，此为肺中冷[2]，必眩，多涎唾，甘草干姜汤[3]以温之。若服汤已渴者，属消渴[4]。

甘草干姜汤方：

甘草四两，炙干姜二两，炮右咀，以水三升，煮取一升五合，去滓。分温再服。

Annotations

[1] *Fei Wei Tuo Xian Mo Er Bu Ke:* Despite the similar symptom of foamy saliva as lung decline, this condition is not lung decline with an absence of cough.

[2] *Yi Niao, Xiao Bian Shuo…Ci Wei Fei Zhong Leng*: This indicates increased urination is a major symptom of retained cold in the lung. It results from the failure of lung qi to control the water in the urinary bladder. It is similar as diabetes insipidus in modern medicine.

[3] *Gan Cao Gan Jiang Tang* (Licorice and Dried Ginger Decoction): A formula to warm the lung and dissipate cold.

[4] *Ruo Fu Tang Yi Ke Zhe, Shu Xiao Ke*: A tentative diagnosis: if patients experience thirst after taking the above formula, they are having wasting and thirsting disorder instead of retained cold in the lung. In summary, increased urination along with thirst is seen in wasting and thirsting disorder, whereas increased urination without thirst is seen in retained cold in the lung.

Interpretations

Retained cold in the lung may cause similar symptom of foamy saliva as lung decline; however, patients do not experience cough or thirst. Their characteristic symptom is increased urination due to lung failing to control the water in the urinary bladder. If patients also experience dizziness and increased foamy saliva, they should take *Gan Cao Gan Jiang Tang* (Licorice and Dried Ginger Decoction) to warm the lung and dissipate cold. If they do not get better afterwards but start to experience thirst, they are having wasting and thirsting disorder instead of retained cold in the lung.

Gan Cao Gan Jiang Tang

[Ingredients]

甘草	*gān cǎo*	4 *liǎng*	Radix et Rhizoma Glycyrrhizae
干姜	*gān jiāng*	2 *liǎng*	Rhizoma Zingiberis

Fry, slice and decoct the two ingredients in three *shēng* of water to get 1.5 *shēng*. Remove the dregs and take when it is warm in two times.

*****

[06] 咳而上气，喉中水鸡声〔1〕，射干麻黄汤〔2〕主之。

射干麻黄汤方：

射干十三枚，一法三两 麻黄四两 生姜四两 细辛 紫菀 款冬花各三两 五味子半升 大枣七枚 半夏大者洗八枚，一法半升 右九味，以水一斗二升，先煮麻黄两沸，去上沫，内诸药，煮取三升。分温三服。

Annotations

[1] *Ke Er Shang Qi, Hou Zhong Shui Ji Sheng:* Cough with panting and frog-like croak sounds in the throat due to phlegm-qi stagnation. It is similar to the wheezing sound in asthma, which is known as "bronchial asthma" or "asthmatic bronchitis" in modern medicine.

[2] *She Gan Ma Huang Tang* (Belamcanda and Ephedra Decoction): A formula to disperse lung qi, soothe panting, dissipate cold, and down-regulate qi.

Interpretations

Cough, panting and frog-like croak sounds in the throat (asthma) should be treated with *She Gan Ma Huang Tang* (Belamcanda and Ephedra Decoction).

She Gan Ma Huang Tang

[Ingredients]

射干	*shè gān*	13 pieces/3 *liǎng*	Rhizoma Belamcandae
麻黄	*má huáng*	4 *liǎng*	Herba Ephedrae
生姜	*shēng jiāng*	4 *liǎng*	Rhizoma Zingiberis Recens
细辛	*xì xīn*	3 *liǎng*	Radix et Rhizoma Asari
紫菀	*zǐ wēi*	3 *liǎng*	Radix et Rhizoma Asteris
款冬花	*kuǎn dōng huā*	3 *liǎng*	Flos Farfarae
五味子	*wǔ wèi zǐ*	0.5 *shēng*	Fructus Schisandrae Chinensis
大枣	*dà zǎo*	7 pieces	Fructus Jujubae
半夏	*bàn xià*	8 pieces/0.5 *shēng*	Rhizoma Pinelliae

First decoct *Ma Huang* in one *dòu* and two *shēng* of water and bring it to a boil twice, skim the froth and add the rest of the ingredients to get 3 *shēng*. Then take the decoction when it is warm in three times.

*****

[07] 咳逆上气，时时唾浊，但坐不得眠〔1〕。皂荚丸〔2〕主之。

皂荚丸方：皂荚八两，刮去皮，用酥炙〔3〕右一味，末之，蜜丸，梧子大。以枣膏和汤〔4〕服三丸，日三夜一服。

Annotations

[1] *Shi Shi Tuo Zhuo, Dan Zuo Bu De Mian:* Profuse thick sputum with an inability to lie flat due to difficulty breathing, which is similar

to orthopnea in modern medicine. It is important to resolve the turbid phlegm in the lung before it accumulates to block the flow of qi.

[2] *Zao Jia Wan* (Gleditsiae Pill): A formula to break and resolve phlegm. As *Zao Jia* (Fructus Gleditsiae) is dry and severely toxic, it is necessay to fry with honey and take in combination with jujube paste and hot water to calm and harmonize the stomach.

[3] *Su Zhi*: A processing method for Chinese materia medica—heat and fry raw medicinals with fat of cow or goat to reduce their toxicity.

[4] *Zao Gao He Tang*: According to the *Jing Fang Shi Yan Lu* (Medical Case Records of Classic Formulas), "In practical use, the *Zao Jia Wan* is taken with prepared Jujube paste and warm water".

Interpretations

Cough, panting, profuse thick sputum with an inability to lie flat should be treated with *Zao Jia Wan* (Gleditsiae Pill).

Zao Jia Wan

[Ingredients]

皂荚	*zào jiá*	8 *liǎng*	Fructus Gleditsiae
蜂蜜	*fēng mì*		Mel

Scrape off the skin of *Zao Jia*, fry with fat of cow or goat and grind into a powder. Mix with honey into pills (the size of firmiana seeds). When in practical use, take three pills for each dose with jujube past mixed with warm water, three times during the day and 1 time at night.

*****

[08] 咳而脉浮〔1〕者，厚朴麻黄汤〔2〕主之

厚朴麻黄汤方：厚朴五两 麻黄四两 石膏如鸡子大 杏仁半升 半夏半升 干姜二两 细辛二两 小麦一斤 五味子半升右九味，以水一斗二升，先煮小麦熟，去滓，内诸药，煮取三升。温服一升，日三服。

[09] 脉沉〔3〕者，泽漆汤〔4〕主之。

泽漆汤方：半夏半升　紫参五两，一作紫菀　泽漆三斤，以东流水[5]五斗，煮取一斗五升　生姜五两　白前五两　甘草　黄芩　人参　桂枝各三两右九味，咀，内泽漆汁中，煮取五升。温服五合，至晚尽〔6〕。

Annotations

[1] *Ke Er Mai Fu:* Cough with a superficial pulse, indicating an exterior syndrome.

[2] *Hou Pu Ma Huang Tang* (Officinal Magnolia Bark and Ephedra Decoction): A modified formula of *Xiao Qing Long Jia Shi Gao Tang* (Minor Blue Green Dragon Decoction Plus Gypsum) by removing *Gui Zhi* (Ramulus Cinnamomi), *Shao Yao* (Radix Paeoniae) and *Gan Cao* (Radix et Rhizoma Glycyrrhizae) and adding *Hou Po* (Cortex Magnoliae Officinalis), *Xing Ren* (Semen Armeniacae Amarum) and *Xiao Mai* (Fructus Tritici). This formula acts to down-regulate qi, resolve phlegm, clear heat and stop coughing.

[3] *Mai Chen*: Cough with a deep pulse, indicating an interior syndrome.

[4] *Ze Qi Tang* (Euphoribiae Helioscopiae Decoction): A formula to down-regulate qi and alleviate panting. This formula uses a large dose of *Ze Qi* to resolve phlegm and clear heat, uses *Shi Jian Chuan* to circulate blood and resolve masses and combines *Ren Shen* and *Gan Cao* to strengthen the spleen. This formula is taken in small doses at short intervals and therefore suitable for patients with a weak constitution.

[5] *Dong Liu Shui*: Rapid flowing, clear water.

[6] *Zhu Qu Wu Sheng, Wen Fu Wu He, Zhi Wan Jin*: A method to take 0.5 *shēng* (half of the normal dose for adults) for each dose and complete the full dosage in ten times by nighttime. This method applies to patients with a weak constitution to resolve phlegm.

Interpretations

Cough with chest fullness and panting and a superficial, rapid pulse (due to phlegm heat accumulating in the lung) should be treated with *Hou Po Ma Huang Tang* (Officinal Magnolia Bark and Ephedra Decoction).

Hou Pu Ma Huang Tang

[Ingredients]

厚朴	*hòu pò*	5 *liǎng*	Cortex Magnoliae Officinalis
麻黄	*má huáng*	4 *liǎng*	Herba Ephedrae
石膏	*shí gāo*	Size of an egg	Gypsum Fibrosum
杏仁	*xìng rén*	0.5 *shēng*	Semen Armeniacae Amarum
半夏	*bàn xià*	0.5 *shēng*	Rhizoma Pinelliae
干姜	*gān jiāng*	2 *liǎng*	Rhizoma Zingiberis
细辛	*xì xīn*	2 *liǎng*	Radix et Rhizoma Asari
小麦	*xiǎo mài*	1 *jīn*	Fructus Tritici
五味子	*wǔ wèi zǐ*	0.5 *shēng*	Fructus Schisandrae Chinensis

First cook *Xiao Mai* thoroughly in one *dòu* and two *shēng* of water, remove the dregs and add the rest of the ingredients to get three *shēng*. Take 1 *shēng* when it is warm for each dose, 3 doses a day.

Chronic cough with fatigue and a deep, weak pulse (due to fluid-heat accumulating in the lung) should be treated with *Ze Qi Tang* (Euphoribiae Helioscopiae Decoction).

Ze Qi Tang

[Ingredients]

泽漆	*zé qī*	3 *jīn*	Herba Euphoribiae Helioscopiae
半夏	*bàn xià*	0.5 *shēng*	Rhizoma Pinelliae
石见穿*	*shí jiàn chuān*	5 *liǎng*	Herba Salviae Chinensis

生姜	shēng jiāng	5 *liǎng*	Rhizoma Zingiberis Recens
白前	*bái qián*	5 *liǎng*	Rhizoma et Radix Cynanchi Stauntonii
甘草	*gān cǎo*	3 *liǎng*	Radix et Rhizoma Glycyrrhizae
黄芩	*huáng qín*	3 *liǎng*	Radix Scutellariae
人参	rén shēn	3 *liǎng*	Radix et Rhizoma Ginseng
桂枝	guì zhī	3 *liǎng*	Ramulus Cinnamomi

*In other texts, this ingredient is *Zi Wan* (Radix et Rhizoma Asteris) (for absence of masses).

Slice and decoct *Ze Qi* in 5 *dòu* of clear, fast flowing water to get 1 *dòu* and 5 *shēng*. Add the rest of the ingredients to decoct to 5 *shēng*. Take 0.5 *shēng* when it is warm for each dose, 10 doses in all by nighttime.

*****

[10] 大逆〔1〕上气，咽喉不利〔2〕。止逆下气〔3〕者，麦门冬汤〔4〕主之。

麦门冬汤方：麦门冬七升 半夏一升 人参二两 甘草二两 粳米三合 大枣十二枚右六味，以水一斗二升，煮取六升。温服一升，日三夜一服。

Annotations

[1] *Da Ni:* This might be a miss spelling of *Huo Ni*, which literally means ascending of deficiency fire.

[2] *Yan Hou Bu Li*: Throat dryness and discomfort, probably accompanied by thirst and cough with foamy saliva.

[3] *Zhi Ni Xia Qi*: A treatment strategy to clear deficiency fire and down-regulate qi.

[4] *Mai Men Dong Tang* (Ophiopogon Decoction): A formula to nourish the lung and stomach and down-regulate qi. It is characterized by the combination of a small dose of *Ban Xia* to benefit the throat with large doses of medicinals to tonify qi and regenerate fluids.

Interpretations

Panting and a dry throat (cough with foamy saliva and thirst) due to ascending of deficiency fire should be treated with *Mai Men Dong Tang* (Ophiopogon Decoction) to down-regulate qi.

Mai Men Dong Tang

[Ingredients]

麦冬	*mài dōng*	5 *shēng*	Radix Ophiopogonis
半夏	*bàn xià*	1 *shēng*	Rhizoma Pinelliae
人参	*rén shēn*	2 *liǎng*	Radix et Rhizoma Ginseng
甘草	*gān cǎo*	2 *liǎng*	Radix et Rhizoma Glycyrrhizae
粳米	*jīng mǐ*	0.3 *shēng*	Oryza Sativa L.
大枣	*dà zǎo*	12 pieces	Fructus Jujubae

Decoct the above 6 ingredients in 1 *dòu* and 2 *shēng* of water to get 6 *shēng*. Take when it is warm, 3 times during the day and once at night.

*****

[11] 肺痈，喘不得卧[1]，葶苈大枣泻肺汤[2]主之。

葶苈大枣泻肺汤方：葶苈熬令黄色，捣丸，如弹子大 大枣十二枚右先以水三升，煮枣取二升，去枣，内葶苈，煮取一升。顿服。

Annotations

[1] *Fei Yong, Chuan Bu De Wo:* Unlike the lung abscess characterized by cough with pus and blood due to wind heat, the "*Fei Yong*" here refers to lung distension due to retained water-fluid, which is characterized by difficulty breathing with an inability to lie flat.

[2] *Ting Li Da Zao Xie Fei Tang* (Lepidium/Descurainiae and Jujube Lung-Draining Decoction): A formula to clear the lung and resolve water retention. This formula is also used for *Zhi Yin* (thoracic fluid retention) in chapter 12.

Interpretations

Difficulty breathing with an inability to lie flat in lung distension due to water-fluid accumulating in the lung should be treated with *Ting Li Da Zao Xie Fei Tang* (Lepidium/Descurainiae and Jujube Lung-Draining Decoction).

Ting Li Da Zao Xie Fei Tang

[Ingredients]

葶苈子	*tíng lì zǐ*		Semen Lepidii; Semen Descurainiae
大枣	*dà zǎo*	12 pieces	Fructus Jujubae

Decoct *Ting Li Zi* until it becomes yellow, grind into a powder and make into pills the size of slingshot balls. Decoct 12 pieces of jujube in 3 *shēng* of water to get 2 *shēng*, remove *Da Zao* and add *Ting Li Zi* to decoct to get 1 *shēng* and drink up at a draught.

*****

[12] 咳而胸满，振寒脉数〔1〕，咽干不渴〔2〕，时出浊唾腥臭，久久吐脓如米粥〔3〕者，为肺痈，桔梗汤〔4〕主之。桔梗汤方亦治血痹：

桔梗一两 甘草二两右二味，以水三升，煮取一升，分温再服，则吐脓血也。

Annotations

[1] *Ke Er Xiong Man, Zhen Han Mai Shuo:* Over time, retained wind heat in the lung may form abscess and result in cough, chest fullness, chills, fever and a slippery, rapid pulse.

[2] *Yan Gan Bu Ke*: A dry throat with severe thirst (instead of no thirst, here it should mean severe thirst).

[3] *Shi Chu Zhuo Tuo Xing Chou, Jiu Jiu Tu Nong Ru Mi Zhou*: Frequent presence of thick, foul smelling sputum containing pus and blood.

[4] *Jie Geng Tang* (Platycodonis Decoction): A formula to drain pus and remove toxins. This formula is not indicated for blood-Bi (impediment).

Interpretations

Cough, chest fullness, (fever), chills, a slippery, rapid pulse, a dry throat, thirst and frequent presence of thick, foul smelling sputum that contains pus and blood are characteristic symptoms of lung abscess. This can be treated with *Jie Geng Tang* (Platycodonis).

Jie Geng Tang

[Ingredients]

桔梗	*jié gěng*	1 *liǎng*	Radix Platycodonis
甘草	*gān cǎo*	2 *liǎng*	Radix et Rhizoma Glycyrrhizae

Decoct the above two ingredients in 3 *shēng* of water to get 1 *shēng*. Take when it is warm in two times. After taking the decoction, patients may cough out pus/blood-contained sputum.

Although the text mentions this formula is also used for blood-Bi (impediment), it doesn't seem right.

*****

[13] 咳而上气，此为肺胀。其人喘，目如脱状[1]，脉浮大[2]者，越婢加半夏汤[3]主之。

越婢加半夏汤方：麻黄六两 石膏半斤 生姜三两 大枣十五枚 甘草二两 半夏半升右六味，以水六升，先煮麻黄，去上沫，内诸药，煮取三升。分温三服。

Annotations

[1] *Mu Ru Tuo Zhuang:* Protrusion of the eyes as if they are about to burst from their sockets. This results from severe panting.

[2] *Mai Fu Da*: A superficial, surging pulse. A superficial pulse indicates an exterior syndrome, and a surging pulse indicates heat. This indicates lung distension results from exposure to wind heat and retention of phlegm-fluid.

[3] *Yue Bi Jia Ban Xia Tang* (Lung-Dispersing Decoction plus Pinellia): A formula to induce sweating, clear heat, disperse the lung and resolve retained fluid.

Interpretations

Cough with panting is a manifestation of lung distension. Protrusion of the eyes due to severe panting and a superficial, surging pulse (due to external contraction of wind heat and internal retention of phlegm fluid) should be treated with *Yue Bi Jia Ban Xia Tang* (Lung-Dispersing Decoction plus Pinellia).

Yue Bi Jia Ban Xia Tang

[Ingredients]

麻黄	*má huáng*	6 *liǎng*	Herba Ephedrae
石膏	*shí gāo*	0.5 *jīn*	Gypsum Fibrosum
生姜	*shēng jiāng*	3 *liǎng*	Rhizoma Zingiberis Recens
大枣	*dà zǎo*	15 pieces	Fructus Jujubae
甘草	*gān cǎo*	2 *liǎng*	Radix et Rhizoma Glycyrrhizae
半夏	*bàn xià*	0.5 *shēng*	Rhizoma Pinelliae

Decoct *Ma Huang* first in 6 *shēng* of water, skim the froth and add the rest of the ingredients to get 3 *shēng*. Take the decoction when it is warm in three times.

*****

[14] 肺胀，咳而上气，烦燥而喘[1]，脉浮者，心下有水[2]，小青龙加石膏汤[3]主之。

小青龙加石膏汤方《千金》证治同，外更加胁下痛引缺盆[4]：

麻黄 芍药 桂枝 细辛 甘草 干姜各三两 五味子 半夏各半升 石膏二两右九味，以水一斗，先煮麻黄，去上沫，内诸药，煮取三升。强人服一升；羸者减之，日三服。小儿服四合。

Annotations

[1] *Fan Zao Er Chuan:* Severe panting or rapid breathing.

[2] *Mai Fu Zhe, Xin Xia You Shui*: Thoracic fluid retention.

[3] *Xiao Qing Long Jia Shi Gao Tang* (Minor Blue Green Dragon Decoction Plus Gypsum): A formula to release the exterior, resolve fluid retention and clear heat. The previous *Yue Bi Jia Ban Xia Tang* acts to induce sweating, clear heat and resolve fluid retention, and is therefore more indicated for panting due to severe interior heat. This formula is more indicated for panting due to severe fluid retention.

[4] *Que Pen*: A body part in Chinese medicine located in the middle of the superior border of the clavicle, i.e., supraclavicual fossa.

Interpretations

Cough with panting and a superficial pulse (exterior syndrome) due to thoracic fluid retention in lung distension should be treated with *Xiao Qing Long Jia Shi Gao Tang* (Minor Blue Green Dragon Decoction Plus Gypsum). The *Qian Jin Yao Fang* (Important Formulas Worth a Thousand Gold Pieces) records the same descriptions plus pain in the subcostal region that radiates toward the supraclavicular fossa.

Xiao Qing Long Jia Shi Gao Tang

[Ingredients]

麻黄	*má huáng*	3 *liǎng*	Herba Ephedrae
芍药	*sháo yào*	3 *liǎng*	Radix Paeoniae
桂枝	*guì zhī*	3 *liǎng*	Ramulus Cinnamomi
细辛	*xì xīn*	3 *liǎng*	Radix et Rhizoma Asari
甘草	*gān cǎo*	3 *liǎng*	Radix et Rhizoma Glycyrrhizae
干姜	*gān jiāng*	3 *liǎng*	Rhizoma Zingiberis
五味子	*wǔ wèi zǐ*	0.5 *shēng*	Fructus Schisandrae Chinensis
半夏	*bàn xià*	0.5 *shēng*	Rhizoma Pinelliae
石膏	*shí gāo*	2 *liǎng*	Gypsum Fibrosum

First cook *Ma Huang* in one *dòu* of water, skim the froth and add the rest of the ingredients to get three *shēng*. For patients with a strong body, take 1 *shēng* for each dose. For patients who are thin and weak, take a smaller dose, 3 times a day. For children, take 0.4 *shēng* for each dose.

*****

Annex Formula # 1 *Zhi Gan Cao Tang*

《外台》炙甘草汤〔1〕：治肺痿，涎唾多，心中温温液液〔2〕者。方见虚劳中。

Annotations

[1] *Zhi Gan Cao Tang* (Honey-Fried Licorice Decoction) from the *Wai Tai Mi Yao* (Arcane Essentials from the Imperial Library): This formula is originally from the *Shang Han Lun* (Treatise on Cold Damage) (No 177) and used for palpitations with a knotted or intermittent pulse. In *Qian Jin Yi Fang* (Supplement to 'Important Formulas Worth a Thousand Gold Pieces'), this formula is used for fatigue, sweating, chest tightness and a hesitant, knotted pulse. For more information, please refer to chapter 6. Here it is used for lung decline, but with a different dosage.

[2] *Xin Zhong Wen Wen Ye Ye*: Nausea and heartburn.

Interpretations

The *Zhi Gan Cao Tang* (Honey-Fried Licorice Decoction) in the *Wai Tai Mi Yao* (Arcane Essentials from the Imperial Library) is used for lung decline (due to deficiency of qi and yin) with cough, foamy sputum, heartburn and nausea. For more information about the formula, see chapter 6.

*****

Annex Formula # 2 *Gan Cao Tang*

《千金》甘草汤〔1〕：

甘草右一味，以水三升，煮减半。分温三服。

Annotations

[1] *Gan Cao Tang* (Licorice Decoction) from the *Qian Jin Yao Fang* (Important Formulas Worth a Thousand Gold Pieces): A single ingredient formula to reduce fire and remove toxins. It does not mention dose and indications. This formula is originally from the *Shang Han Lun* (Treatise on Cold Damage) (No 311) and used for dry and sore throat. Here it is used for mild lung decline.

Interpretations

The *Gan Cao Tang* (Licorice Decoction) in the *Qian Jin Yao Fang* (Important Formulas Worth a Thousand Gold Pieces) is used for mild lung decline with profuse foamy sputum and dry, sore throat. Method: Decoct *Gan Cao* in 3 *shēng* of water to get 1.5 *shēng* and take when it is warm in three times.

*****

Annex Formula # 3 *Sheng Jiang Gan Cao Tang*

《千金》生姜甘草汤〔1〕，治肺痿，咳唾涎沫不止，咽燥而渴〔2〕。

生姜五两 人参三两 甘草四两 大枣十五枚右四味，以水七升，煮取三升。分温三服。

Annotations

[1] *Sheng Jiang Gan Cao Tang* (Fresh Ginger and Licorice Decoction) from the *Qian Jin Yao Fang* (Important Formulas Worth a Thousand Gold Piece): A modified *Zhi Gan Cao Fang* to tonify spleen qi, moisten the lung and regenerate fluids.

[2] *Ke Tuo Xian Mo Bu Zhi, Yan Zao Er Ke*: Persistent foamy saliva and dry, sore throat.

Interpretations

The *Sheng Jiang Gan Cao Tang* (Fresh Ginger and Licorice Decoction) in the *Qian Jin Yao Fang* (Important Formulas Worth a Thousand Gold Pieces) is used for lung decline with profuse foamy sputum, which over time may consume body fluids and result in dry throat and thirst.

Sheng Jiang Gan Cao Tang

[Ingredients]

生姜	*shēng jiāng*	5 *liǎng*	Rhizoma Zingiberis Recens
人参	*rén shēn*	3 *liǎng*	Radix et Rhizoma Ginseng
甘草	*gān cǎo*	4 *liǎng*	Radix et Rhizoma Glycyrrhizae
大枣	*dà zǎo*	15 pieces	Fructus Jujubae

Decoct the four ingredients in 7 *shēng* of water to get 3 *shēng*. Take when it is warm in three times.

*****

Annex Formula # 4 *Gui Zhi Qu Shao Yao Jia Zao Jia Tang*

《千金》桂枝去芍药加皂荚汤[1]，治肺痿吐涎沫[2]。

桂枝 生姜各三两 甘草二两 大枣十枚 皂荚一枚去皮子，炙焦右五味，以水七升，微微火煮取三升。分温三服。

Annotations

[1] *Gui Zhi Qu Shao Yao Jia Zao Jia Tang* (Cinnamon Twig Decoction Minus Peony and Plus Gleditsiae Decoction) from the *Qian Jin Yao Fang* (Important Formulas Worth a Thousand Gold Piece): A modified *Gui Zhi*

Tang (Cinnamon Twig Decoction) plus *Zao Jia Wan* (Gleditsiae Pill) to harmonize the *Ying*-nutrients and *Wei*-defense and drain phlegm.

[2] *Zhi Fei Wei Tu Xian Mo*: Lung decline with foamy saliva.

Interpretations

The *Gui Zhi Qu Shao Yao Jia Zao Jia Tang* (Cinnamon Twig Decoction Minus Peony and Plus Gleditsiae Decoction) in the *Qian Jin Yao Fang* (Important Formulas Worth a Thousand Gold Pieces) is used for lung decline with foamy saliva (cough, panting and thick phlegm).

Gui Zhi Qu Shao Yao Jia Zao Jia Tang

[Ingredients]

桂枝	*guì zhī*	3 *liǎng*	Ramulus Cinnamomi
生姜	*shēng jiāng*	3 *liǎng*	Rhizoma Zingiberis Recens
皂荚	*zào jiá*	1 piece	Fructus Gleditsiae (remove skin and seeds and fry with honey)
甘草	*gān cǎo*	2 *liǎng*	Radix et Rhizoma Glycyrrhizae
大枣	*dà zǎo*	10 pieces	Fructus Jujubae

Decoct the five ingredients in 7 *shēng* of water with mild fire to get 3 *shēng*. Take when it is warm in three times.

*****

Annex Formula # 5 *Jie Geng Bai San*

《外台》桔梗白散[1]：治咳而胸满，振寒脉数[2]，咽干不渴，时出浊唾腥臭，久久吐脓如米粥[3]者，为肺痈。桔梗　贝母各三分　巴豆一分去皮，熬，研如脂　右三味，为散。强人饮服半钱匕；羸者减之。病在膈上者，吐脓血；膈下者，泻出。若下多不止，饮冷水一杯则定。

Annotations

[1] *Jie Geng Bai San* (Platycodonis White Powder) from the *Wai Tai Mi Yao* (Arcane Essentials from the Imperial Library): A formula to remove toxins, eliminate boils, resolve phlegm and drain pus. This formula is referred to as "*Bai San* (white powder)" in the *Shang Han Lun* (Treatise on Cold Damage) (No 141).

[2] *Ke Er Xiong Man, Zhen Han Mai Shuo*: Initial symptoms of lung abscess.

[3] *Yan Gan Bu/Pi Ke*: Severe lung abscess with a dry throat with strong thirst and profuse thick, foul-smelling sputum.

Interpretations

The *Jie Geng Bai San* (Platycodonis White Powder) in the *Wai Tai Mi Yao* (Arcane Essentials from the Imperial Library) is used for cough, chest tightness, chills, a slippery, rapid pulse, a dry throat, thirst and presence of thick, foul smelling sputum. Over time, patients may have thick sputum like rice porridge. These symptoms are indicative of lung abscess.

Jie Gen Bai San

[Ingredients]

桔梗	*jié gěng*	3 *fēn*	Radix Platycodonis
贝母	*bèi mǔ*	3 *fēn*	Bulbus Fritillaria
巴豆	*bā dòu*	1 *fēn*	Fructus Crotonis (remove skin, simmer and remove fat)

Grind the three ingredients into a fine powder. For patients with a strong body, take half a spoon with warm water. Patients who are thin and weak take half the dose. If abscess affects the chest and diaphragm, patients may expectorate pus or blood-contained sputum. If abscess affects the abdomen, patients may have pus-contained stools. In case of persistent diarrhea, a glass of cold water may help.

*****

Annex Formula # 6 *Wei Jing Tang*

《千金》苇茎汤[1]，治咳有微热、烦满、胸中甲错[2]，是为肺痈。

苇茎二升　薏苡仁半升　桃仁五十枚　瓜瓣半升　右四味，以水一斗，先煮苇茎，得五升，去滓，内诸药，煮取二升。服一升，再服，当吐如脓。

Annotations

[1] *Wei Jing Tang* (Phragmites Stem Decoction) from the *Qian Jin Yao Fang* (Important Formulas Worth a Thousand Gold Piece): A formula (for lung abscess) to clear the lung, resolve phlegm, eliminate boils and drain pus.

[2] *Xiong Zhong Jia Cuo*: Dry, crusted and scaly skin on the chest and abdomen due to malnourishment (by qi and blood).

Interpretations

The *Wei Jing Tang* (Phragmites Stem Decoction) in the *Qian Jin Yao Fang* (Important Formulas Worth a Thousand Gold Piece) is used for cough, low-grade fever, restlessness, dry, crusted and scaly skin on the chest and abdomen. These symptoms are indicative of lung abscess.

Wei Jing Tang

[Ingredients]

苇茎	*wěi jìng*	3 *shēng*	Rhizoma Phragmitis
薏苡仁	*yì yǐ rén*	0.5 *shēng*	Semen Coicis
桃仁	*táo rén*	50 pieces	Semen Persicae
瓜瓣	*guā bàn*	0.5 *shēng*	Wax gourd seeds

First decoct *Wei Jing* in 1 *dòu* of water to get 5 *shēng*, remove dregs and add the rest of the ingredients to decoct and get 2 *shēng*. Take 1 *shēng* for each dose. Patients may expectorate thick sputum after the second dose.

*****

[15] 肺痈，胸满胀，一身面目浮肿〔1〕，鼻塞清涕出，不闻香臭酸辛〔2〕，咳逆上气，喘鸣迫塞〔3〕，葶苈大枣泻肺汤主之。方见上。三日一剂，可至三四剂。此先服小青龙汤一剂，乃进〔4〕。小青龙方见咳嗽门中。

Annotations

[1] *Fei Yong, Xiong Man Zhang, Yi Shen Mian Mu Fu Zhong*: Lung abscess due to water-fluid retention. Exogenous pathogens may block lung qi and affect its function in regulating the waterway, causing chest fullness and general edema.

[2] *Bi Sai Qing Ti Chu, Bu Wen Xiang Chou Suan Xin*: Exogenous wind cold may block the nose, causing runny, stuffy nose and an inability to perceive odor.

[3] *Ke Ni Shang Qi, Chuan Ming Po Sai*: Severe coughing, panting or difficulty breathing due to retained water in the lung obstructing the flow of qi.

[4] *Xian Fu Xiao Qing Long Tang Yi Ji, Nai Jin*: It's advisable to take *Xiao Qing Long Tang* (Minor Green Dragon Decoction) to release the exterior and resolve water retention, followed by *Ting Li Da Zao Xie*

Fei Tang (Lepidium/Descurainiae and Jujube Lung-Draining Decoction) to clear the lung and further resolve water retention.

Interpretations

For lung abscess (due to retained water in the lung plus exposure to exogenous pathogens) with chest fullness, general edema, stuffy, runny nose, inability to perceive odor, coughing, panting and rapid breathing with a wheezing sound, it's advisable to take 1 dose of *Xiao Qing Long Tang* (Minor Green Dragon Decoction) (see chapter 12) before taking *Ting Li Da Zao Xie Fei Tang* (Lepidium/Descurainiae and Jujube Lung-Draining Decoction) (see the formula in this chapter).

奔豚气病脉证治第八
Chapter 8 Running Piglet Qi—Pulses, Patterns and Treatment

Overview

This chapter discusses the patterns and treatment for *Ben Tun Qi* (running piglet qi). The word *Ben* means running or rushing. The word *Tun* means piglets. The term *Ben Tun* was first recorded in Chapter 4, *Ling Shu* (Spiritual Pivot), *Huang Di Nei Jing* (Yellow Emperor's Inner Classic) as "a condition characterized by heaviness, coldness and poor mobility of the lower limbs resulting from pathogenic factors affecting the kidney". It was later described in the 56th difficult issue, *Nan Jing* (The Classic of Difficult Issues) as one of the five masses, "the kidney mass is known as a running piglet, which arises from the lower abdomen, rushes up to the chest with such ferocity that the patient feels he is close to death. It attacks and then remits. It may cause panting, limb weakness and shortness of breath". Running piglet qi is associated with the heart, liver and kidney. The *Mai Jing* (The Pulse Classic) combines this condition with chest-Bi impediment into "Chest-Bi impediment with chest pain, shortness of breath and running piglet".

*****

[01] 师曰：病有奔豚〔1〕，有吐脓〔2〕，有惊怖〔3〕，有火邪〔4〕，此四部病，皆从惊发得之〔5〕。师曰：奔豚病，从少腹起，上冲咽喉，发作欲死，复还止，皆从惊恐得之[6]。

Annotations

[1] *Ben Tun:* A paroxysmal condition that qi rushing from the lower abdomen to the chest, even to the throat. It attacks and then remits.

[2] *Tu Nong*: Expectoration of pus or blood-contained sputum.

[3] *Jing Bu*: Panic.

[4] *Huo Xie*: Excess fire that may aggravate the disease condition.

[5] *Ci Si Bu Bing, Jie Cong Jing Fa De Zhi*: Running piglet, expectoration of pus or blood-contained sputum, panic and excess fire are all induced by fright.

[6] *Jie Cong Jing Kong De Zhi*: Running piglet results from fear and fright and is associated with the heart and kidney.

Interpretations

The Master says, "Running piglet, expectoration of pus or blood-contained sputum, panic and excess fire are all induced by fright (heart). The Master also says, "Running piglet qi arises from the lower abdomen and rushes up to the throat with such ferocity that the patient feels he is so close to death. It attacks and then remits. This condition is associated with fear (kidney) and fright (heart).

*****

[02] 奔豚气上冲胸，腹痛，往来寒热〔1〕，奔豚汤〔2〕主之。

奔豚汤方：甘草 芎䓖 当归各二两 半夏四两 黄芩二两 生葛五两 芍药二两 生姜四两 甘李根白皮一升 右九味，以水二斗，煮取五升。温服一升，日三夜一服。

Annotations

[1] *Fu Tong, Wang Lai Han Re:* Pain in the chest and rib area, along with alternating chills and fever due to stagnant heat in the liver.

[2] *Ben Tun Tang* (Running Piglet-Alleviating Decoction): A formula (using *Gan Li Gen Bai Pi* as the monarch ingredient) to clear the liver, down-regulate qi, alleviate spasm and stop pain.

Interpretations

Running piglet qi rushing up to the chest, pain in the chest and rib area and alternating chills and fever can be treated with *Ben Tun Tang* (Running Piglet-Alleviating Decoction).

Ben Tun Tang

[Ingredients]

甘李根白皮	*gān lǐ gēn bái pí*	1 *shēng*	Cortex Radicis Pruni Salicinae
甘草	*gān cǎo*	2 *liǎng*	Radix et Rhizoma Glycyrrhizae
川芎	*chuān xiōng*	2 *liǎng*	Rhizoma Chuanxiong
当归	*dāng guī*	2 *liǎng*	Radix Angelicae Sinensis
半夏	*bàn xià*	4 *liǎng*	Rhizoma Pinelliae
黄芩	*huáng qín*	2 *liǎng*	Radix Scutellariae
葛根	*gé gēn*	5 *liǎng*	Radix Puerariae Lobatae
芍药	*sháo yào*	2 *liǎng*	Radix Paeoniae
生姜	*shēng jiāng*	4 *liǎng*	Rhizoma Zingiberis Recens

Decoct the nine ingredients in one *dòu* of water to get 5 *shēng*. Take one *shēng* when it is warm for each dose, 3 times during the day and once at night.

*****

[03] 发汗后〔1〕，烧针令其汗，针处被寒，核起而赤者〔2〕，必发贲豚〔3〕，气从小腹上至心，灸其核上各一壮〔4〕，与桂枝加桂汤〔5〕主之。

桂枝加桂汤方：

桂枝五两 芍药三两 甘草二两，炙 生姜三两 大枣十二枚 右五味，以水七升，微火煮取三升，去滓。温服一升。

Annotations

[1] *Fa Han Hou:* It literally means "after sweating", however, there is no such three words in *Shang Han Lun* (Treatise on Cold Damage) and *Yu Han Jing* (Jade Case Classic).

[2] *Shao Zhen Ling Qi Han...He Qi Er Chi Zhe*: A method to inducing sweating with warming needle.

[3] *Ben Tun*: Running piglet.

[4] *Jiu Qi He Shang Ge Yi Zhuang*: Apply an ignited moxa cone to elevated red bumps.

[5] *Gui Zhi Jia Gui Tang* (Cinnamon Twig Decoction with extra Cinnamon): A formula to release the exterior and down-regulate qi.

Interpretations

After inducing sweating with warming needle therapy (for patients with Taiyang disease), red elevated bumps may occur on the needling sites upon exposure to cold. This may induce running piglet qi rushing up from the lower abdomen to the chest. This condition requires applying moxibustion to the red bumps and taking *Gui Zhi Jia Gui Tang* (Cinnamon Twig Decoction with extra Cinnamon) orally.

Gui Zhi Jia Gui Tang

[Ingredients]

桂枝	*guì zhī*	5 *liǎng*	Ramulus Cinnamomi
芍药	*sháo yào*	3 *liǎng*	Radix Paeoniae
炙甘草	*zhì gān cǎo*	2 *liǎng*	Radix et Rhizoma Glycyrrhizae Praeparata cum Melle
生姜	*shēng jiāng*	4 *liǎng*	Rhizoma Zingiberis Recens
大枣	*dà zǎo*	12 pieces	Fructus Jujubae

Decoct the five ingredients in 7 *shēng* of water to get 3 *shēng* and remove dregs. Take one *shēng* when it is warm for each dose.

*****

[04] 发汗后，脐下悸〔1〕者，欲作贲豚，茯苓桂枝甘草大枣汤〔2〕主之。

茯苓桂枝甘草大枣汤方：

茯苓半斤 甘草二两，炙 大枣十五枚 桂枝四两 右四味，以甘烂水一斗，先煮茯苓，减二升，同诸药，煮取三升，去滓。温服一升，日三服。甘烂水法：取水二斗，置大盆内，以杓扬之，水上有珠子五六千颗相逐，取用之。

Annotations

[1] *Qi Xia Ji:* Rapid pulsations below the umbilicus due to heart yang damage by profuse sweating.

[2] *Fu Ling Gui Zhi Gan Cao Da Zao Tang* (Poria, Cinnamon Twig, Licorice and Jujube Decoction): A formula (with a large dose of poria) to promote urination and resolve fluid retention.

Interpretations

After inducing sweating with warming needle therapy (for patients with Taiyang disease), rapid pulsations below the umbilicus is indicative of a likely onset of running piglet. This should be treated with *Fu Ling Gui Zhi Gan Cao Da Zao Tang* (Poria, Cinnamon Twig, Licorice and Jujube Decoction).

Fu Ling Gui Zhi Gan Cao Da Zao Tang

[Ingredients]

茯苓	*fú líng*	0.5*jīn*	Poria
炙甘草	*zhì gān cǎo*	2 *liǎng*	Radix et Rhizoma Glycyrrhizae Praeparata cum Melle
桂枝	*guì zhī*	4 *liǎng*	Ramulus Cinnamomi
大枣	*dà zǎo*	12 pieces	Fructus Jujubae

Decoct *Fu Ling* first in 1 *dòu* of *Gan Lan Shui* (specially prepared water) to get 8 *shēng* and then add the other three ingredients to decoct and get 3 *shēng*. Remove the dregs and take one *shēng* when it is warm for each dose, 3 doses a day. Preparation of *Gan Lan Shui*: Pour 2 *dòu* of water into a large basin, lift it continuously with a ladle. The water is ready for use when there are 5000-6000 globules on the surface of the water.

胸痹心痛短气病脉证治第九
Chapter 9 Chest-Bi Impediment, Chest Pain and Shortness of Breath—Pulses, Patterns and Treatment

Overview

This chapter is exclusively dedicated to chest-Bi impediment. Chest pain and shortness of breath are two symptoms of this condition.

*****

[01] 师曰：夫脉当取太过不及〔1〕。阳微阴弦，即胸痹而痛〔2〕，所以然者，责其极虚〔3〕也。今阳虚知在上焦〔4〕，所以胸痹、心痛者，以其阴弦故也〔5〕。

Annotations

[1] *Mai Dang Qu Tai Guo Bu Ji:* The first word *Mai* literally means pulse; however, here it refers to all examination methods, not limited to the pulse diagnosis. It is essential to differentiate deficiency or excess of yin and yang in diagnosing medical conditions.

[2] *Yang Wei Yin Xuan, Ji Xiong Bi Er Tong*: A faint pulse felt at the *Cun* position indicates yang qi deficiency; and a wiry pulse at the *Chi* position indicates (interior) yin excess. (Interior) yin excess may block chest yang and result in chest pain and shortness of breath.

[3] *Ji Xu*: The first word *Ji* literally means extreme; however, it does not mean extreme deficiency, just deficiency.

[4] *Jin Yang Xu Zhi Zai Shang Jiao*: Yang qi deficiency manifests in the chest area alone, which is similar to myocardial ischemia in modern medicine.

[5] *Suo Yi Xiong Bi Xin Tong Zhe, Yi Qi Yin Xuan Gu Ye*: The root cause of chest-Bi impediment is excess (interior) yin.

Interpretations

The Master said, "It is essential to differentiate the deficiency or excess of yin and yang in diagnosing medical conditions. Yang qi deficiency and (interior) yin excess may cause chest-Bi impediment with chest pain. This is caused by yang deficiency; however, yang defiency in this condition only manifests in the chest, the root cause of chest pain in chest-Bi impediment is (interior) yin excess.

*****

[02] 平人〔1〕，无寒热〔2〕，短气不足以息〔3〕者，实也。

Annotations

[1] *Ping Ren:* It does not mean healthy people, but patients with normal appetite.

[2] *Wu Han Re*: No chills or fever (seen in an exterior syndrome).

[3] *Duan Qi Bu Zu Yi Xi*: A major symptom of chest-Bi impediment—shortness of breath.

Interpretations

Shortness of breath or rapid breathing in patients who seem healthy and have no chills or fever indicates an excess syndrome of chest-Bi impediment.

*****

[03] 胸痹之病，喘息咳唾，胸背痛，短气〔1〕，寸口脉沉而迟，关上小紧数〔2〕，栝蒌薤白白酒汤〔3〕主之。

栝蒌薤白白酒汤方：

栝蒌实一枚，捣 薤白半升 白酒〔4〕七升右三味，同煮，取二升。分温再服。

Annotations

[1] *Chuan Xi Ke Tuo, Xiong Bei Tong, Duan Qi*: Typical symptoms of chest-Bi impediment: panting, chest pain that may radiate to the back and cough with foamy saliva due to retained phlegm-fluid blocking chest yang.

[2] *Cun Kou Mai Chen Er Chi, Guan Shang Xiao Jin Shuo:* A complicated pulse condition in chest-Bi impediment: a deep, slow and weak pulse in the *Cun* position (indicating yang deficiency) with a small, tight and rapid pulse in the *Guan* position (indicating yin excess). According to the *Jin Kui Zheng Yi* (Annotations on the 'Essentials from the Golden Cabinet'), "A deep, slow, small and tight pulse indicates yin excess; whereas a rapid pulse indicates yang, a rapid pulse at the *Guan* position suggests that chest yang fails to distribute over the lower *jiao* but get trapped in between the chest and diaphragm by yin excess, thus leading to chest pain that radiates to the back".

[3] *Gua Lou Xie Bai Bai Jiu Tang* (Trichosanthes, Chinese Chive and White Wine Decoction): A formula to unblock yang.

[4] *Bai Jiu*: It literally means white wine; however, here it refers to rice vinegar made of sorghum, rice, barley, millet or low-degree liquor.

Interpretations

The *Gua Lou Xie Bai Bai Jiu Tang* (Trichosanthes, Chinese Chive and White Wine Decoction) is indicated for chest-Bi impediment with panting, cough with foamy saliva, chest pain radiating to the back, shortness of breath and a deep, slow pulse at the *Cun* position and a mildly tight and rapid pulse at the *Chi* position.

Gua Lou Xie Bai Bai Jiu Tang

[Ingredients]

栝蒌	*guā lóu*	1 piece	Fructus Trichosanthis (crushed)
薤白	*xiè bái*	0.5 *shēng*	Bulbus Allii Macrostemi
米醋	*mǐ cù*	7 *shēng*	Rice vinegar

Decoct the three ingredients to get 2 *shēng*, take when it is warm in two times.

*****

[04] 胸痹不得卧[1]，心痛彻背[2]者，栝蒌薤白半夏汤[3]主之。

栝蒌薤白半夏汤方：栝蒌实一枚薤白三两 半夏半斤 白酒一斗右四味，同煮，取四升。温服一升，日三服。

Annotations

[1] *Xiong Bi Bu De Wo:* Symptoms of chest-Bi impediment: shortness of breath, panting and an inability to lie flat.

[2] *Xin Tong Che Bei:* Severe chest pain radiating to the back.

[3] *Gua Lou Xie Bai Ban Xia Tang* (Trichosanthes, Chinese Chive and Pinellia Decoction): A modified formula of *Gua Lou Xie Bai Bai Jiu Tang* plus *Ban Xia* (Rhizoma Pinelliae). It acts to unblock yang, resolve fluid retention and down-regulate qi.

Interpretations

Chest-Bi impediment with an inability to lie flat and severe chest pain radiating to the back should be treated with *Gua Lou Xie Bai Ban Xia Tang* (Trichosanthes, Chinese Chive and Pinellia Decoction).

Gua Lou Xie Bai Ban Xia Tang

[Ingredients]

栝蒌	*guā lóu*	1 piece	Fructus Trichosanthis (crushed)
薤白	*xiè bái*	3 *liǎng*	Bulbus Allii Macrostemi
半夏	*bàn xià*	0.5 *shēng*	Rhizoma Pinelliae
米醋	*mǐ cù*	1 *dòu*	Rice vinegar

Decoct the four ingredients to get 4 *shēng*, take 1 *shēng* for each dose when it is warm, 3 doses a day.

*****

[05] 胸痹心中痞，留气结在胸，胸满，胁下逆抢心〔1〕，枳实薤白桂枝汤〔2〕主之；人参汤〔3〕亦主之。

枳实薤白桂枝汤方：

枳实四枚 厚朴四两 薤白半斤 桂枝一两 栝蒌一枚，捣 右五味，以水五升，先煮枳实、厚朴，取二升，去滓，内诸药，煮数沸。分温三服。

人参汤方：

人参 甘草 干姜 白术各三两 右四味，以水八升，煮取三升。温服一升，日三服。

Annotations

[1] *Xiong Bi Xin Zhong Pi...Xie Xia Ni Qiang Xin*: Chest-Bi impediment mainly characterized by chest fullness and tightness. This is actually more severe than chest pain. Qi stagnates in the chest and causes chest discomfort and stuffiness. In addition, patients may experience a sensation of qi ascending from the subcostal region to the heart. These manifestations can be diagnosed into deficiency or excess. In addition to chest discomfort, stuffiness, and counterflow of qi, (interior) yin excess due to spleen yang deficiency may also cause a pale complexion, sweats on the soles and palms, cold sweating and a faint, thready pulse.

[2] *Zhi Shi Xie Bai Gui Zhi Tang* (Immature Bitter Orange, Chinese Chive and Cinnamon Twig Decoction): A modified formula of *Gua Lou*

Xie Bai Bai Jiu Tang by removing (i.e., rice vinegar) and adding *Zhi Shi* (Fructus Aurantii Immaturus), *Hou Po* (Cortex Magnoliae Officinalis) and *Gui Zhi* (Ramulus Cinnamomi). This formula acts to unblock yang, dissipate masses, down-regulate qi and alleviate fullness. It is indicated for the excess pattern of chest-Bi impediment characterized by chest discomfort and tightness.

[3] *Ren Shen Tang* (Ginseng Decoction): A formula that contains same ingredients as *Li Zhong Tang/Wan* (Middle Jiao-Regulating Decoction/ Pill), please refer to the *Shangh Han Lun* (Treatise on Cold Damage) (No 396). This formula acts to warm the spleen and stomach, tonify qi, and supplement yang. It is indicated for the deficiency pattern of chest-Bi impediment characterized by chest discomfort and tightness.

Interpretations

Chest-Bi impediment with chest discomfort and tightness, qi stagnation in the chest, chest stuffiness and a sensation of qi ascending from the subcostal region to the heart (due to phlegm-fluid obstructing the flow of qi) should be treated with *Zhi Shi Xie Bai Gui Zhi Tang* (Immature Bitter Orange, Chinese Chive and Cinnamon Twig Decoction) to unblock yang. The presence of deficiency symptoms (a pale complexion, cold limbs, cold sweating and a faint, thready pulse) should be treated with *Ren Shen Tang* (Ginseng Decoction) to tonify qi.

Zhi Shi Xie Baio Gui Zhi Tang

[Ingredients]

枳实	*zhǐ shí*	4 pieces	Fructus Aurantii Immaturus
栝蒌	*guā lóu*	1 piece	Fructus Trichosanthis (crushed)
薤白	*xiè bái*	0.5 *jīn*	Bulbus Allii Macrostemi
厚朴	*hòu pò*	4 *liǎng*	Cortex Magnoliae Officinalis
桂枝	*guì zhī*	1 *liǎng*	Ramulus Cinnamomi

Decoct *Zhi Shi* and *Hou Po* first in 5 *shēng* of water to get 2 *shēng*, remove the dregs and add the rest of the ingredients and bring to a boil for a couple of times. Take when it is warm in three times.

Ren Shen Tang

[Ingredients]

人参	*rén shēn*	3 *liǎng*	Radix et Rhizoma Ginseng
甘草	*gān cǎo*	3 *liǎng*	Radix et Rhizoma Glycyrrhizae
干姜	*gān jiāng*	3 *liǎng*	Rhizoma Zingiberis
白术	*bái zhú*	3 *liǎng*	Rhizoma Atractylodis Macrocephalae

Decoct the four ingredients in 8 *shēng* of water to get 3 *shēng*. Take 1 *shēng* for each dose when it is warm, 3 times a day.

*****

[06] 胸痹，胸中气塞，短气〔1〕，茯苓杏仁甘草汤〔2〕主之；橘枳姜汤〔3〕亦主之。

茯苓杏仁甘草汤方：茯苓三两杏仁五十个甘草一两　右三味，以水一斗，煮取五升。温服一升，日三服。不差，更服。

橘枳姜汤方：

橘皮一斤枳实三两生姜半斤　右三味，以水五升，煮取二升。分温再服。《肘后》、《千金》云：治胸痹，胸中愊愊如满〔4〕，噎塞习习如痒，喉中涩唾燥沫〔5〕。

Annotations

[1] *Xiong Bi, Xiong Zhong Qi Sai, Duan Qi*: Symptoms of chest-Bi impediment in remissive stages. Chest stuffiness indicates qi stagnation, wheres shortness of breath indicates fluid retention.

[2] *Fu Ling Xing Ren Gan Cao Tang* (Poria, Apricot Kernel and Licorice Decoction): A formula to move fluids and resolve fluid retention.

[3] *Ju Zhi Jiang Tang* (Tangerine Peel, Immature Bitter Orange and Ginseng Decoction): A formula to down-regulate and move qi.

[4] *Xiong Zhong Fu Fu Ru Man*: Severe chest stuffiness.

[5] *Ye Sai Xi Xi Ru Yang, Hou Zhong Se Tuo Zao Mo*: A sense of dry saliva stuck in the throat.

Interpretations

Chest-Bi impediment with chest stuffiness and shortness of breath can be treated with *Fu Ling Xing Ren Gan Cao Tang* (Poria, Apricot Kernel and Licorice Decoction) or *Ju Zhi Jiang Tang* (Tangerine Peel, Immature Bitter Orange and Ginseng Decoction).

Zhi Shi Xie Baio Gui Zhi Tang

[Ingredients]

枳实	*zhǐ shí*	4 pieces	Fructus Aurantii Immaturus
栝蒌	*guā lóu*	1 piece	Fructus Trichosanthis (crushed)
薤白	*xiè bái*	0.5 *jīn*	Bulbus Allii Macrostemi
厚朴	*hòu pò*	4 *liǎng*	Cortex Magnoliae Officinalis
桂枝	*guì zhī*	1 *liǎng*	Ramulus Cinnamomi

Decoct *Zhi Shi* and *Hou Po* first in 5 *shēng* of water to get 2 *shēng*, remove the dregs and add the rest of the ingredients and bring to a boil for a couple of times. Take when it is warm in three times.

Ren Shen Tang

[Ingredients]

茯苓	*fú líng*	3 *liǎng*	Poria
杏仁	*xìng rén*	50 pieces	Semen Armeniacae Amarum
甘草	*gān cǎo*	1 *liǎng*	Radix et Rhizoma Glycyrrhizae

Decoct the three ingredients in 1 *dòu* of water to get 5 *shēng*. Take 1 *shēng* for each dose when it is warm, 3 times a day. Continue taking the formula if necessary.

Ju Zhi Jiang Tang

[Ingredients]

橘皮	*jú pí*	1 *jīn*	Pericarpium Citri Reticulatae
枳实	*zhǐ shí*	3 *liǎng*	Fructus Aurantii Immaturus
生姜	*shēng jiāng*	0.5 *jīn*	Rhizoma Zingiberis Recens

Decoct the three ingredients in 5 *shēng* of water to get 2 *shēng*, and take when it is warm in two times. According to the *Zhou Hou Bei Ji Fang* (Emergency Formulas to Keep Up One's Sleeve) and *Qian Jin Yao Fang* (Important Formulas Worth a Thousand Gold Pieces), this formula can also be used to treat chest-Bi impediment with chest stuffiness and a sense of dry saliva stuck in the throat.

*****

[07] 胸痹缓急〔1〕者，薏苡仁附子散〔2〕主之。

薏苡附子散方：

薏苡仁十五两大附子十枚，炮 右二味，杵为散。服方寸匕，日三服。

Annotations

[1] *Xiong Bi Huan Ji*: Severe attack of chest-Bi impediment due to yin cold obstructing chest yang. Symptoms may include chest pain, shortness of breath and panting, etc.

[2] *Yi Yi Ren Fu Zi San* (Coix and Aconite Powder): A formula to warm the spleen and stomach, dissipate cold, alleviate spasm and stop pain.

Interpretations

Severe attacks of chest-Bi impediment (with chest pain, shortness of breath and panting) can be treated with *Yi Yi Ren Fu Zi San* (Coix and Aconite Powder).

Yi Yi Ren Fu Zi San

[Ingredients]

薏苡仁	*yì yǐ rén*	15 *liǎng*	Semen Coicis
附子	*fù zǐ*	10 pieces	Radix Aconiti Lateralis Praeparata

Grind the two ingredients into a fine powder and take 1 square-inch spon for each dose, 3 doses a day.

*****

[08] 心中痞，诸逆〔1〕心悬痛〔2〕，桂枝生姜枳实汤〔3〕主之。

桂姜枳实汤方：

桂枝生姜各三两 枳实五枚 右三味，以水六升，煮取三升。分温三服。

Annotations

[1] *Xin Zhong Pi, Zhu Ni*: Mild pattern of chest-Bi impediment. Symptoms may include chest stuffiness or a sense of qi ascending from the subcostal region to the heart.

[2] *Xuan Tong:* Referred pain.

[3] *Gui Zhi Sheng Jiang Zhi Shi Tang* (Cinnamon Twig, Fresh Ginger and Immature Bitter Orange Decoction): A formula to unblock yang, down-regulate qi, resolve masses and eliminate fluid retention.

Interpretations

Chest-Bi impediment with chest stuffiness/discomfort, a sense of qi ascending from the subcostal region to the heart and referred pain below the heart can be treated with *Gui Zhi Sheng Jiang Zhi Shi Tang* (Cinnamon Twig, Fresh Ginger and Immature Bitter Orange Decoction).

Gui Zhi Sheng Jiang Zhi Shi Tang

[Ingredients]

桂枝	*guì zhī*	3 *liǎng*	Ramulus Cinnamomi
生姜	*shēng jiāng*	3 *liǎng*	Rhizoma Zingiberis Recens
枳实	*zhǐ shí*	5 pieces	Fructus Aurantii Immaturus

Decoct the three ingredients in 6 *shēng* of water to get 3 *shēng*, take when it is warm in three times.

*****

[09] 心痛彻背，背痛彻心〔1〕。乌头赤石脂丸〔2〕主之。

赤石脂丸方：

蜀椒一两，一法二分乌头一分，炮 附子半两，炮，一法一分 干姜一两，一法一分 赤石脂一两，一法二分 右五味，末之，蜜丸，如梧子大。先食服一丸，日三服。不知，稍加服。

Annotations

[1] *Xin Tong Che Bei, Bei Tong Che Xin*: Severe symptoms of chest-Bi impediment—Persistent, intense pain in the chest that radiates to the back due to retained yin cold, which is similar to angina pectoris in modern medicine.

[2] *Wu Tou Chi Shi Zhi Wan* (Aconite Main Tuber and Halloysite Pill): A formula to warm yang, dissipate cold and stop pain.

Interpretations

Chest-Bi impediment with intense pain in the chest that radiates to the back (probably coupled with cold sweatins and cold hands/feet) can be treated with *Wu Tou Chi Shi Zhi Wan* (Aconite Main Tuber and Halloysite Pill).

Wu Tou Chi Shi Zhi Wan

[Ingredients]

蜀椒	*huā jiāo*	1 *liǎng*/2 *fēn*	Pericarpium Zanthoxyli
乌头	*wū tóu*	1 *fēn*	Radix Aconiti Preparata
附子	*fù zǐ*	0.5 *liǎng*	Radix Aconiti Lateralis Praeparata
干姜	*gān jiāng*	1 *liǎng*/1 *fēn*	Rhizoma Zingiberis
赤石脂	*chì shí zhī*	1 *liǎng*/2 *fēn*	Halloysitum Rubrum

Grind the five ingredients into a powder and mix with honey to make into pills the size of firmiana seeds. Take 1 pill for each dose before meals, 3 doses a day. If the effect is not noticeable, gradually increase the dose.

*****

九痛丸〔1〕，治九种心痛〔2〕。

附子三两，炮生狼牙一两，炙香　巴豆一两，去皮心，熬，研如脂人参干姜吴茱萸各一两 右六味，末之，炼蜜丸如梧子大。酒下。强人初服三丸，日三服；弱者二丸。兼治卒中恶〔3〕，腹胀痛，口不能言。又治连年积冷，流注心胸痛〔4〕，并冷肿上气，落马坠车血疾〔5〕等皆主之。忌口如常法。

Annotations

[1] *Jiu Tong Wan* (Pill for Nine Pains): A formula for nine types of chest pain or a variety of pain in the chest, stomach and abdomen due to cold retention, qi stagnation, parasitesm, phlegm-fluid or stagnant blood. It acts to dissipate cold, eliminate masses, kill parasites and unblock yang.

[2] *Jiu Zhong Xin Tong*: According the *Qian Jin Yao Fang* (Important Formulas Worth a Thousand Gold Pieces), the nine types of chest pain are respectively associated with parasites, weird spirits/ghosts, wind, fear/fright, indigestion, fluid-retention, cold limbs, or heat; and one type of pain is intermittent.

[3] *Zhong Wu*: Sudden onset due to exposure to exogenous pathogens.

[4] *Liu Zhu Xin Xiong Tong*: Migrating chest pain.

[5] *Luo Ma Zhui Che Xue Ji*: Stagnant blood due to falls

Interpretations

The *Jiu Tong Wan* (Pill for Nine Pains) can be used to treat nine types of chest pain.

Jiu Tong Wan

[Ingredients]

附子	*fù zǐ*	3 *liǎng*	Radix Aconiti Lateralis Praeparata
生狼牙	*shēng láng yá*	1 *liǎng*	Radix Euphorbiae Fischerianae (fried)
巴豆	*bā dòu*	1 *liǎng*	Fructus Crotonis (remove the skin and kernel, stew to remove the fat)
人参	*rén shēn*	1 *liǎng*	Radix et Rhizoma Ginseng
干姜	*gān jiāng*	1 *liǎng*	Rhizoma Zingiberis
吴茱萸	*wú zhū yú*	1 *liǎng*	Fructus Evodiae

Grind the six ingredients into a powder, mix with the stewed honey and make into pills the size of firmiana seeds. Take with wine. Patients with a strong body start from 3 pills for each dose, 3 doses a day. Patients who are thin and weak start with 2 pills for each dose. This formula is also indicated for sudden, unexplained distension and pain in the chest and abdomen or migratory chest pain due to cold retention, along with cough, panting and edema as well as stagnant blood due to falls from a horse or cart. Patients need to follow routine dietary contraindications.

腹满寒疝宿食病脉证治第十

Chapter 10 Abdominal Fullness, Cold-Induced Abdominal Pain and Retained Food in the Stomach—Sequences, Pulses and Patterns

Overview

This chapter discusses abdominal fullness, cold-induced abdominal pain and retained food in the stomach together, since they share the symptoms of abdominal distension, fullness and pain. These conditions are similar to acute abdomen in surgery that requires urgent and specific diagnosis.

*****

[01] 趺阳脉微弦〔1〕，法当腹满〔2〕，不满者必便难〔3〕，两胠疼痛〔4〕，此虚寒从下上也〔5〕，当以温药服之。

Annotations

[1] *Fu Yang Mai Wei Xian*: A faint, wiry pulse felt at the point Chongyang (ST 42). A faint pulse indicates yang deficiency, and a wiry pulse indicates cold or pain. A faint, wiry *Fu Yang* pulse is indicative of abdominal fullness or pain.

[2] *Fu Man*: Abdominal distension, fullness or pain.

[3] *Bu Man Zhe Bi Bian Nan*: Abdominal fullness is often accompanied by difficult bowel movements. The first word *Bu* does not mean "*No*" but "Very".

[4] *Liang Qu Teng Tong*: Pain in the subcostal region.

[5] *Ci Xu Han Cong Xia Shang Ye*: Deficiency cold is the cause of abdominal fullness or constipation.

Interpretations

A faint, wiry pulse felt at Chongyang (ST 42) in often seen in patients with abdominal fullness, distension and pain, along with difficult bowel movements and pain in the subcostal region. These symptoms are caused by ascending of intangible cold qi, and therefore should be treated with warming medicinals (to drain downward and dissipate cold).

*****

[02] 病者腹满，按之不痛为虚，痛者为实[1]，可下之。舌黄未下者，下之，黄自去。

Annotations

[1] *An Zhi Bu Tong Wei Xu, Tong Zhe Wei Shi*: An examination method to palpate the abdomen to differentiate deficiency from excess according to pain upon pressure, known as abdominal examination in modern medicine.

Interpretations

For patients with abdominal fullness, an absence of pain upon pressure indicates (qi) deficiency and presence of pain upon pressure indicates excess (i.e, retained food in the stomach). The excess pattern needs to be treated with medicinals to drain downward. Before treatment, patients with abdominal fullness present with a yellow tongue coating due to excess heat. After treatment, the yellow coating disappears as the heat is cleared through the downward-draining method.

*****

[03] 腹满时减，复如故，此为寒[1]，当与温药。

Annotations

[1] *Fu Man Shi Jian, Fu Ru Gu, Ci Wei Han*: Abdominal fullness that alleviates and returns indicates cold.

Interpretations

Abdominal fullness that sometimes alleviates but later comes back (with paroxysmal abdominal pain) is caused by cold and should be treated with warming medicinals (to warm, unblock and drain downward).

*****

[04] 病者痿黄，躁而不渴〔1〕，胸中寒实〔2〕，而利不止者，死〔3〕。

Annotations

[1] *Bing Zhe Wei Huang, Zao Er Bu Ke*: A critical sign of abdominal fullness—dark, yellowish skin, restlessness and thirst.

[2] *Xiong Zhong Han Shi*: Interior excess cold in the abdomen.

[3] *Si*: Life-threatening

Interpretations

For patients with abdominal fullness, presence of jaundice (dark, yellowish skin), restlessness and thirst indicates interior excess cold. Additional loose stools with persistent diarrhea can be life threatening.

*****

[05] 寸口脉弦者，即胁下拘急而痛〔1〕，其人啬啬〔2〕恶寒也。

Annotations

[1] *Cun Kou Mai Xian Zhe, Ji Xie Xia Ju Ji Er Tong*: A wiry pulse felt at the *Cunkou* position is often seen in upper right abdominal spasm and pain.

[2] *Se Se:* chills, shivering.

Interpretations

For patients with abdominal fullness, a wiry pulse at the *Cunkou* position is often accompanied by spasm and pain in the upper right abdomen, (fever) and shivering.

*****

[06] 夫中寒家〔1〕，喜欠〔2〕，其人清涕出，发热色和者，善嚏。

Annotations

[1] *Zhong Han Jia*: People who are susceptible to contract wind cold.

[2] *Xi Qian:* Stretch with a yawn, often seen in patients with a weak constitution.

Interpretations

Patients who are more susceptible to contract wind cold frequently (feel tired) and yawn. Upon exposure to exogenous pathogenic factors, they may have a normal facial complexion but experience runny nose with clear nasal discharge, fever, and sneezing.

*****

[07] 中寒，其人下利〔1〕，以里虚也。欲嚏不能，此人肚中寒。一云痛。

Annotations

[1] *Zhong Han, Qi Ren Xia Li*: Diarrhea due to exposure to external cold.

Interpretations

Diarrhea (or in combination with abdominal pain) upon exposure to external cold is actually associated with interior cold due to yang deficiency. Absence of sneezing is also related to deficiency cold.

*****

[08] 夫瘦人绕脐痛，必有风冷〔1〕。谷气不行〔2〕，而反下之，其气必冲〔3〕。不冲〔4〕者，心下则痞也。

Annotations

[1] *Shou Ren Rao Qi Tong, Bi You Feng Leng*: Major symptoms and causative factors of cold-induced abdominal pain. The word *Shou Ren* here does not mean "thin people" but people without abdominal fullness. *Rao Qi Tong* means pain around the umbilicus (lower abdomen). It is caused by wind cold.

[2] *Gu Qi Bu Xing*: Qi blockage of the fu organs, referring to constipation.

[3] *Er Fan Xia Zhi, Qi Qi Bi Chong*: Draining downward method cannot be used for cold-induced abdominal pain; otherwise, pathogenic qi may rush up.

[4] *Bu Chong*: The *Bu* here does not mean "No". *Bu Chong* actually means rushing up.

Interpretations

For patients without abdominal fullness, pain around the umbilicus indicates retained wind cold. The wrong use of draining downward method for constipation may damage stomach yang and cause the cold to rush up, resulting in epigastric stuffiness or discomfort.

*****

[09] 病腹满，发热十日，脉浮而数〔1〕，饮食如故〔2〕，厚朴七物汤〔3〕主之。

厚朴七物汤方：

厚朴半斤 甘草大黄各三两 大枣十枚枳实五枚 桂枝二两 生姜五两右七味，以水一斗，煮取四升。温服八合，日三服。呕者加半夏五合；下利去大黄；寒多者加生姜至半斤。

Annotations

[1] *Bing Fu Man, Fa Re Shi Ri, Mai Fu Er Shuo:* A pulse condition for abdominal fullness due to excess heat. Fever lasting days, a superficial, rapid pulse indicates unresolved exterior syndrome. Abdominal fullness includes abdominal distension, pain and constipation.

[2] *Yin Shi Ru Gu*: It does not mean normal food ingestion but means an absence of vomiting, because the disorder is in the intestine instead of the stomach.

[3] *Hou Po Qi Wu Tang* (Officinal Magnolia Bark Seven Ingredients Decoction): A basic formula for abdominal fullness due to excess heat, consisting of *Xiao Cheng Qi Tang* (Minor Purgative Decoction) to move qi and *Gui Zhi Tang* (Cinnamon Twig Decoction) to release the exterior and harmonize the *Ying*-nutrients and *Wei*-defense.

Interpretations

For paitents with abdominal fullness (distension or pain), fever lasting days (chills), a superficial, rapid pulse and eating without vomiting should be treated with *Hou Po Qi Wu Tang* (Officinal Magnolia Bark Seven Ingredients Decoction).

Hou Po Qi Wu Tang

[Ingredients]

厚朴	*hòu pò*	3 *liǎng*	Cortex Magnoliae Officinalis
甘草	*gān cǎo*	3 *liǎng*	Radix et Rhizoma Glycyrrhizae
大黄	*dà huáng*	3 *liǎng*	Radix et Rhizoma Rhei
大枣	*dà zǎo*	10 pieces	Fructus Jujubae
枳实	*zhǐ shí*	5 pieces	Fructus Aurantii Immaturus
桂枝	*guì zhī*	3 *liǎng*	Ramulus Cinnamomi
生姜	*shēng jiāng*	3 *liǎng*	Rhizoma Zingiberis Recens

Decoct the seven ingredients in 1 *dòu* of water to get 4 *shēng*. Take 0.8 *shēng* for each dose when it is warm, 3 doses a day. For vomiting due to fluid retention in the stomach, add 0.5 *shēng* of *Ban Xia* (Rhizoma Pinelliae) to resolve the retained fluid. For diarrhea, remove *Da Huang*. For severe chills, increase the dose of *Sheng Jiang* (Rhizoma Zingiberis Recens) to 0.5 *jīn* to dissipate cold.

*****

[10] 腹中寒气〔1〕，雷鸣切痛〔2〕，胸胁逆满，呕吐〔3〕，附子粳米汤〔4〕主之。

附子粳米汤方：

附子一枚，炮半夏半升甘草一两大枣十枚粳米半升右五味，以水八升，煮米熟，汤成，去滓。温服一升，日三服。

Annotations

[1] *Fu Zhong Han Qi*: Abdominal fullness due to upward flow of cold qi.

[2] *Lei Ming Qie Tong*: Thunderous bowel sounds (hyperactive bowel sounds in modern medicine) with sharp, stabbing abdominal pain. This is caused by retained cold qi in the stomach and intestines.

[3] *Xiong Xie Ni Man, Ou Tu*: Abdominal fullness and distension due to upward flow of cold qi. Vomting is caused by retained water fluid. This is similar to intestinal obstruction in modern medicine.

[4] *Fu Zi Jing Mi Tang* (Aconite and Non-glutinous Rice Decoction): A formula to warm the spleen and stomach, dissipate cold, down-regulate qi and stop vomiting.

Interpretations

For paitents with abdominal fullness, presence of loud, noisy bowel sounds, sharp, stabbing abdominal pain, abdominal distension and vomiting should be treated with *Fu Zi Jing Mi Tang* (Aconite and Non-glutinous Rice Decoction).

Fu Zi Jing Mi Tang

[Ingredients]

附子	*fù zǐ*	1 piece	Radix Aconiti Lateralis Praeparata
半夏	*bàn xià*	0.5 *shēng*	Rhizoma Pinelliae
甘草	*gān cǎo*	1 *liǎng*	Radix et Rhizoma Glycyrrhizae
大枣	*dà zǎo*	10 pieces	Fructus Jujubae
粳米	*jīng mǐ*	0.5 *shēng*	Oryza Sativa L.

Decoct the five ingredients in 8 *shēng* of water until the non-glutinous rice is fully cooked. Remove the dregs and take 1 *shēng* for each dose when it is warm, 3 doses a day.

*****

[11] 痛而闭〔1〕者，厚朴三物汤〔2〕主之。

厚朴三物汤方：

厚朴八两大黄四两　枳实五枚　右三味，以水一斗二升，先煮二味，取五升，内大黄，煮取三升。温服一升，以利为度。

Annotations

[1] *Tong Er Bi*: Abdominal distension, fullness and pain as well as constipation due to excess heat. The word *Bi* here means qi blockage of stomach and intestines without flatus.

[2] *Hou Po San Wu Tang* (Officinal Magnolia Bark Three Ingredients Decoction): A formula to move qi and alleviate abdominal fullness. It shares the same ingredients with *Xiao Cheng Qi Tang* (Minor Purgative Decoction); however, they are different in monarch ingredient and dosage. The *Xiao Cheng Qi Tang* uses *Da Huang* as the monarch and mainly acts to promote bowel movements, while this formula uses *Hou Po* as the monarch.

Interpretations

Abdominal (fullness, distension) pain with constipation should be treated with *Hou Po San Wu Tang* (Officinal Magnolia Bark Three Ingredients Decoction).

Hou Po San Wu Tang

[Ingredients]

厚朴	*hòu pò*	8 *liǎng*	Cortex Magnoliae Officinalis
大黄	*dà huáng*	4 *liǎng*	Radix et Rhizoma Rhei
枳实	*zhǐ shí*	5 pieces	Fructus Aurantii Immaturus

Decoct *Hou Po* and *Zhi Shi* in 1 *dòu* and 2 *shēng* of water to get 5 *shēng*, add *Da Huang* and decoct to get 3 *shēng*. Remove the dregs and take 1 *shēng* for each dose and stop taking the formula when the bowel movement is normal.

*****

[12] 按之心下满痛〔1〕者，此为实也，当下之，宜大柴胡汤〔2〕。

大柴胡汤方：

柴胡半斤黄芩三两芍药三两半夏半升，洗枳实四枚，炙 大黄二两大枣十二枚 生姜五两右八味，以水一斗二升，煮取六升，去滓，再煎。温服一升，日三服。

Annotations

[1] *An Zhi Xin Xia Man Tong Zhe*: Upper abdominal fullness and tenderness, a common abdominal diagnosis method in modern surgery.

[2] *Da Chai Hu Tang* (Major Bupleurum Decoction): A formula to clear heat and drain downward. It is now commonly used for acute cholecystitis, gall stones and pancreatitis.

Interpretations

Abdominal fullness due to interior excess heat may cause upper abdominal fullness and tenderness (fever, vomiting or jaundice may also be present). This should be treated with *Da Cheng Qi Tang* (Major Bupleurum Decoction) to drain downward and clear heat.

Da Chai Hu Tang

[Ingredients]

柴胡	*chái hú*	0.5 *jīn*	Radix Bupleuri
黄芩	*huáng qín*	3 *liǎng*	Radix Scutellariae
芍药	*sháo yào*	3 *liǎng*	Radix Paeoniae
半夏	*bàn xià*	0.5 *shēng*	Rhizoma Pinelliae (washed)
枳实	*zhǐ shí*	4 pieces	Fructus Aurantii Immaturus (fried)
大黄	*dà huáng*	2 *liǎng*	Radix et Rhizoma Rhei
大枣	*dà zǎo*	12 pieces	Fructus Jujubae
生姜	*shēng jiāng*	5 *liǎng*	Rhizoma Zingiberis Recens

Decoct the eight ingredients in 1 *dòu* and 8 *shēng* of water to get 6 *shēng*. Remove the dregs and re-decoct to get 3 *shēng*. Take 1 *shēng* for each dose when it is warm, 3 doses a day.

*****

[13] 腹满不减，减不足言[1]，当须下之，宜大承气汤[2]。

大承气汤方：

大黄四两，酒洗 厚朴半斤，去皮炙 枳实五枚，炙 芒硝三合右四味，以水一斗，先煮二物，取五升，去滓，内大黄，煮取二升，内芒硝，更上火微一二沸。分温再服。得下，余勿服。

Annotations

[1] *Fu Man Bu Jian, Jian Bu Zu Yan*: Persistent abdominal fullness without alleviation due to retained heat in the intestines. *Jian Bu Zu Yan* means sometimes the symptom get slightly better but not enough for alleviation.

[2] *Da Cheng Qi Tang* (Major Purgative Decoction): See chapter 2.

Interpretations

Persistent abdominal fullness (with constipation due to interior excess heat), even though sometimes get slightly better but not alleviated at all, should be treated with *Da Cheng Qi Tang* (Major Purgative Decoction).

Da Cheng Qi Tang

[Ingredients]

大黄	*dà huáng*	4 *liǎng*	Radix et Rhizoma Rhei (soaked in wine)
厚朴	*hòu pò*	0.5 *jīn*	Cortex Magnoliae Officinalis
枳实	*zhǐ shí*	5	Fructus Aurantii Immaturus Praeparata
芒硝	*máng xiāo*	3 *gě*	Natrii Sulfas

Decoct *Hou Po* and *Zhi Shi* in 1 *dòu* of water to get 5 *shēng*. Remove the dregs and add *Da Huang* to decoct and get 2 *shēng*. Then add *Mang Xiao* and decoct to bring it to boil (once or twice). Take the decoction when it is warm in two times (doses). Stop taking the formula as soon as the constipation is alleviated.

*****

[14] 心胸中大寒痛〔1〕，呕不能饮食〔2〕，腹中寒，上冲皮起，出见有头足〔3〕，上下痛而不可触近〔4〕。大建中汤〔5〕主之。

大建中汤方：

蜀椒二合，去汗干姜四两 人参二两右三味，以水四升，煮取二升，去滓，内胶饴一升，微火煎取一升半。分温再服。如一炊顷，可饮粥二升，后更服，当一日食糜〔6〕，温覆之。

Annotations

[1] *Xin Xiong Zhong Da Han Tong*: Extensive, severe abdominal fullness and pain due to cold retention in the spleen and stomach.

[2] *Ou Bu Neng Yin Shi:* Frequent nausea and vomiting with an inability to eat or drink due to retained cold qi in the stomach. This is similar to intestinal obstruction in modern medicine.

[3] *Fu Zhong Han, Shang Chong Pi Qi, Chu Jian You Tou Zu*: Abdomen inspection—bulging of the skin that resembles the shape of a head or feet, which is similar to the bulging of the skin that resembles the shape of a part of intestine in acute abdomen.

[4] *Shang Xia Tong Er Bu Ke Chu Jin*: Abdomen palpation—Tenderness of the entire abdomen.

[5] *Da Jian Zhong Tang* (Major Middle Jiao-Fortifying Decoction): A formula to warm the spleen and stomach, dissipate cold, and fortify qi of the spleen and stomach.

[6] *Ru Yi Chui Qi Qing...Dang Yi Ri Shi Mi*: Intake of half-liquid food all day long.

Interpretations

Intense abdominal pain (due to cold retention in the middle *jiao*), frequent vomiting, an inability to eat or drink, bulging of the abdominal skin that resembles the shapes of a head or feet due to acent of cold qi, and tenderness on the whole abdomen should be treated with *Da Jian Zhong Tang* (Major Middle Jiao—Fortifying Decoction).

Da Jian Zhong Tang

[Ingredients] *shǔ jiāo*

蜀椒	*huā jiāo*	4 *liǎng*	Pericarpium Zanthoxyli (oil removed)
干姜	*gān jiāng*	4 *liǎng*	Rhizoma Zingiberis
人参	*rén shēn*	2 *liǎng*	Radix et Rhizoma Ginseng

Decoct the three ingredients in 4 *shēng* of water to get 2 *shēng*. Remove the dregs and add 1 *shēng* of malt sugar to decoct with mild fire to get 1.5 *shēng*. Take when it is warm in two times. After the time it takes to cook a meal, eat 2 *shēng* of congee. It is advisable to eat congee all day long and stay warm.

*****

[15] 胁下偏痛〔1〕、发热〔2〕，其脉紧弦，此寒也〔3〕。以温药下之，宜大黄附子汤〔4〕。

大黄附子汤方：

大黄三两附子三枚，炮细辛二两右三味，以水五升，煮取二升。分温三服。若强人煮取二升半〔5〕。分温三服。服后如人行四五里，进一服。

Annotations

[1] *Xie Xia Pian Tong*: Pain on the right subcostal region.

[2] *Fa Re:* Fever. This word was not recorded in the *Mai Jing* (The Pulse Classic).

[3] *Mai Jin Xian, Ci Han Ye*: Retained interior cold in the subcostal region.

[4] *Da Huang Fu Zi Tang* (Rhubarb and Aconite Decoction): A formula (consisting of both cold- and warm-property medicinals) to drain downward, dissipate cold and stop pain.

[5] *Qiang Ren Zhu Qu Er Sheng Ban*: Decoct to get 2.5 *shēng* for patients with a strong body to get a stronger purgative effect of *Da Huang*.

Interpretations

Pain on the right subcostal region, fever (or in combination with chills, vomiting and constipation), and a tight, wiry pulse indicates retained excess cold in the subcostal region. This should be treated with *Da Huang Fu Zi Tang* (Rhubarb and Aconite Decoction) to warm and drain downward.

Da Huang Fu Zi Tang

[Ingredients]

大黄	*dà huáng*	3 *liǎng*	Radix et Rhizoma Rhei
附子	*fù zǐ*	3 pieces	Radix Aconiti Lateralis Praeparata
细辛	*xì xīn*	2 *liǎng*	Radix et Rhizoma Asari

Decoct the three ingredients in 5 *shēng* of water to get 2 *shēng*. Remove the dregs and take when it is warm in three times. For patients with a strong body, decoct a shorter period of time to get 2.5 *shēng*, remove the dregs and take whent it is warm in three times. The time interval between two doses is the time it takes to walk 2-2.5 kilometers.

*****

[16] 寒气厥逆[1]，赤丸[2]主之。

赤丸方：

茯苓四两　半夏四两洗，一方用桂[3]乌头二两，炮细辛一两，《千金》作人参[4]右六味，末之，内真朱为色，炼蜜丸，如麻子大。先食酒饮下三丸，日再夜一服。不知，稍增之，以知为度。

Annotations

[1] *Han Qi Jue Ni*: Upward flow of cold qi that carries water-fluid. Patients may experience abdominal pain, vomiting and cold hands/feet.

[2] *Chi Wan*: A formula to dissipate cold, stop pain, resolve fluid retention and down-regulate qi.

[3] *Yi Fang Yong Gui*: *Gui Zhi* (Cinnamon Twig) is used in another formula instead of *Ban Xia*.

[4] *Qian Jin Zuo Ren Shen*: *Ren Shen* (Ginseng) is used in *Qian Jin Yao Fang* instead of *Xi Xin*; however, it's not appropriate because *Ren Shen* tonifies qi, whereas *Xi Xin* dissipates cold.

Interpretations

Upward flow of cold qi that carries water fluid (with abdominal pain, vomiting or cold hands/feet) can be treated with *Chi Wan* (Red Pill).

Chi Wan

[Ingredients]

茯苓	*fú líng*	3 *liǎng*	Poria
半夏	*bàn xià*	4 *liǎng*	Rhizoma Pinelliae (washed)
乌头	*wū tóu*	2 *liǎng*	Radix Aconiti Kusnezoffii
细辛	*xì xīn*	1 *liǎng*	Radix et Rhizoma Asari

Grind the four ingredients into a powder and add cinnabar to make into red color. Mix the powder with honey to make into pills the size of hemp seeds. Take three pills with wine before meals, twice during the day and once at night. If there is no efficacy, gradually increase the dose.

*****

[17] 腹痛〔1〕，脉弦而紧。弦则卫气不行，即恶寒，紧则不欲食。邪正相搏，即为寒疝〔2〕。寒疝绕脐痛，若发则白汗出，手足厥冷〔3〕，其脉沉弦〔4〕者。大乌头煎〔5〕主之。

乌头煎方：乌头大者五枚，熬，去皮，不㕮咀

右以水三升，煮取一升，去滓，内蜜二升，煎令水气尽，取二升。强人服七合，弱人服五合。不差，明日更服，不可一日再服〔6〕。

Annotations

[1] *Fu Tong*: Abdominal pain. In *Mai Jing* (the Pulse Classic), these two words are *Cunkou* instead.

[2] *Han Shan*: Paroyxsmal intense abdominal pain due to cold qi stagnation.

[3] *Ruo Fa Ze Bai Han Chu, Shou Zu Jue Ling*: Intense abdominal pain causing cold sweats and cold limbs due to stagnant cold qi blocking yang qi.

[4] *Qi Mai Chen Xian*: A deep, wiry pulse. In other text, it is said a deep, tight pulse.

[5] *Da Wu Tou Jian* (Major Aconiti Kusnezoffii Decoction): A formula to dissipate cold, break masses and stop pain. Since *Wu Tou* (Radix Aconiti Kusnezoffii) is toxic, its decoction needs to be taken with caution. It's advisable that *Wu Tou* (without being chopped) is decocted with honey to reduce its toxicity. In addition, the dose varies from person to person.

[6] *Bu Ke Yi Ri Zai Fu*: One cannot take two doses in one day.

Interpretations

Abdominal pain with a wiry, tight pulse is associated with cold. Blocked flow of yang qi may cause chills and no desire to eat. Cold qi stagnation may cause intense pain in the lower abdomen (around the umbilicus), cold sweats, cold limbs and a deep, wiry pulse. This should be treated with *Da Wu Tou Jian* (Major Aconiti Kusnezoffii Decoction).

Method: Decoct 5 pieces of skin-removed *Wu Tou* (Radix Aconiti Kusnezoffii) in 3 *shēng* of water to get 1 *shēng*. Remove the dregs, add 2 *shēng* of honey to decoct and get 2 *shēng*. Patients with a strong body take 0.7 *shēng*, whereas patients who are thin and weak take 0.5 *shēng*. If there is no efficacy, take another dose the next day. One cannot take two doses in one day.

*****

[18] 寒疝腹中痛，及胁痛里急〔1〕者，当归生姜羊肉汤〔2〕主之。

当归生姜羊肉汤方：

当归三两生姜五两羊肉一斤　右三味，以水八升，煮取三升。温服七合，日三服。若寒多者，加生姜成一斤；痛多而呕者，加橘皮二两，白术一两。加生姜者，亦加水五升，煮取三升二合。服之。

Annotations

[1] *Ji Xie Tong Li Ji*: Mild pain in the subcostal region due to blood deficiency. In severe cases, pain occurs around the umbilicus.

[2] *Dang Gui Sheng Jiang Yang Rou Tang* (Chinese Angelica, Fresh Ginger, and Goat Meat Decoction): A formula to circulate blood, dissipate cold, reinforce the body and stop pain. This formula can also be used for women after childbirth.

Interpretations

Cold qi stagnation usually causes pain around the umbilicus. Mild pain in the subcostal region should be treated with *Dang Gui Sheng Jiang Yang Rou Tang* (Chinese Angelica, Fresh Ginger, and Goat Meat Decoction).

Chi Wan

[Ingredients]

当归	*dāng guī*	3 *liǎng*	Radix Angelicae Sinensis
生姜	*shēng jiāng*	5 *liǎng*	Rhizoma Zingiberis Recens
羊肉	*yáng ròu*	1 *jīn*	Goat meat

Decoct the three ingredients in 8 *shēng* of water to get 3 *shēng*. Take 0.7 *shēng* for each dose, 3 doses a day. For severe cold, increase the dose of fresh ginger to 1 *jīn* and add 5 *shēng* of water and decoct to get 3.2 *shēng*. For severe pain in the subcostal pain with vomiting, add 2 *liǎng* of *Ju Pi* (Pericarpium Citri Reticulatae) and 1 *liǎng* of *Bai Zhu* (Rhizoma Atractylodis Macrocephalae).

*****

[19] 寒疝腹中痛，逆冷，手足不仁。若身疼痛，灸刺诸药不能治〔1〕，抵当乌头桂枝汤〔2〕主之。

乌头桂枝汤方：

乌头　　右一味，以蜜二斤，煎减半，去滓，以桂枝汤五合解之〔3〕，令得一升后。初服二合。不知，即服三合。又不知，复加至五合。其知者，如醉状，得吐者，为中病〔4〕。

桂枝汤方：

桂枝三两去皮　芍药三两甘草二两，炙　生姜三两　大枣十二枚右五味，锉，以水七升，微火煮取三升，去滓。

Annotations

[1] *Jiu Ci Zhu Yao Bu Neng Zhi*: Acupuncture alone or medicinals that warm the interior and release the exterior may not work.

[2] *Wu Tou Gui Zhi Tang* (Aconiti Kusnezoffii and Cinnammon Twig Decoction): A formula to dissipate cold in both the exterior and interior. It consists of *Wu Tou San* (Major Aconiti Kusnezoffii Powder) (to dissipate interior cold) and *Gui Zhi Tang* (Cinnamon Twig Decoction) (to release the exterior).

[3] *Yi Gui Zhi Tang Wu He Jie Zhi*: To dissolve the mixed *Wu Tou* powder and honey with 0.5 *shēng* of *Gui Zhi Tang* (Cinnamon Twig Decoction).

[4] *Qi Zhi Zhe...Wei Zhong Bing*: It's advisable to start with a smaller dose and then gradually increase. If patients appear drunk or began vomiting, it means they are almost poisoned and require care and caution.

Interpretations

For (interior) cold-induced abdominal pain, cold and numb hands and feet indicate exterior cold. If patients experience symptoms of an exterior syndrome like body ache, simple acupuncture or medicinals (to warm the interior and release the exterior) may not work. This has to be treated with *Wu Tou Gui Zhi Tang* (Aconiti Kusnezoffii and Cinnammon Twig Decoction).

Decoct *Wu Tou* (Radix Aconiti Kusnezoffii) in two *jīn* of honey to get 1 *jīn*, remove the dregs and dissolve it with 0.5 *shēng* of *Gui Zhi Tang* (Cinnamon Twig Decoction) and get 1 *shēng*. Take 0.2 *shēng* for the first dose; if no efficacy, take 0.3 *shēng*; if still no efficacy, take 0.5 *shēng*. If patients appear drunk or began vomiting, it is a sign that the formula starts to take effect.

Gui Zhi Tang

[Ingredients]

桂枝	*guì zhī*	3 *liǎng*	Ramulus Cinnamomi (skin removed)
芍药	*sháo yào*	3 *liǎng*	Radix Paeoniae
炙甘草	*zhì gān cǎo*	2 *liǎng*	Radix et Rhizoma Glycyrrhizae Praeparata cum Melle
生姜	*shēng jiāng*	3 *liǎng*	Rhizoma Zingiberis Recens
大枣	*dà zǎo*	12 pieces	Fructus Jujubae

Grind the five ingredients into a powder and decoction in 7 *shēng* of water with mild fire to get 3 *shēng*, remove the dregs.

*****

[20] 其脉数而紧乃弦，状如弓弦，按之不移〔1〕。脉数弦者，当下其寒；脉紧大而迟者，必心下坚；脉大而紧者，阳中有阴〔2〕，可下之。

Annotations

[1] *Mai Shuo Er Jin Nai Xian, Zhuang Ru Gong Xian, An Zhi Bu Yi*: The pulse is rapid and tight. It feels wiry, stringlike and immobile upon pressure.

[2] *Yang Zhong You Yin*: A rapid and large pulse indicates yang (excess); a wiry, tight and slow pulse indicates yin (interior or cold). A rapid, wiry, tight, large and slow indicates yin within yang.

Interpretations

A rapid and tight pulse is felt like wiry, stringlike, forceful (presence of epigastric masses), and immobile upon pressure. A rapid pulse indicates excess cold in the stomach, which should be treated by draining downward. A tight, large and slow pulse or a large and tight pulse indicates yin within yang, which can also be treated by draining downward.

*****

Annex Formula # 1 *Wu Tou Tang* (Aconiti Kusnezoffii Decoction)

《外台》乌头汤[1]：治寒疝腹中绞痛，贼风入攻五脏[2]，拘急不得转侧，发作有时，使人阴缩，手足厥逆[3]。

Annotations

[1] *Wai Tai Wu Tou Tang*: *Wu Tou Tang* (Aconiti Kusnezoffii Decoction) in the *Wai Tai Mi Yao* (Arcane Essentials from the Imperial Library)—a formula for cold-induced abdominal pain.

[2] *Han Shan Fu Zhong Jiao Tong, Zei Feng Ru Gong Wu Zang*: Acute colic as if the zang-fu organs are attacked by wind.

[3] *Ju Ji Bu De Zhuan Ce...Shou Zu Jue Ni*: Severe abdominal pain causing abdominal contracture (hypertonicity) with an inability to turn over the body, paroxysmal abdominal pain, retraction of the genitals and cold hands/feet. This is similar to renal colic in modern medicine.

Interpretations

The *Wu Tou Tang* (Aconiti Kusnezoffii Decoction) from the *Wai Tai Mi Yao* (Arcane Essentials from the Imperial Library) is indicated for acute cold-induced colic as if the zang-fu organs are attacked by wind, abdominal contracture, inability to turn over the body, paroxysmal, intense abdominal pain, and in severe cases, retraction of the genitals and cold hands/feet (cold sweats).

*****

《外台》柴胡桂枝汤[1]方：治心腹卒中痛者。柴胡四两黄芩人参芍药桂枝生姜各一两半甘草一两　半夏二合半大枣六枚　右九味，以水六升，煮取三升。温服一升，日三服。

Annex Formula # 2 *Chai Hu Gui Zhi Tang* (Bupleurum and Cinnamon Twig Decoction)

Annotations

[1] *Chai Hu Gui Zhi Tang* (Bupleurum and Cinnamon Twig Decoction): It is originally from the *Shang Han Lun* (Treatise on Cold Damage). Despite the same ingredients and dose, it has different indications. The formula in *Shang Han Lun* is indicated for fever, mild chills, joitn pain, nausea, and epigastric masses. Here it is indicated for acute abdominal pain. It consists of *Xiao Chai Hu Tang* (Minor Bupleurum Decoction) (to haromize the exterior and interior and clear interior heat) and *Gui Zhi Tang* (Cinnamon Twig Decoction) (to harmonize the *Ying*-nutrients and *Wei*-defense).

Interpretations

The *Chai Hu Gui Zhi Tang* (Bupleurum and Cinnamon Twig Decoction) from the *Wai Tai Mi Yao* (Arcane Essentials from the Imperial Library) is indicated for acute chest or abdominal pain.

Chai Hu Gui Zhi Tang

[Ingredients]

柴胡	*chái hú*	4 *liǎng*	Radix Bupleuri
黄芩	*huáng qín*	1.5 *liǎng*	Radix Scutellariae
人参	*rén shēn*	1.5 *liǎng*	Radix et Rhizoma Ginseng
芍药	*sháo yào*	1.5 *liǎng*	Radix Paeoniae

Chai Hu Gui Zhi Tang

[Ingredients]

桂枝	*guì zhī*	1.5 *liǎng*	Ramulus Cinnamomi
生姜	*shēng jiāng*	1.5 *liǎng*	Rhizoma Zingiberis Recens
甘草	*gān cǎo*	1 *liǎng*	Radix et Rhizoma Glycyrrhizae
半夏	*bàn xià*	0.25 *shēng*	Rhizoma Pinelliae (washed)
大枣	*dà zǎo*	6 pieces	Fructus Jujubae

Decoct the nine ingredients in 6 *shēng* of water to get 3 *shēng*. Take 1 *shēng* when it is warm for each dose, 3 doses a day.

*****

《外台》走马汤〔1〕：治中恶〔2〕心痛腹胀，大便不通。

巴豆二枚，去皮、心，熬 杏仁二枚右二味，以绵缠，捶令碎，热汤二合，捻取白汁。饮之。当下。老少量之。通治飞尸鬼击病〔3〕。

Annex Formula # 3 *Zou Ma Tang* (Galloping Horse Decoction)

Annotations

[1] *Zou Ma Tang* (Galloping Horse Decoction): Known as *Zhang Zhong Jing Liao Fei Shi Zou Ma Tang* in the *Wai Tai Mi Yao* (Arcane Essentials from the Imperial Library) to describe its rapid efficacy like a gallop horse. This formula uses *Ba Dou* (Fructus Crotonis) to break masses and *Xing Ren* (Semen Armeniacae Amarum) to unblock qi.

[2] *Zhong E*: A sudden feeling of epigastric or abdominal distension and pain.

[3] *Fei Shi Guai Ji Bing*: Acute epigastric pain or panting due to contraction of weird qi like flying corpse or demons.

Interpretations

The *Zou Ma Tang* (Galloping Horse Decoction) from the *Wai Tai Mi Yao* (Arcane Essentials from the Imperial Library) is indicated for abdominal pain, distension and constipation due to contraction of weird qi.

Zou Ma Tang

[Ingredients]

巴豆	*bā dòu*	2 pieces	Fructus Crotonis (skin/kernel removed)
杏仁	*xìng rén*	2 pieces	Semen Armeniacae Amarum

Wrap the two ingredients in cotton cloth and pound into pieces with a hammer. Place in 0.2 *shēng* of warm water and twist the cloth to squeeze into white juice. Patients may have bowel movements after drinking the decoction. The elderly and children may take a smaller dose. This formula is indicated for acute abdominal pain and constipation due to contraction of weird qi.

*****

[21] 问曰：人病有宿食〔1〕，何以别之？师曰：寸口脉浮而大，按之反涩，尺中亦微而涩〔2〕，故知有宿食。大承气汤主之。

Annotations

[1] *Su Shi*: Food injury or food retention. Food retention in the stomach or intestines may cause abdominal fullness and pain.

[2] *Cun Kou Mai Fu Er Da, An Zhi Fan Se*: A superficial, large and hesitant pulse indicates chronic food retention.

Interpretations

Question: How can we tell one patient has food retention?

Answer: If the pulse is supererficial, large and forceful but hesitant upon heavy pressure at the *Cunkou* positon and faint, hesitant at the *Chi* positon, it indicates chronic food retention and qi stagnation in the stomach and intestines (symptoms may include abdominal distension, fullness and pain or constipation). This should be treated with *Da Cheng Qi Tang* (Major Purgative Decoction) to promote bowel movements.

*****

[22] 脉数而滑者，实也，此有宿食〔1〕。下之愈，宜大承气汤。

Annotations

[1] *Mai Shuo Er Hua Zhe, Shi Ye, Ci You Su Shi*: A rapid, slippery pulse indicates food retention. Previously, a hesitant pulse indicates chronic food retention, and the hesitant pulse is caused by qi blockage of the stomach and intestine. Here a rapid, slippery pulse is caused by acute food retention. Chronic food reetntion needs to be dealt with immediately and therefore should be treated with *Da Cheng Qi Tang* (Major Purgative Decoction). The acute food retention needs to be managed by draining downward, but not necessarily by a harsh-property formula, and therefore it is stated "*Da Cheng Qi Tang* (Major Purgative Decoction) is recommended".

Interpretations

A rapid, slippery pulse indicates stomach excess with food retention (symptoms may include abdominal distension, belching, acid reflux and constipation). *Da Cheng Qi Tang* (Major Purgative Decoction) is recommended to drain downward for this condition. Patients may recover once the retained food is cleared.

*****

[23] 下利〔1〕不饮食〔2〕者，有宿食也，当下之。宜大承气汤。大承气汤方见前痉病中。

Annotations

[1] *Xia Li:* Watery diarrhea in people with retained food in the intestines.

[2] *Bu Yin Shi*: No desire to eat due to food retention. Associated symptoms may include stomach discomfort/stuffiness, a foul breath, and acid reflux.

Interpretations

Water diarrhea and no desire to eat (probably in combination with stomach discomfort/stuffiness, a foul breath and acid reflux) in patients with food retention should be treated with *Da Cheng Qi Tang* (Major Purgative Decoction) to drain downward. For more information about the formula, see chapater 2.

*****

[24] 宿食在上脘，当吐之〔1〕，宜瓜蒂散〔2〕。

瓜蒂散方：瓜蒂一分，熬黄赤小豆一分，煮 右二味，杵为散，以香豉七合煮取汁。和散一钱匕。温服之。不吐者，少加之，以快吐为度而止。亡血及虚者，不可与之。

Annotations

[1] *Su Shi Zai Shang Wan, Dang Tu Zhi*: Retained food in the stomach may cause stomach distension and nausea. This should be treated by inducing vomiting.

[2] *Gua Di San* (Melon Stalk Powder): A formula to induce vomiting.

Interpretations

Retained food in the stomach should be treated with *Gua Di San* (Melon Stalk Powder) to induce vomiting.

Gua Di San

[Ingredients]

瓜蒂	*guā dì*	1 *fēn*	Pedicellus Melo
赤小豆	*chì xiǎo dòu*	1 *fēn*	Semen Phaseoli
香豉	*xiāng chǐ*	0.7 *shēng*	Semen Sojae Praeparatum

Decoct the *Gua Di* and *Chi Xiao Dou* into a powder. Decoct *Xiang Chi* in water and mix the decoction with 1 square inch-spoon powder. Take when it is warm. Slightly increase the dose if patients do not vomit and stop taking it when they vomit. It is contraindicated for patients with blood loss or a weak constitution.

*****

[25] 脉紧如转索无常者〔1〕，有宿食也。

Annotations

[1] *Mai Jin Ru Zhuan Suo Wu Chang Zhe*: A tight pulse like a twisting rope.

Interpretations

A tight, slippery pulse that feels like a twisting rope indicates retained food.

*****

[26] 脉紧，头痛，风寒；腹中有宿食[1]不化也。

Annotations

[1] *Mai Jin...Fu Zhong You Su Shi*: A tight pulse with headache indicates an exterior wind cold syndrome; a tight pulse with watery diarrhea, no desire to eat, and abdominal fullness/pain indicates retained food.

Interpretations

A tight pulse with headache is seen in exterior wind cold syndrome. A tight pulse with abdominal pain and fullness (constipation or watery diarrhea) indicates food retention (it's essential to diagnose by combining pulse and symptoms).

五脏风寒积聚病脉证并治第十一
Chapter 11 Wind-Cold in the Five-Zang Organs and Chronic Stagnation—Pulses, Patterns and Treatment

Overview

This chapter discusses wind-cold attacking the five-zang organs, chronic stagnation (of qi, blood, phlegm, food or water) and critical pulse conditions. The *Jin Gui Yu Han Yao Lüè Shu Yi* (Elaborations on Essentials from the Jade Case Classic of the Golden Cabinet) states, "Wind stroke or cold stroke in this text is different from that in cold damage or stroke with hemiplegia". Unlike external wind or cold attacking meridians, this chapter focuses on wind cold attacking the zang-organs. According to *Gao Zhu Jin Gui Yao Lüè* (Gao's Annotations to 'Essentials of the Golden Cabinet'), "This chapter discusses the varying degrees of wind cold affecting different zang-organs, which are not covered in *Shang Han Lun* (Treatise on Cold Damage)". As problems caused by wind cold affecting the five-zang organs are difficult to be treated, they are discussed together with chronic stagnation and critical pulse conditions related to the five-zang organs. However, this chapter did not include wind stroke of the kidney, cold stroke of the kidney and cold stroke of the spleen.

Chronic stagnation here refers to gradual retention of qi, blood, phlegm, food and water, instead of masses, accumulations or gatherings. The *Jin Gui Yao Lüè Lun Zhu* (Annotated 'Essentials from the Golden Cabinet') mentions, "the word *Ji* does not mean masses or not necessarily tangible retention". The *Jin Gui Yao Lüè Zheng Yi* (Annotations on the 'Essentials from the Golden Cabinet') states, "Over time, coagulated or retained yin cold may form into stagnation...stagnation in the chest like chest-Bi impediment...phlegm-qi stagnation in the throat like globus hystericus...stagnation in the lower abdomen like cold abdominal pain...stagnation in Qichong (ST 30) like painful abdominal masses". This chapter included three conditions due to wind cold affecting the zang-fu organs—liver stagnation (*Gan Zhuo*), spleen deficiency-induced constipation (*Pi Yue*), and kidney stagnation (*Shen Zhuo*).

The critical pulse conditions of the five-zang organs are also known as true zang-organ pulses. The *Su Wen Yu Ji Zhen Zang Lun* (Chapter 19, the Basic Questions) states, "The true zang-organ pulses are life-threatening signs indicative of qi collapse of the zang-organs".

*****

[01] 肺中风〔1〕者，口燥而喘，身运〔2〕而重，冒而肿胀。〔3〕

Annotations

[1] *Fei Zhong Feng*: Wind strike of the lung. Patients may experience panting, dizziness and body swelling. It is similar to pulmonary heart disease, pulmonary and cerebral syndrome or failure of respiratory circulation in modern medicine.

[2] *Shen Yun*: Dizziness.

[3] *Mao Er Zhong Zhang*: Body heaviness and swelling.

Interpretations

Wind strike of the lung may cause a dry mouth, panting, dizziness, blurred vision, and body swelling and heaviness.

*****

[02] 肺中寒〔1〕，吐浊涕〔2〕。

Annotations

[1] *Fei Zhong Han*: Cold strike of the lung. Patients may experience cough with thick, sticky sputum. It is similar to pulmonary abscess or infection secondary to bronchiectasis.

[2] *Tu Zhuo Ti*: Thick, sticky sputum.

Interpretations

Cold strike of the lung may cause coughing with thick, sticky sputum.

*****

[03] 肺死脏〔1〕，浮之虚，按之弱如葱叶下无根者〔2〕，死。

Annotations

[1] *Fei Si Zang*: Critical pulse condition of the lung.

[2] *Fu Zhi Xu, An Zhi Ruo Ru Cong Ye Xia Wu Gen Zhe*: The pulse is deficient with light pressure, but weak like a scallion leaf and rootless with heavy pressure.

Interpretations

The pulse indicating a life-threatening condition of the lung is deficient with gentle pressure and weak like a scallion leaf and rootless with heavy pressure.

*****

[04] 肝中风〔1〕者，头目、两胁痛，行常伛〔2〕，令人嗜甘。

Annotations

[1] *Gan Zhong Feng*: Wind strike of the liver. Patients may experience involuntary head movement, pain in the subcostal region and walking with a hunched posture.

[2] *Xing Chang Yu*: Walking with a hunched posture.

Interpretations

Wind strike of the liver may cause involuntary head movement, pain in the subcostal region, walking with a hunched posture, and a preference for sweet food.

*****

[05] 肝中寒〔1〕者，两臂不举，舌本燥，喜太息〔2〕，胸中痛，不得转侧，食则吐而汗出也。《脉经》、《千金》云：时盗汗，咳，食已吐其汁。

Annotations

[1] *Gan Zhong Han*: Cold strike of the liver. Patients may experience difficulty raising arms, a dry mouth and tongue, sighing, pain in the subcostal region with an inability to turn over in bed, and vomiting after eating food.

[2] *Shan Tai Xi*: Sighing (long, deep breath).

Interpretations

Cold strike of the liver may cause difficulty raising arms, a dry mouth and tongue, frequent sighing, pain in the subcostal region with an inability to turn over in bed, and vomiting with sweating after eating food. The *Mai Jing* (the Pulse Classic) and *Qian Jin Fang* (Important Formulas Worth a Thousand Gold Pieces) state,

"(Cold strike of the liver) may cause frequent night sweats, cough and vomiting up watery vomitus after eating food".

*****

[06] 肝死脏〔1〕，浮之弱，按之如索不来，或曲如蛇行〔2〕者，死。

Annotations

[1] *Gan Si Zang*: Critical pulse condition of the liver.

[2] *Fu Zhi Ruo, An Zhi Ruo Ru Suo Bu Lai, Huo Qu Ru She Xing*: The pulse is weak with light pressure, but ropy, intermittent or sinuous like a snake moving with heavy pressure. In modern medicine, it indicates cardiac arrhythmias and is often seen in atrial or ventricular premature heart beats.

Interpretations

The pulse indicating a life-threatening condition of the liver is weak with light pressure and ropy, intermittent or sinuous like a snake moving with heavy pressure (indicating absence of stomach qi and collapse of liver qi).

*****

[07] 肝着〔1〕，其人常欲蹈其胸上〔2〕，先未苦时，但欲饮热〔3〕，旋复花汤〔4〕主之。

Annotations

[1] *Gan Zhuo*: Stagnation of liver qi and blood. Patients may experience tightness and discomfort in the subcostal region.

[2] *Chang Yu Dao Qi Xiong Shang*: Frequently pounding the chest with hands to alleviate chest tightness and discomfort.

[3] *Xian Wei Ku Shi, Dan Yu Yin Re*: Preference for hot water before appearance of chest tightness or discomfort.

[4] *Xuan Fu Hua Tang* (Inula Decoction): A formula to move qi, circulate blood, unblock yang, and resolve masses. For more information about this formula, see chapter 22. This formula can also be used to treat miscarriage and slight but persistent uterine bleeding.

Interpretations

Patients with liver stagnation frequently pound the chest with hands to alleviate chest tightness. They prefer to drink hot water before the appearance of chest discomfort. Liver stagnation can be treated with *Xuan Fu Hua Tang* (Inula Decoction).

*****

[08] 心中风[1]者，翕翕发热[2]，不能起，心中饥[3]，食即呕吐。

Annotations

[1] *Xin Zhong Feng*: Wind strike of the heart (stomach). Patients may experience fever, upset stomach and vomiting after eating food. It is similar to acute gastritis in modern medicine.

[2] *Xi Xi Fa Re*: High-grade fever.

[3] *Xin Zhong Ji*: Hunger in the stomach, i.e., fast hunger due to stomach heat.

Interpretations

Wind strike of the heart (stomach) may cause a high-grade fever, an inability to get out of bed, upset stomach, hunger and vomiting after eating food.

*****

[09] 心中寒〔1〕者，其人苦病，心如啖蒜状〔2〕。剧者心痛彻背，背痛彻心，譬如蛊注〔3〕。其脉浮〔4〕者，自吐乃愈。

Annotations

[1] *Xin Zhong Han*: Cold strike of the heart (stomach). Patients may experience heartburn and stomach pain.

[2] *Ku Bing Xin Dan Suan Zhuang*: Heartburn like from eating garlic.

[3] *Gu Zhu*: Abdominal pain caused by parasitic roundworms. It is similar to biliary ascariasis in modern medicine.

[4] *Mai Fu*: A superficial pulse. Here it indicates that cold retained in the heart (stomach).

Interpretations

Cold strike of the heart (stomach) may cause heartburn like from eating garlic and intense pain in the chest and back as if there were parasitic roundworms in the abdomen. If the pulse is superficial (cold retained in the heart/stomach), the abdominal pain alleviates after vomiting.

*****

[10] 心伤〔1〕者，其人劳倦，即头面赤而下重，心中痛而自烦，发热，当脐跳〔2〕，其脉弦，此为心藏伤所致也。

Annotations

[1] *Xin Shang*: Damage to the heart by excessive fatigue. Patients may experience a burning sensation and pain in the chest, facial redness and leg heaviness.

[2] *Qi Tiao*: A subjective throbbing sensation around the umbilicus. It is similar to pulsation of the abdominal aorta.

Interpretations

Damage to the heart by excessive fatigue may cause facial redness, leg heaviness, pain and a burning sensation in the chest, and throbbing around the umbilicus. A wiry pulse is caused by damage to the heart.

*****

[11] 心死脏[1]，浮之实如麻豆，按之益躁疾者[2]，死。

Annotations

[1] *Xin Si Zang*: Critical pulse condition of the heart.

[2] *Fu Zhi Shi Ru Ma Dou, An Zhi Yi Zao Ji Zhe*: The pulse is as solid as a soybean with light pressure, but rapid and abrupt with heavy pressure (similar to atrial fibrillation in modern medicine).

Interpretations

The pulse indicating a life-threatening condition of the heart is solid like a soybean with light pressure and rapid and abrupt with heavy pressure (indicating collapse of heart qi).

*****

[12] 邪哭[1]使魂魄不安者，血气少也。血气少者属于心[2]，心气虚者，其人则畏，目欲眠，梦远行而精神离散，魂魄妄行[3]。阴气衰者为癫，阳气衰者为狂[4]。

Annotations

[1] *Xie Ku*: Unexplained crying spells.

[2] *Xue Qi Shao Zhe Shu Yu Xin*: Deficiency of qi and blood in the heart (brain). It is similar to insufficient blood supply to the brain in modern medicine.

[3] *Hun Po Wang Xing*: Mental disorder with frenetic, impulsive behaviors.

[4] *Yin Qi Shuai Zhe Wei Dian, Yang Qi Shuai Zhe Wei Kuang*: Depletion of yin qi results in depression, whereas depletion of yang qi results in mania. The "yin" and "yang" here refer to blood and qi. In addition to depression and mania, *Dian Kuang* in Chinese medicine also covers dementia or schizophrenia.

Interpretations

Unexplained crying spells that disturb the mind are often caused by deficiency of qi and blood. Deficiency of qi and blood is most closely associated with the heart (brain). Patients with deficiency of heart qi and blood may experience fear. When they close their eyes and try to sleep, they dream of traveling far away. They may develop mental disorder with frenetic behaviors. In addition, yin qi depletion may cause depression, whereas yang qi depletion may cause mania.

*****

[13] 脾中风〔1〕者，翕翕发热，形如醉人，腹中烦重〔2〕，皮目〔3〕瞤而短气。〔4〕

Annotations

[1] *Pi Zhong Feng*: Wind strike of the spleen. Patients may experience fever, abdominal fullness and heaviness.

[2] *Fu Zhong Fan Zhong*: Abdominal fullness and heaviness.

[3] *Pi Mu*: It literally means skin and eyes. The *Mai Jing* (the Pulse Classic) and *Qian Jin Fang* (Important Formulas Worth a Thousand Gold Pieces) record *Pi Rou* (skin and muscles).

[4] *Duan Qi*: Shortness of breath.

Interpretations

Wind strike of the spleen may cause a high-grade fever and facial redness that resembles flushing from drinking alcohol, along with abdominal distension, fullness and heaviness, twitching of the skin and muscles and shortness of breath.

*****

[14] 脾死脏〔1〕，浮之大坚，按之如覆杯洁洁，状如摇〔2〕者，死。臣亿等详五脏各有中风、中寒，今脾只载中风，肾中风、中寒俱不载者，以古文简乱极多，去古既远，无文可以补缀也。

Annotations

[1] *Pi Si Zang*: Critical pulse condition of the spleen.

[2] *Fu Zhi Da Jian, An Zhi Ru Fu Bei Jie Jie, Zhuang Ru Yao*: The pulse is large and solid with light pressure, but like an inverted, empty and shaking cup with heavy pressure.

Interpretations

The pulse indicating a life-threatening condition of the spleen is large and solid with light pressure, and like an inverted, empty and shaking cup. Chen Yi et al believes that the contents regarding wind-cold strike of the five-zang organs are incomplete, because there is no cold strike of the spleen or wind/cold strike of the kidney.

*****

[15] 趺阳脉浮而涩，浮则胃气强，涩则小便数，浮相抟，大便则坚〔1〕，其脾为约〔2〕，麻子仁丸〔3〕主之。

麻子仁丸方：麻子仁二升 芍药半斤 枳实一斤 大黄一斤 厚朴一尺 杏仁一升 右六味，末之，炼蜜和丸，梧子大。饮服十丸，日三。以知为度。

Annotations

[1] *Fu Ze Wei Qi Qiang, Se Ze Xiao Bian Shuo…Da Bian Ze Jian*: A superficial pulse felt at Chongyang (ST 42) indicates stomach heat and excess stomach qi. A hesitant pulse is caused by insufficiency of spleen yin due to frequent urination. As a result, yin fluids fail to moisten the intestines and cause hard stools.

[2] *Qi Pi Wei Yue*: Difficulty passing (hard) stools due to insufficiency of spleen yin.

[3] *Ma Zi Ren Wan* (Cannabis Fruit Pill): A formula to nourish yin, moisten dryness, clear heat and promote bowel movements.

Interpretations

When the pulse felt at Chongyang (ST 42) is superficial and hesitant—the superficial pulse indicates stomach heat and excess stomach qi, whereas the hesitant pulse indicates frequent urination (due to insufficient spleen yin). With excess stomach qi and insufficient spleen yin, patients may experience difficulty passing stools. This is called spleen deficiency-induced constipation and can be treated with *Ma Zi Ren Wan* (Cannabis Fruit Pill).

Ma Zi Ren Wan

[Ingredients]

麻仁	*má rén*	2 *shēng*	Fructus Cannabis
芍药	*sháo yào*	0.5 *jīn*	Radix Paeoniae
枳实	*zhǐ shí*	1 *jīn*	Fructus Aurantii Immaturus (fried)
大黄	*dà huáng*	1 *jīn*	Radix et Rhizoma Rhei (skin removed)
厚朴	*hòu pò*	1 *chǐ* (23cm)	Cortex Magnoliae Officinalis (fried and skin removed)
杏仁	*xìng rén*	1 *shēng*	Semen Armeniacae Amarum (tip and skin removed, boiled)

Grind the six ingredients into a powder and blend with processed honey to make into pills the size of firmiana seeds. Take ten pills for each dose, 3 doses a day. The dose can be gradually increased until the efficacy is established.

*****

[16] 肾着〔1〕之病，其人身体重〔2〕，腰中冷，如坐水中，形如水状，反不渴，小便自利，饮食如故〔3〕，病属下焦。身劳汗出，衣一作表里冷湿，久久得之，腰以下冷痛，腹重〔4〕如带五千钱。甘姜苓术汤〔5〕主之。

甘草干姜茯苓白术汤方：

甘草白术各二两干姜茯苓各四两　　右四味，以水五升，煮取三升。分温三服。腰中即温。

Annotations

[1] *Shen Zhuo*: Kidney stagnation characterized by cold, pain and heaviness in the lower back due to retained cold and dampness.

[2] *Shen Ti Zhong*: Heaviness in the low back.

[3] *Xiao Bian Zi Li, Yin Shi Ru Gu*: Normal urination (indicating there is no water-damp retention) and normal appetite (indicating normual functioning of the spleen and stomach).

[4] *Fu Zhong*: Here it means low back (instead of abdomen) heaviness.

[5] *Gan Jiang Ling Zhu Tang* (Licorice, Dried Ginger, Poria and Atractylodes Macrocephala Decoction): A formula to warm meridians, dissipate cold, strengthen the spleen and resolve dampness. The *Jin Gui Yu Han Yao lüè Fang Lun Shi Yi* (Explanations of Formulas from 'Essentials from the Golden Cabinet') states, "This is a modified formula of *Li Zhong Tang* (Middle Jiao-Regulating Decoction) by removing *Ren Sheng* (Radix et Rhizoma Ginseng) and adding *Fu Ling* (Poria), *Ren Shen* is removed because the problem is located in the lower jiao. In the modified formula, instead of using ingredients for the kidney, *Fu Ling* (Poria) and *Bai Zhu* (Rhizoma Atractylodis Macrocephalae) are used to drain dampness, *Gan Cao* (Radix et Rhizoma Glycyrrhizae) and *Gan*

Jiang (Rhizoma Zingiberis) to warm meridians and dissipate cold, since kidney stagnation does not mean that cold or damp actually retain in the kidney."

Interpretations

Patients with kidney stagnation may experience heaviness and a cold sensation below the low back. The heaviness appears like water-damp retention, the cold sensation feels as if sitting in water. However, patients do not feel thirsty and have normal urination and appetite. The problem is located in the lower *jiao*. It gradually develops from cold, wet clothes upon sweating from physical labor. Patients complain of cold, pain and heaviness in the low back. The heaviness feels as if carrying five thousand coins. This condition can be treated with *Gan Jiang Ling Zhu Tang* (Licorice, Dried Ginger, Poria and Atractylodes Macrocephala Decoction).

Gan Cao Gan Jiang Fu Ling Bai Zhu Tang

[Ingredients]

甘草	*gān cǎo*	2 *liǎng*	Radix et Rhizoma Glycyrrhizae
白术	*bái zhú*	2 *liǎng*	Rhizoma Atractylodis Macrocephalae
干姜	*gān jiāng*	4 *liǎng*	Rhizoma Zingiberis
茯苓	*fú líng*	4 *liǎng*	Poria

Decoct the four ingredients in 5 *shēng* of water to get 3 *shēng*. Take when it is warm in three times, and patients can feel warm in the low back immediately.

*****

[17] 肾死脏〔1〕，浮之坚，按之乱如转丸，益下入尺中〔2〕者，死。

Annotations

[1] *Shen Si Zang*: Critical pulse condition of the kidney.

[2] *Fu Zhi Jian, An Zhi Luan Ru Zhuan Wan, Yi Xia Ru Chi Zhong*: The pulse is solid with light pressure, but chaotic like spinning pellets with heavy pressure; and the rapid, chaotic feeling extends to the *Chi* position.

Interpretations

The pulse indicating a life-threatening condition of the spleen is solid with light pressure, but chaotic like spinning pellets, and the rapid chaotic feeling extends to the *Chi* position (indicating depletion of kidney qi).

*****

[18] 问曰：三焦竭[1]部，上焦竭，善噫[2]，何谓也？师曰：上焦受中焦气未和，不能消谷[3]，故能噫耳。下焦竭，即遗溺失便[4]，其气不和，不能自禁制，不须治[5]，久则愈。

Annotations

[1] *San Jiao Jie*: Functional failure of the upper, middle and lower *jiao*.

[2] *Ai*: Belching. It occurs as a result of upward flow of stomach qi and is often seen after eating food.

[3] *Xiao Gu*: Digestion.

[4] *Yi Ni Shi Bian*: Bowel and bladder incontinence.

[5] *Bu Xu Zhi*: It's not necessary to treat the upper and lower jiao, but focus on the middle jiao.

Interpretations

Question: Speaking of functional failure of the upper, middle and lower jiao, patients with functional failure of the upper jiao often present with belching. Why is that?

Answer: The upper jiao is affected by the middle jiao. Belching occurs when stomach qi becomes disharmonized and fails to digest food. Functional failure of the lower jiao may cause bladder and bowel incontinence due to failure of stomach qi to control bladder and bowel movements. As a result, it's not necessary to treat the upper and lower jiao, but focus on the middle jiao, and these symptoms may gradually disappear.

*****

[19] 师曰：热在上焦者，因咳为肺痿；热在中焦者，则为坚〔1〕；热在下焦者，则尿血，亦令淋秘不通〔2〕。大肠有寒者，多鹜溏；有热者，便肠垢。小肠有寒〔3〕者，其人下重便血；有热者，必痔。

Annotations

[1] *Jian*: Hard stools.

[2] *Lin Mi Bu Tong*: Dribbing, hesitant and painful urination, and urine retention.

[3] *Da Chang You Han...Xiao Chang You Han*: According to the *Jin Gui Yao Lüè Shu Yi* (Explanations on 'Essentials from the Golden Cabinet'), "The position of the small intestine should be replaced with the large intestine, and vice versa".

Interpretations

The Master said, "Heat retained in the upper jiao (lung) may cause cough and, over time, lung decline. Heat retained in the middle jiao (stomach) may cause hard stools (over time, spleen deficiency-induced constipation). Heat retained in the lower jiao may cause bloody urine. Alternatively, it may also cause dribbling, hesitant urination or urine retention. Cold retained in the small intestine may cause loose stools like duck droppings. Heat retained in the small intestine may cause mucus in stool. Cold retained in the large intestine may cause rectal prolapse and bloody stools. Heat retained in the large intestine may cause hemorrhoids.

*****

[20] 问曰：病有积，有聚，有谷气〔1〕，何谓也？师曰：积者，藏病也，终不移〔2〕。聚者，府病也，发作有时，展转痛移〔3〕，为可治。谷气者，胁下痛，按之则愈，复发为谷气〔4〕。诸积大法，脉　来细而附骨〔5〕者，乃积也。寸口，积在胸中；微出寸口，积在喉中。关上，积在脐傍；上关上，积在心下；微下关，积在少腹。尺中，积在气冲〔6〕。脉出左，积在左；脉出右，积在右。脉两出，积在中央。各以其部处之。

Annotations

[1] *Bing Yu Ji, You Ju, You Gu Qi*: Three causative factors of abdominal pain—*Ji* (immobile masses), *Ju* (mobile masses) and *Gu Qi* (stagnation of spleen/stomach qi). The *Ji* is chronic and associated with the zang-organs (long in duration, deep in location and more severe). The *Ju* is temporary and associated with the fu-organs (short in duration, shallow in location and less severe). The *Gu Qi* refers to pain in subcostal region due to qi stagnation of the spleen and stomach.

[2] *Zhong Bu Yi*: A distinctive feature of *Ji*—persistent abdominal pain with a fixed location.

[3] *Fa Zuo You Shi, Zhan Zhuan Tong Yi*: A distinctive feature of *Ju*—parayxosmal, miagratory abdominal pain (without a fixed location).

[4] *An Zhi Ze Yu, Fu Fa Wei Gu Qi*: Abdominal pain alleviates with pressure and comes back when the pressure is released. This is caused by qi stagnation of the spleen and stomach.

[5] *Mai Lai Xi Er Fu Gu*: A thready, small, deep and hidden pulse.

[6] *Qi Chong*: A stomach meridian point ST 30 (location: 2 cun lateral to the median line of the abdomen in the upper inguinal region, medial to the common iliac artery). Here it refers the bilateral, lower abdomen.

Interpretations

Question: Abdominal pain can be caused by three factors—*Ji* (immobile masses), *Ju* (mobile masses) and *Gu Qi* (qi stagnation of the spleen and stomach). How do you differentiate one from another?

Answer: *Ji* (immobile masses) is associated with the zang-organs and causes persistent abdominal pain with a fixed location. *Ju* (mobile masses) is associated with the fu-organs and causes parayxosmal abdominal pain without a fixed location. This type of abdominal pain is easy to manage. Bilateral lower abdominal pain due to *Gu Qi* (qi stagnation of the spleen and stomach) alleviates with pressure and returns when the pressure is released.

A thready, small, deep and hidden pulse often indicates *Ji* (immobile masses). Specific locations of *Ji* (immobile masses) can be determined according to the postion of the pulse. Feeling at the *Cun* position means it affects the chest, feeling above the *Cun* position means it affects the throat, feeling at the *Guan* position means it affects the peri-umbilical area, feeling above the *Guan* position means it affects the area below the heart, feeling slightly below the *Guan* position means it affects the lower abdomen, feeling at the *Chi* position means it affects the area below the lower abdomen—left *Chi* position indicates the left side, right *Chi* position indicates the right side, and both left and right *Chi* positions indicates the middle area.

痰饮咳嗽病脉证并治第十二
Chapter 12 Phlegm-Fluid Retention and Coughing—Pulses, Patterns and Treatment

Overview

This chapter discusses phlegm-fluid retention and one of its symptoms—cough. Cough due to other causes is not included in this chapter. The phlegm-fluid is known as *Tan Yin* in Chinese or *Dan Yin* in the *Mai Jing* (The Pulse Classic), which literally means water moving. The *Jin Gui Jiang Yi* (Explanatory Notes to 'Essentials from the Golden Cabinet') states, "Zhang Zhongjing had a reason to choose the word *Yin*: the liquid to ingest into the body is called water, whereas liquid that retains in the body is called fluid retention". As a result, phlegm-fluid is also known as water-fluid. Phlegm-fluid or water-fluid may retain in the intestines, subcostal regions, four limbs, below the heart, the lung, or the spleen. The difference between phlegm-fluid and water-qi is that the former retains in specific body parts and the latter reaches all over the body.

*****

[01] 问曰：夫饮有四〔1〕，何谓也？师曰：有痰饮〔2〕，有悬饮〔3〕，有溢饮〔4〕，有支饮〔5〕。

[02] 问曰：四饮何以为异？师曰：其人素盛今瘦，水走肠间，沥沥有声，谓之痰饮；饮后水流在胁下，咳唾引痛，谓之悬饮；饮水流行，归于四肢，当汗出而不汗出，身体疼重，谓之溢饮；咳逆倚息，短气不得卧，其形如肿，谓之支饮。

Annotations

[1] *Fu Yin You Si:* There are four types of phlegm-fluid: *Tan Yin* (water-fluid retention in the intestines), *Xuan Yin* (water-fluid retention in the subcostal region), *Yi Yin* (water-fluid retention over the surface of the body) and *Zhi Yin* (water-fluid retention in the lung).

[2] *Tan Yin:* Literally means phlegm-fluid. In a broad sense, it refers to disorders caused by retained phlegm and fluid. In a narrow sense, it specifically refers to water-fluid retention in the intestines caused by dysfunctions of the lung, spleen and kidney. It is mainly characterized by weight loss and gurgling bowel sounds (similar to shifting dullness in ascites in modern medicine).

[3] *Xuan Yin*: Literally means suspended fluid, referring to water-fluid retention in the subcostal region. It is mainly characterized by cough with sputum and cough-induced pain in the subcostal region.

[4] *Yi Yin*: Literally means overflow fluid, referring to water-fluid retention affecting the surface of the body. It is mainly characterized by body ache and absence of sweating.

[5] *Zhi Yin*: Throacic fluid retention, referring to water-fluid retention in the heart and lung. It is mainly characterized by cough, panting, shortness of breath with an inability to lie flat and generalized swelling.

Interpretations

Question: What are the four types of phlegm-fluid?

Answer: *Tan Yin* (phlegm fluid retention), *Xuan Yin* (suspended fluid retention), *Yi Yin* (overflow fluid retention) and *Zhi Yin* (thoracic fluid retention).

Question: How can we differentiate one from another?

Anwer: When a previously healthy and strong person experience weight loss and gurgling bowel sounds due to water fluid running in the intestines, this is called *Tan Yin* (phlegm fluid retention). When water fluid flows to the subcostal region and causes cough with sputum and cough-induced pain in the subcostal region, this is called *Xuan Yin* (suspended fluid retention). When water fluid flows over the four limbs and causes absence of sweating, body ache and heaviness, this is called *Yi Yin* (overflow fluid retention). When water fluid causes cough, panting, shortness of breath with an inability to lie flat and generalized swelling, this is called *Zhi Yin* (thoracic fluid retention).

*****

[03] 水在心〔1〕，心下坚筑〔2〕，短气，恶水不欲饮。
[04] 水在肺〔3〕，吐涎沫，欲饮水。
[05] 水在脾〔4〕，少气身重。
[06] 水在肝〔5〕，胁下支满，嚏而痛〔6〕。
[07] 水在肾〔7〕，心下悸。〔8〕

Annotations

[1] *Shui Zai Xin:* Water-fluid affecting the heart, i.e., *Tan Yin* (phlegm fluid retention).

[2] *Xin Xia Jian Zhu:* Hardness below the heart.

[3] *Shui Zai Fei*: Water-fluid affecting the lung, i.e., *Zhi Yin* (thoracic fluid retention).

[4] *Shui Zai Pi*: Water-fluid affecting the spleen, i.e, *Yi Yin* (overflow fluid retention).

[5] *Shui Zai Gan*: Water-fluid affecting the liver, i.e., *Xuan Yin* (suspended fluid retention).

[6] *Ti Er Tong*: Cough-induced pain in the subcostal region.

[7] *Shui Zai Shen*: Water-fluid affecting the kidney.

[8] *Xin Xia Ji*: Literally means palpitations; however, it should be a wrong spelling of rapid pulsations below the umbilicus.

Interpretations

Water fluid in the heart may cause hardness below the heart, shortness of breath and no desire to drink water. Water fluid in the lung may cause cough with thin sputum and thirst with a desire to drink water. Water fluid in the spleen may cause lassitude, body heaviness and edema. Water fluid in the liver may cause distension, fullness and cough-induced pain in the subcostal region. Water fluid in the kidney may cause rapid pulsations below the umbilicus.

*****

[08] 夫心下有留饮[1]，其人背寒冷如手大。

[09] 留饮者，胁下痛引缺盆[2]，咳嗽则辄已[3]一作转甚。

[10] 胸中有留饮，其人短气而渴，四肢历节痛。脉沉[4]者，有留饮。

Annotations

[1] *Liu Yin:* Retained water fluid, indicating an early stage of phlegm fluid.

[2] *Que Pen*: A body part in Chinese medicine located in the middle of the superior border of the clavicle.

[3] *Ke Sou Ze Zhe Yi*: The pain alleviates on coughing.

[4] *Mai Chen*: A deep pulse, indicating interior and water retention.

Interpretations

Patients with retained water fluid below the heart may experience a cold sensation on a palm-sized (corresponding) area on the back. Retained water fluid may cause pain in the subcostal region that radiates to the supraclavical fossa and alleviates (aggravates in other texts) on coughing. Retained water fluid in the chest may cause shortness of breath, thrist, and joint pain. A deep pulse often indicates retained water fluid.

*****

[11] 膈上[1]病痰，满喘咳吐。发则寒热，背痛腰疼，目泣自出[2]，其人振振身瞤剧[3]，必有伏饮。[4]

Annotations

[1] *Ge Shang:* Literally means above the diaphragm, referring to the chest.

[2] *Mu Qi Zi Chu*: Watery eyes due to severe cough. The *Mai Jing* (The Pulse Classic) mentions "blurred vision" instead of watery eyes.

[3] *Zhen Zhen Shen Shun Ju*: Raising of the shoulders and twitching of the body due to severe dyspnea.

[4] *Fu Yin*: Prolonged, deep-lying fluid retention, similar to asthematic bronchitis or bronchial asthma in modern medicine.

Interpretations

Retained phlegm fluid in the chest may cause chest fullness, panting, and cough with sputum. During acute attacks, patients may experience fever, chills, backache, watery eyes due to severe cough and raised shoulders with twitching of the entire body due to severe dyspnea. This is an episode of prolonged, deep-lying fluid retention.

*****

[12] 夫病人饮水多，必暴喘满〔1〕。凡食少饮多，水停心下。甚者则悸，微者短气〔2〕。脉双弦者寒也，皆大下后虚；脉偏弦者饮也〔3〕。

Annotations

[1] *Bing Ren Yin Shui Duo, Bi Bao Chuan Man:* Drinking too much water in a short period of time may cause fluid retention with panting and chest fullness. It is similar to pulmonary edema in modern medicine.

[2] *Shi Shao Yin Duo, Shui Ting Xin Xia. Shen Zhe Ze Ji, Wei Zhe Duan Qi*: Eat a small amount of food due to spleen/stomach weakness but drink a large amount of water may impair the transportation and transformation, resulting in fluid retention below the heart. In severe cases, retained fluid may affect the heart and cause palpitations. In mild

cases, retained fluid may obstruct the flow of qi and cause shortness of breath.

[3] *Mai Shuan Xian Zhe Han Ye ... Mai Pian Xian Zhe Yin Ye*: A wiry pulse on both hands indicates deficiency cold, whereas a wiry pulse on one side indicates fluid retention (in the subcostal region).

Interpretations

Drinking too much water in a short period of time may cause sudden rapid breathing and chest fullness or tightess. Eat a small amount of food (due to weakness of the spleen and stomach) plus too much water drinking may cause retained fluid below the heart. In severe cases, palpitations may be present; in mild cases, shortness of breath may be present. A wiry pulse on both hands indicates general deficiency cold due to aggressive use of purgative method. A wiry pulse on onse side indicates retained fluid (in the subcostal region).

*****

[13] 肺饮〔1〕不弦，但苦喘短气。

[14] 支饮亦喘而不能卧，加短气，其脉平也〔2〕。

Annotations

[1] *Fei Yin:* Water fluid affecting the lung.

[2] *Mai Ping*: Literally means a normal pulse; however, it is not the case here. It merely means the pulse is not wiry.

Interpretations

Water fluid affecting the lung may not cause a wiry pulse. Patients may experience severe paning and shortness of breath. Water fluid in the subcostal region may also cause panting, an inability to lie flat, shortness of breath, and a similar pulse in other types of water fluid.

*****

[15] 病痰饮者，当以温药[1]和之。

Annotations

[1] *Wen Yao:* Warm-property medicinals to activate yang qi to transport and resolve water-fluid (not to tonify or reinforce).

Interpretations

Phlegm-fluid should be treated with yang-warming medicinals to resolve fluid retention and promote urination.

*****

[16] 心下有痰饮[1]，胸胁支满，目眩，苓桂术甘汤[2]主之。

茯苓桂枝白术甘草汤方：

茯苓四两桂枝白术各三两甘草二两 右四味，以水六升，煮取三升。分温三服。小便则利。

Annotations

[1] *Xin Xia You Tan Yin*: Water-fluid below the heart. The *Jin Gui Yu Han Yao Lüè Shu Yi* (Elaborations on Essentials from the Jade Case Classic of the Golden Cabinet) states, "Stagnant phlegm-fluid causes fullness in the subcostal region, which in turn obstructs the ascending of clear yang and results in blurred vision".

[2] *Ling Gui Zhu Gan Tang* (Poria, Cinnamon Twig, Atractylodes Macrocephala and Licorice Decoction): A formula to warm yang, resolve fluid retention, fortify the spleen and promote urination. It is indicated for phlegm-fluid (in a narrow sense).

Interpretations

Retained water-fluid below the heart may cause distension and fullness in the subcostal region, dizziness and blurred vision (possibly in combination with shortness of breath and dysuria). This can be treated with *Ling Gui Zhu Gan Tang* (Poria, Cinnamon Twig, Atractylodes Macrocephala and Licorice Decoction).

Ling Gui Zhu Gan Tang

[Ingredients]

Monarch	茯苓	*fú líng*	4 *liǎng*	Poria
Minister	桂枝	*guì zhī*	3 *liǎng*	Ramulus Cinnamomi
Assistant	白术	*bái zhú*	3 *liǎng*	Rhizoma Atractylodis Macrocephalae
Guide	甘草	*gān cǎo*	2 *liǎng*	Radix et Rhizoma Glycyrrhizae

Decoct the four ingredients in 6 *shēng* of water to get 3*shēng*. Remove the dregs and take when it is warm in three times, and patients can have normal urination afterwards.

*****

[17] 夫短气有微饮〔1〕，当从小便去之，苓桂术甘汤主之方见上。肾气丸亦主之。方见脚气中〔2〕。

Annotations

[1] *Wei Yin*: Mild phlegm fluid or remissive stage of phlegm fluid.

[2] For detailed information of *Shen Qi Wan* (Kidney Qi Pill), see *Cai Shi Ba Wei Wan* (Cui's Eight Ingredient Pill) in chapter 5 or *Shen Qi Wan* (Kidney Qi Pill) in chapter 22.

Interpretations

The treatment strategy for mild phlegm-fluid with shortness of breath (and dysuria) is to promote urination; however, it's essential to differentiate whether it's associated with the kidney or the spleen. Phlegm-fluid associated with the spleen can be treated with *Ling Gui Zhu Gan Tang* (Poria, Cinnamon Twig, Atractylodes Macrocephala and Licorice Decoction) and phlegm-fluid associated with the kidney can be treated with *Shen Qi Wan* (Kidney Qi Pill) (see chapter 22).

*****

[18] 病者脉伏〔1〕，其人欲自利，利反快，虽利，心下续坚满，此为留饮欲去故也，甘遂半夏汤〔3〕主之。

甘遂半夏汤方：

甘遂大者三枚半夏十二枚，以水一升，煮取半升，去滓。芍药五枚甘草如指大，一枚，炙，一本作无。右四味，以水二升，煮取半升，去滓，以蜜半升，和药汁，煎取八合。顿服之。

Annotations

[1] *Mai Fu:* A severe deep pulse.

[2] *Gan Sui Ban Xia Tang* (Kansui and Pinellia Decoction): A formula to break masses and resolve water retention.

Interpretations

Patients with a deep pulse (with hardness, distension and fullness below the heart and dysuria) may experience spontaneous diarrhea. Abdominal fullness slightly alleviates after diarrhea, because the retained water fluid was discharged along with the bowel movements. However, hardness and fullness below the heart may remain and can be treated with *Gan Sui Ban Xia Tang* (Kansui and Pinellia Decoction).

Gan Sui Ban Xia Tang

[Ingredients]

Monarch	甘遂	*gān suì*	3 pieces	Radix Kansui (it is harsh and toxic, and therefore only used for patient with a strong body).
Minister	半夏	*bàn xià*	12 pieces	Rhizoma Pinelliae
Assistant	芍药	*sháo yào*	5 pieces	Radix Paeoniae
Guide	甘草	*gān cǎo*	1 piece	Radix et Rhizoma Glycyrrhizae (fried) (not included in other texts).

Decoct the four ingredients in 2 *shēng* of water to get 0.5 *shēng*. Remove the dregs and mix with 0.5 *shēng* of honey and decoct to get 0.8 *shēng*. Drink up the decoction at a draught.

*****

[19] 脉浮而细滑，伤饮[1]。
[20] 脉弦数，有寒饮[2]，冬夏难治。

Annotations

[1] *Mai Fu Er Xi Hua, Shang Yin*: A superficial, thready and slippery pulse indicates damage by external fluids. Patients with water fluid often have a deep pulse.

[2] *Mai Xian Shuo, You Han Yin*: A wiry, rapid pulse with cold fluid (the pulse does not match with the syndrome) is hard to treat in winter

or summer. According to the *Jin Gui Yu Han Jing Er Zhu* (Supplementary Annotations to 'The Jade Case Classic of the Golden Cabinet'), "In summer, warm-property medicinals to resolve fluid may aggravate the rapid pulse. In winter, cold-property medicinals to clear heat may aggravate the cold fluid. That's why it is hard to treat in winter and summer".

Interpretations

A superficial, thready and slippery pulse can be seen in sudden damage by external fluid. A wiry, rapid pulse with retained cold fluid (inconsistency between the pulse and syndrome) is hard to treat in winter or summer.

*****

[21] 脉沉而弦者，悬饮内痛〔1〕。

[22] 病悬饮者，十枣汤〔2〕主之。

十枣汤方：

芫花熬 甘遂大戟各等分 右三味，捣筛，以水一升五合，先煮肥大枣十枚，取八合，去滓，内药末。强人服一钱匕，羸人服半钱，平旦温服之〔3〕。不下者，明日更加半钱，得快下后，糜粥自养。

Annotations

[1] *Mai Chen Er Xian Zhe, Xuan Yin Nei Tong*: A deep, wiry pulse indicates suspended fluid and pain. A deep pulse suggests fluid retention and a wiry pulse suggests pain.

[2] *Shi Zao Tang* (Ten Jujubes Decoction): A formula to dispel water retention. It consists of three ingredients to aggressively resolve water retention: *Yuan Hua* (Flos Genkwa), *Gan Sui* (Radix Kansui) and *Da Ji* (Radix Euphorbiae Pekinensis) and uses 10 jujubes as the monarch ingredient. As harsh-property ingredients may damage healthy qi, the jujubes also act to regulate the spleen and stomach and moderate the toxicity of the other ingredients.

[3] *Ping Dan Wen Fu Zhi*: Take the decoction between 4 and 5 am.

Interpretations

A deep, wiry pulse indicates fluid retention in the subcostal region, along with referred pain. Patients with this condition should be treated with *Shi Zao Tang* (Ten Jujubes Decoction).

Shi Zao Tang

[Ingredients]

大枣	*dà zǎo*	Fructus Jujubae (10 pieces)
芫花	*yuán huā*	Flos Genkwa (boiled)
大戟	*dà jǐ*	Radix Euphorbiae Pekinensis
甘遂	*gān suì*	Radix Kansui

Grind equal amounts of *Yuan Huan*, *Da Ji* and *Gan Sui* into a fine powder. Frist decoct 10 jujubes in 1.5 *shēng* of water to get 0.8 *shēng*. Remove the dregs and mix with the powder. Patients with a strong body take one square inch-spoon (approximately 2g), and patients who are thin and weak take half the dose. Take it warm between 4 and 5 am. If patients have no bowel movements the next day, increase the dose by half a spoon. Patients can take congree after bowel movements.

*****

[23] 病溢饮者，当发其汗〔1〕，大青龙汤〔2〕主之，小青龙汤〔3〕亦主之。

大青龙汤方：

麻黄六两，去节桂枝二两，去皮 甘草二两，炙 杏仁四十个，去皮、尖 生姜三两大枣十二枚石膏如鸡子大碎 右七味，以水九升，先煮麻黄，减二升，去上沫，内诸药，煮取三升，去滓。温服一升，取微似汗。汗多者，温粉粉之〔4〕。

小青龙汤方：

麻黄三两，去节芍药三两 五味子半升干姜三两甘草三两，炙细辛三两桂枝三两，去皮 半夏半升，汤洗 右八味，以水一斗，先煮麻黄，减二升，去上沫，内诸药，煮取三升，去滓。温服一升。

Annotations

[1] *Bing Yi Yin Zhe, Dang Fa Qi Han*: Retained fluid coupled with exposure to exogenous pathogenic factors may block the flow of lung qi and affect the surface of the body. In addition to edema and body heaviness, patients may also experience fever and absence of sweating. Therefore the treatment strategy is to induce sweating. The *Yi Zong Jin Jian* (Golden Mirror of the Medical Tradition) states, "water-fluid retention over the surface of the body needs to be treated by sweating; however, it is necessary to differentiate cold from heat. Heat-property water-fluid should be treated with *Da Qing Long Tang* (Major Green Dragon Decoction) and cold-property water-fluid with *Xiao Qing Long Tang* (Minor Green Dragon Decoction)".

[2] *Da Qing Long Tang* (Major Green Dragon Decoction): A formula to induce sweating, resolve water retention and clear interior heat. It is indicated for water-fluid retention with exterior symptoms and interior heat. For more information, see *Shang Han Lun* (Treatise on Cold Damage) No 38.

[3] *Xiao Qing Long Tang* (Minor Green Dragon Decotion): A formula to induce sweating, release the exterior and warm and resolve water retention. It is indicated for water-fluid retention with exteriro cold. For more information, see *Shang Han Lun* (Treatise on Cold Damage) No 40.

[4] *Wen Fen Fen Zhi*: Sprinkle medicinal powder to the body. The powder is made from *Chuan Xiong* (Rhizoma Chuanxiong), *Bai Zhi* (Radix Angelicae Dahuricae), *Gao Ben* (Rhizoma Ligustici), and rice flour.

Interpretations

Patients with overflow of water fluid should be treated with sweating method. Severe interior heat with restlessness (in addition to body ache, absence of sweating, fever and chills) should be treated with *Da Qing Long Tang* (Major Green Dragon Decoction); and severe interior fluid retention with cough and panting should be treated with *Xiao Qing Long Tang* (Minor Green Dragon Decoction).

Da Qing Long Tang

[Ingredients]

麻黄	*má huáng*	6 *liǎng*	Herba Ephedrae (nodes removed)
桂枝	*guì zhī*	2 *liǎng*	Ramulus Cinnamomi (skin removed)
甘草	*gān cǎo*	2 *liǎng*	Radix et Rhizoma Glycyrrhizae (fried)
杏仁	*xìng rén*	40 pieces	Semen Armeniacae Amarum (tip and skin removed)
生姜	*shēng jiāng*	3 *liǎng*	Rhizoma Zingiberis Recens
大枣	*dà zǎo*	12 pieces	Fructus Jujubae
石膏	*shí gāo*	The size of a chicken egg	Gypsum Fibrosum (crushed)

Decoct *Ma Huang* first in 9 *shēng* of water to get 7 *shēng*. Skim the foam and add the other ingredients to decoct and get 3 *shēng*. Remove the dregs and take 1 *shēng* when it is warm to cause mild but persistent sweating. For too much sweating, sprinkle some medicinal powder.

Xiao Qing Long Tang

[Ingredients]

麻黄	*má huáng*	3 *liǎng*	Herba Ephedrae (nodes removed)
芍药	*sháo yào*	3 *liǎng*	Radix Paeoniae

五味子	*wǔ wèi zǐ*	0.5 *shēng*	Fructus Schisandrae Chinensis
干姜	*gān jiāng*	3 *liǎng*	Rhizoma Zingiberis
甘草	*gān cǎo*	3 *liǎng*	Radix et Rhizoma Glycyrrhizae (fried)
细辛	*xì xīn*	3 *liǎng*	Radix et Rhizoma Asari
桂枝	*guì zhī*	3 *liǎng*	Ramulus Cinnamomi (skin removed)
半夏	*bàn xià*	0.5 *shēng*	Rhizoma Pinelliae (washed)

Decoct *Ma Huang* first in 1 *dòu* of water to get 8 *shēng*. Skim off the foam and add the other ingredients to decoct and get 3 *shēng*. Remove the dregs and take 1 *shēng* when it is warm for each dose.

*****

[24] 膈间支饮〔1〕，其人喘满，心下痞坚，面色黧墨，其脉沉紧，得之数十日，医吐下之不愈〔2〕，木防己汤〔3〕主之。虚者即愈，实者三日复发。复与不愈者〔4〕，宜木防己汤去石膏加茯苓芒硝汤〔5〕主之。

木防己汤方：

木防己三两石膏十二枚，如鸡子大桂枝二两人参四两右四味，以水六升，煮取二升。分温再服。

木防己加茯苓芒硝汤方：

木防己桂枝各二两 人参四两芒硝三合茯苓四两 右五味，以水六升，煮取二升，去滓，内芒硝，再微煎。分温再服。微利则愈。

Annotations

[1] *Ge Jian Zhi Yin*: Water fluid in the chest or diaphragm.

[2] *Yi Tu Xia Zhi Bu Yu*: Patients do not respond to the wrong use of vomiting or draining downward method.

[3] *Mu Fang Ji Tang* (Cocculi Decoction): A formula to move water, dissipate masses, reinforce the body and down-regualte qi. The formula uses *Mu Fang Ji* (Radix Cocculi Trilobi) as the monarch ingredient to

move water and resolve water retention, *Gui Zhi* (Ramulus Cinnamomi) to unblock yang and dissipate masses, *Ren Shen* (Radix et Rhizoma Ginseng) to tonify qi and *Shi Gao* (Gypsum Fibrosum) to alleviate panting.

[4] *Xu Zhe Ji Yu, Shi Zhe San Ri Fu Fa, Fu Yu Bu Yu Zhe*: The *Xu* (deficiency) and *Shi* (excess) here refer to the severity of water fluid retention—*Xu* means mild water fluid retention and *Shi* means severe water fluid retention. As a result, mild water fluid retention responds immediately to the decoction; severe water-fluid retention may return three days later. The previous formula needs to be modified.

[5] *Mu Fang Ji Tang Qu Shi Gao Jia Fu Ling Mang Xiao Tang* (Cocculi Decoction Minus Gypsum Plus Poria and Mirabilite): A modified formula of *Mu Fang Ji Tang* (Cocculi Decoction). *Fu Ling* is added to promote urination and resolve water retention and *Mang Xiao* to soften and dissipate masses. As *Shi Gao* works more on the qi phase, it is replaced by *Mang Xiao* to work on the blood.

Interpretations

Fluid retention in the chest or diagphram in patients (with preexisting phlegm-fluid) may cause panting, chest fullness, hardness and discomfort below the heart, a dark, gray complexion, and a deep, tight pulse (due to retained water fluid). This condition may last dozens of days and will not respond to vomiting or draining downward method. It should be treated with *Mu Fang Ji Tang* (Cocculi Decoction) to promote urination and resolve water retention. Mild fluid retention may respond immediately; however, severe fluid retention may return three days later. The recurrent condition may not respond to the previous formula and should be treated with modified *Mu Fang Ji Qu Shi Gao Jia Fu Ling Mang Xiao Tang* (Cocculi Decoction Minus Gypsum Plus Poria and Mirabilite) (to enhance the efficacy of promoting urination and breaking masses).

Mu Fang Ji Tang

[Ingredients]

木防己	*mù fáng jǐ*	3 *liǎng*	Radix Cocculi Trilobi
石膏	*shí gāo*	12 pieces	Gypsum Fibrosum (the size of a chicken egg)
桂枝	*guì zhī*	2 *liǎng*	Ramulus Cinnamomi
人参	*rén shēn*	2 *liǎng*	Radix et Rhizoma Ginseng

Decoct the four ingredients in 6 *shēng* of water to get 2 *shēng*. Take when it is warm in two times.

Mu Fang Ji Jia Fu Ling Mang Xiao Tang

[Ingredients]

木防己	*mù fáng jǐ*	2 *liǎng*	Radix Cocculi Trilobi
桂枝	*guì zhī*	2 *liǎng*	Ramulus Cinnamomi
人参	*rén shēn*	4 *liǎng*	Radix et Rhizoma Ginseng
芒硝	*máng xiāo*	0.3 *shēng*	Natrii Sulfas
茯苓	*fú líng*	4 *liǎng*	Poria

Decoct *Mu Fang Ji*, *Gui Zhi*, *Ren Shen* and *Fu Ling* in 6 *shēng* of water to get 2 *shēng*. Remove the dregs and add *Mang Xiao* to decoct for a little while. Take when it is warm in two times. Patients may have normal bowel and bladder movements afterwards and get better.

*****

[25] 心下有支饮，其人苦冒眩〔1〕，泽泻汤〔2〕主之。

泽泻汤方：

泽泻五两白术二两 右二味，以水二升，煮取一升。分温再服。

Annotations

[1] *Xin Xia You Zhi Yin, Qi Ren Ku Mao Xuan*: Patients with fluid retention below the heart may experience severe dizziness or vertigo. As vomiting may also be present, some believe the water fluid affects the spleen and stomach. The *Jin Gui Yao Lüè Jin Shi* (Modern Interpretation of the 'Essentials from the Golden Cabinet') states, "the water retains in the stomach and manifests in the brain". It is now known as vertigo syndrome.

[2] *Ze Xie Tang* (Alisma Decoction): A formula to promote urination and resolve water retention.

Interpretations

Fluid retention below the heart may cause severe dizziness or vertigo. This should be treated with *Ze Xie Tang* (Alisma Decoction).

Ze Xie Tang

[Ingredients]

泽泻	*zé xiè*	5 *liǎng*	Rhizoma Alismatis
白术	*bái zhú*	2 *liǎng*	Rhizoma Atractylodis Macrocephalae

Decoct the two ingredients in 2 *shēng* of water to get 1 *shēng*. Take when it is warm in two times.

*****

[26] 支饮胸满〔1〕者，厚朴大黄汤〔2〕主之。

厚朴大黄汤方：厚朴一尺　大黄六两枳实四枚右三味，以水五升，煮取二升。分温再服。

Annotations

[1] *Zhi Yin Xiong Man*: Fluid retention in the subcostal region with abdominal fullness. The *Xiong* (chest) by Zhang Zhongjing covers *Fu*

(abdomen). Abdominal fullness is often caused by excess stomach heat, patients also experience abdominal pain or constipation.

[2] *Hou Po Da Huang Tang* (Officinal Magnolia Bark and Rhubarb Decoction): This formula has the same ingredients as *Xiao Cheng Qi Tang* (Minor Purgative Decoction) in chapter 17 or *Hou Po San Wu Tang* (Officinal Magnolia Bark Three Ingredients Decoction) in chapter 10. It uses *Hou Po* (Cortex Magnoliae Officinalis) as the monarch ingredient to move qi, relieve fullness, and clear heat in the fu organs.

Interpretations

Fluid retention in the subcostal region with abdominal fullness (or constipation) can be treated with *Hou Po Da Huang Tang* (Officinal Magnolia Bark and Rhubarb Decoction).

Hou Po Da Huang Tang

[Ingredients]

厚朴	*hòu pò*	1 *chǐ* (23cm)	Cortex Magnoliae Officinalis
大黄	*dà huáng*	6 *liǎng*	Radix et Rhizoma Rhei
枳实	*zhǐ shí*	4 pieces	Fructus Aurantii Immaturus

Decoct the three ingredients in 5 *shēng* of water to get 2 *shēng*. Take when it is warm in two times.

*****

[27] 支饮不得息〔1〕，葶苈大枣泻肺汤〔2〕主之。方见肺痈中。

Annotations

[1] *Zhi Yin Bu De Xi*: Shortness of breath with an inability to lie flat due to water fluid accumulating in the lung.

[2] *Ting Li Da Zao Xie Fei Tang* (Lepidium/Descurainiae and Jujube Lung-Draining Decoction): See chapter 7.

Interpretations

Shortness of breath with an inability to lie flat due to retained fluid in the heart and lung should be treated with *Ting Li Da Zao Xie Fei Tang* (Lepidium/Descurainiae and Jujube Lung-Draining Decoction). For formula ingredients and usage, see chapter 7.

*****

[28] 呕家本渴，渴者为欲解〔1〕。今反不渴，心下有支饮故也〔2〕，小半夏汤〔3〕主之。《千金》云：小半夏加茯苓汤。

小半夏汤方：

半夏一升　生姜半斤　右二味，以水七升，煮取一升半。分温再服。

Annotations

[1] *Ou Jia Ben Ke, Ke Zhe Wei Yu Jie*: As vomiting damages body fluids, after vomiting, patients often feel thirsty. The presence of thirst indicates the stopping of vomiting.

[2] *Jin Fan Bu Ke, Xin Xia You Zhi Yin Gu Ye*: Patients do not feel thirst after vomiting due to fluid retention. Absence of thirst following vomiting indicates retained water fluid in the stomach. As a result, vomiting without thirst is a distinctive feature of vomiting due to phlegm fluid.

[3] *Xiao Ban Xia Tang* (Minor Pinelliae Decoction): A formula to resolve water retention and stop vomiting.

Interpretations

Generally, patients feel thirsty after vomiting. The presence of thirst indicates the imminent stopping of vomiting. However, patients with phlegm fluid do not feel thirsty after vomiting because of retained water fluid in the stomach. This condition should be treated with *Xiao Ban Xia Tang* (Minor Pinelliae Decoction). The

Qian Jin Yao Fang (Important Formulas Worth a Thousand Gold Pieces) records *Xiao Ban Xia Jia Fu Ling Tang* (Minor Pinelliae Decoction plus Poria).

Xiao Ban Xian Tang

[Ingredients]

半夏	*bàn xià*	1 *shēng*	Rhizoma Pinelliae
生姜	*shēng jiāng*	0.5 *jīn*	Rhizoma Zingiberis Recens

Decoct the two ingredients in 7 *shēng* of water to get 1.5 *shēng*. Take when it is warm in two times.

*****

[29] 腹满，口舌干燥，此肠间有水气〔1〕，己椒苈黄丸〔2〕主之。

防己椒目葶苈大黄丸方：

防己椒目葶苈熬大黄各一两 右四味，末之，蜜丸如梧子大。先食饮服一丸，日三服。稍增，口中有津液。渴者加芒硝半两。

Annotations

[1] *Chang Jian You Shui Qi*: Water-qi retention in the abdomen, causing abdominal fullness or difficult urination.

[2] *Ji Jiao Li Huang Wan* (Stephaniae Tetrabdraem, Zanthoxyli, Lepidii and Rhubarb Pill): A formula to resolve water fluid through promoting bowel and bladder movements.

Interpretations

Abdominal fullness (gurgling bowel sounds and difficult urination) and a dry mouth and tongue indicate retained water in the abdomen and should be treated with *Ji Jiao Li Huang Wan* (Stephaniae Tetrabdraem, Zanthoxyli, Lepidii and Rhubarb Pill).

Fang Ji Jiao Mu Ting Li Da Huang Wan

[Ingredients]

防己	*fáng jǐ*	1 *liǎng*	Radix Stephaniae Tetrandrae
椒目	*jiāo mù*	1 *liǎng*	Semen Zanthoxyli
葶苈	*tíng lì*	1 *liǎng*	Semen Lepidii (boiled)
大黄	*dà huáng*	1 *liǎng*	Radix et Rhizoma Rhei

Grind the four ingredients into a fine powder and mix with honey to make into pills the size of firmiana seeds. Take one pill for each dose with water before meals, 3 doses a day. Increase the dose gradually until there is saliva in the mouth. If patients still feel thirsty after taking the decoction, add 0.5 *liǎng* of *Mang Xiao* (Natrii Sulfas) to soften masses and resolve retained water in the abdomen.

*****

[30] 卒呕吐〔1〕，心下痞，膈间有水，眩悸〔2〕者，半夏加茯苓汤〔3〕主之。

小半夏加茯苓汤方：

半夏一升 生姜半斤茯苓三两，一法四两 右三味，以水七升，煮取一升五合。分温再服。

Annotations

[1] *Cu Ou Tu*: Sudden vomiting (due to water fluid below the heart)

[2] *Xuan Ji*: Dizziness and palpitations. The *Jin Gui Yao Lüè Ben Yi* (Original Meanings of the 'Essentials from the Golden Cabinet') states, "Retained water fluid in the stomach and intestines may impair

the normal flow of qi. Upflow of stomach qi causes vomiting. Stagnation of stomach qi causes fullness below the heart. Failure of clear yang to ascend causes dizziness. Water fluid may ascend to affect the heart and result in palpitations".

[3] *Xiao Ban Xia Jia Fu Ling Tang* (Minor Pinellia Decoction plus Poria): A formula to move water, resolve water fluid, harmonize the stomach and down-regulate qi.

Interpretations

Sudden vomiting with fullness and discomfort below the heart indicate retained water fluid in the middle *jiao*. Dizziness and palpitations may also be present. These symptoms are more severe than those indicated by *Xiao Ban Xia Tang* (Minor Pinellia Decoction) and therefore, should be treated with *Xiao Ban Xia Jia Fu Ling Tang* (Minor Pinellia Decoction plus Poria).

Xiao Ban Xia Jia Fu Ling Tang

[Ingredients]

半夏	*bàn xià*	1 *shēng*	Rhizoma Pinelliae
椒目	*jiāo mù*	0.5 *jīn*	Semen Zanthoxyli
茯苓	*fú líng*	3 *liǎng*	Poria (4 *liǎng* in another text)

Grind the four ingredients in 7 *shēng* of water to get 1.5 *shēng*, and drink when it is warm in two times.

*****

[31] 假令瘦人〔1〕脐下有悸〔2〕，吐涎沫而癫眩〔3〕，此水也。五苓散〔4〕主之。

五苓散方：

泽泻一两一分 猪苓三分，去皮 茯苓三分白术三分桂二分，去皮

右五味，为末。白饮服方寸匕，日三服。多饮暖水，汗出愈。

Annotations

[1] *Shou Ren*: Patients without edema.

[2] *Qi Xia You Ji*: Rapid pulsations below the umbilicus. Retained water fluid in the lower jiao may impair the qi transformation of the urinary bladder and cause difficult urination. The *Yi Zong Jin Jian* (Golden Mirror of the Medical Tradition) states, "Palpations indicate water fluid below the heart; umbilical pulsations indicate water fluid below the umbilicus".

[3] *Dian Xuan*: Dizziness. The first word *Dian* means the top of the head and the second word *Xuan* means dizziness.

[4] *Wu Ling San* (Five Ingredients Powder with Poria): A formula to move qi and promote urination. Among the ingredients, *Ze Xie* (Rhizoma Alismatis), *Zhu Ling* (Polyporus) and *Fu Ling* (Poria) promote urination, *Bai Zhu* (Rhizoma Atractylodis Macrocephalae) fortifies the spleen and promotes urination, and *Gui Zhi* (Ramulus Cinnamomi) unblocks yang and down-regulates qi.

Interpretations

For patients without retained water-dampness, rapid pulsations below the umbilicus, vomiting of foamy saliva, and dizziness indicate internal retention of water fluid and should be treated with *Wu Ling San* (Five Ingredients Powder with Poria).

Wu Ling San

[Ingredients]

泽泻	*zé xiè*	11 *fēn*	Rhizoma Alismatis
猪苓	*zhū líng*	3 *fēn*	Polyporus (skin removed)
茯苓	*fú líng*	3 *fēn*	Poria
白术	*bái zhú*	3 *fēn*	Rhizoma Atractylodis Macrocephalae
桂枝	*guì zhī*	2 *fēn*	Ramulus Cinnamomi (skin removed)

Grind the five ingredients into a fine powder. Take one square inch-spon of the powder for each dose with warm water, 3 doses a day. Drink plenty of water afterwards, and sweating is good for the recovery.

Annex Formula *Fu Ling Yin* (Poria Decoction)

《外台》茯苓饮[1]：治心胸中有停痰宿水[2]，自吐出水后，心胸间虚、气满不能食，清痰气，令能食。

茯苓人参白术各三两枳实二两橘皮二两半生姜四两　右六味，水六升，煮取一升八合。分温三服。如人行八九里进之。

Annotations

[1] *Wai Tai Fu Ling Yin* (Poria Decoction): A formula recorded in the *Wai Tai Mi Yao* (Arcane Essentials from the Imperial Library) to fortify the spleen, regulate qi and resolve phlegm. It is an aftercare formula for patients with phlegm fluid.

[2] *Xin Xiong Zhong You Ting Tan Su Shui*: Water fluid retaining in the middle jiao.

Interpretations

Fu Ling Yin (Poria Decoction) in the *Wai Tai Mi Yao* (Arcane Essentials from the Imperial Library) is indicated for abdominal distension/fullness and no appetite (due to deficiency of the spleen and stomach) after vomiting of water. It helps to resolve phlegm, regulate qi and thus restore the patients' appetite.

Fu Ling Yin

[Ingredients]

茯苓	*fú líng*	3 *liǎng*	Poria
人参	*rén shēn*	3 *liǎng*	Radix et Rhizoma Ginseng

Fu Ling Yin

[Ingredients]

白术	*bái zhú*	3 *liǎng*	Rhizoma Atractylodis Macrocephalae
枳实	*zhǐ shí*	2 *liǎng*	Fructus Aurantii Immaturus
橘皮	*jú pí*	2.5 *liǎng*	Pericarpium Citri Reticulatae
生姜	*shēng jiāng*	4 *liǎng*	Rhizoma Zingiberis Recens

Decoct the six ingredients in 6 *shēng* of water to get 1.8 *shēng*. Take when it is warm in three times. The time interval between two doses is the time it takes to walk 4-4.5 kilometers.

*****

[32] 咳家〔1〕其脉弦〔2〕，为有水，十枣汤主之。

Annotations

[1] *Ke Jia:* Patients with chronic cough.

[2] *Mai Xian:* A wiry pulse, referring to suspended fluid retention (in the subcostal region).

Interpretations

Cough-induced chest pain in patients with chronic cough indicates retained water fluid and should be treated with *Shi Zao Tang* (Ten Jujubes Decoction). For ingredients and usage of the formula, see line 22 in this chapter.

*****

[33] 夫有支饮家〔1〕，咳烦胸中痛〔2〕者，不卒死，至一百日或一岁〔3〕，宜十枣汤。方见上。

Annotations

[1] *Zhi Yin Jia:* Patients with chronic fluid retention (similar to chronic bronchitis).

[2] *Ke Fan Xiong Zhong Tong*: Frequent coughing and cough-induced pain in the subcostal region.

[3] *Bu Cu Si, Zhi Yi Bai Ri Huo Yi Sui*: Despite there is no threat of imminent death, without timely treatment, the disease may linger months or a year.

Interpretations

Frequent coughing and cough-induced chest pain in patients with chronic fluid retention should be treated with *Shi Zao Tang* (Ten Jujubes Decoction). For ingredients and usage of the formula, see line 22 in this chapter.

*****

[34] 久咳数岁，其脉弱者可治，实大数者死[1]。其脉虚者必苦冒，其人本有支饮在胸中故也。治属饮家。

Annotations

[1] *Jiu Ke Shu Sui...Shi Da Shu Zhe Si:* For patients with chronic cough, a weak pulse indicates mild pathogenic qi and a favorable prognosis; a large, replete and large pulse indicates deficiency of healthy qi and excess of pathogenic qi and an unfavorable prognosis.

Interpretations

For patients with years of coughing, a weak pulse indicates mild pathogenic qi and a favorable prognosis; a replete, surging and large, or slippery and rapid pulse indicates deficiency of healthy qi and excess of pathogenic qi and an unfavorable prognosis. A weak pulse (in patients with chronic cough) with noticeable dizziness and blurred vision (this cannot be mistaken for deficiency) is caused by retained water fluid in the chest. As a result, the treatment should be focused on resolving phlegm fluid.

*****

[35] 咳逆倚息〔1〕不得卧，小青龙汤〔2〕主之。方见上及肺痈中〔3〕。

Annotations

[1] *Ke Ni Yi Xi*: Shortness of breath when lying flat. It is similar to ortheopenia in modern medicine.

[2] *Xiao Qing Long Tang* (Minor Green Dragon Decoction): A formula to release the exterior, dissipate cold and resolve fluid retention. As it contains *Ma Huang* (Herba Ephedrae) and *Xi Xin* (Radix et Rhizoma Asari) that are warm and pungent, this formula is not indicated for patients with chronic fluid retention due to kidney yang deficiency.

[3] For ingredients and usage of *Xiao Qing Long Tang* (Minor Green Dragon Decoction), see line 23 in this chapter.

Interpretations

Cough and shortness of breath with an inability to lie flat can be be treated with *Xiao Qing Long Tang* (Minor Green Dragon Decoction).

*****

[36] 青龙汤下已，多唾口燥，寸脉沉，尺脉微〔1〕，手足厥逆，气从小腹上冲胸咽，手足痹，其面翕热如醉状〔2〕，因复下流阴股〔3〕，小便难，时复冒者，与茯苓桂枝五味子甘草汤〔4〕，治其气冲。

桂苓五味甘草汤方：

桂枝四两，去皮茯苓四两甘草三两，炙 五味子半斤右四味，以水八升，煮取三升，去滓。分三温服。

Annotations

[1] *Cun Mai Chen, Chi Mai Wei*: The pulse is deep at the *Cun* position and faint at the *Chi* positon before taking *Xiao Qing Long Tang* (Minor Green Dragon Decoction). The pulsation at the *Cun* position tells the condition of the lung, a deep pulse at this position indicates fluid retention. The pulsation at the *Chi* position tells the condition of the kidney, a faint pulse at this position indicates kidey yang deficiency. To sum up, before taking the decoction, patients had fluid retention in the lung with kidney yang deficiency.

[2] *Mian Xi Re Ru Zui Zhuang*: A hot sensation on the face as if one was drunk.

[3] *Yin Gu*: Medial side of the thigh. Here it refers to the lower *jiao*.

[4] *Gui Ling Wu Wei Gan Cao Tang* (Cinnamon Twig, Poria, Schisandra, and Licorice Decoction): A formula to supplement yang, astringe yin, fortify the spleen and stomach and resolve fluid retention.

Interpretations

After taking *Xiao Qing Long Tang* (Major Green Dragon Decotion), patients have increased sputum but experienced a dry mouth and tongue. Since the patients previously had a deep pulse at the *Cun* position (indicating fluid retention in the lung) and a faint pulse at the *Chi* position (indicating kidney yang deficiency), and cold limbs, after taking the decoction, they experienced uprush of qi, numbness in hands/feet, and a hot sensation on the face as if they were drunk. In addition, the pathogenic qi tends to flow downward to the lower jiao and cause difficulty urination, along with occasional dizziness. In this case, *Gui Ling Wu Wei Gan Cao Tang* (Cinnamon Twig, Poria, Schisandra, and Licorice Decoction) should be used to deal with variations of qi uprush.

Gui Ling Wu Wei Gan Cao Tang

[Ingredients]

桂枝	*guì zhī*	4 *liǎng*	Ramulus Cinnamomi (skin removed)
茯苓	*fú líng*	4 *liǎng*	Poria
甘草	*gān cǎo*	3 *liǎng*	Radix et Rhizoma Glycyrrhizae (fried)
五味子	*wǔ wèi zǐ*	0.5 *shēng*	Fructus Schisandrae Chinensis

Decoct the seven ingredients in 8 *shēng* of water to get 3 *shēng*. Remove the dregs and take 0.5 *shēng* when it is warm for each dose, 3 doses a day.

*****

[37] 冲气即低〔1〕，而反更咳，胸满者，用桂苓五味甘草汤去桂加干姜、细辛〔2〕，以治其咳满。

苓甘五味姜辛汤方：

茯苓四两甘草干姜细辛各三两五味子半升　右五味，以水八升，煮取三升，去滓。温服半升，日三。

Annotations

[1] *Chong Qi Ji Di*: Relief of uprush of qi.

[2] *Gui Ling Wu Wei Gan Cao Tang Qu Gui Jia Gan Jiang, Xi Xin* (Cinnamon Twig, Poria, Schisandra, and Licorice Decoction minus Cinnamon Twig plus Dried Ginger and Asarum): A modified formula of *Gui Ling Wu Wei Gan Cao Tang* (Cinnamon Twig, Poria, Schisandra, and Licorice Decoction) by removing *Gui Zhi* (Ramulus Cinnamomi) and adding *Gan Jiang* (Rhizoma Zingiberis) and *Xi Xin* (Radix et Rhizoma Asari) to resolve fluid retention and stop coughing.

Interpretations

After taking the decoction, the uprush of qi alleviated; however, the cough worsened and patients started to experience chest fullness and discomfort. In such case, *Gui Zhi* (Ramulus Cinnamomi) should be removed from the previous formula and *Gan Jiang* (Rhizoma Zingiberis) and *Xi Xin* (Radix et Rhizoma Asari) added to stop coughing and eliminate fullness.

Fu Gan Wu Wei Jia Gan Jiang Xi Xin Tang

[Ingredients]

茯苓	*fú líng*	4 *liǎng*	Poria
甘草	*gān cǎo*	3 *liǎng*	Radix et Rhizoma Glycyrrhizae
五味子	*wǔ wèi zǐ*	0.5 *shēng*	Fructus Schisandrae Chinensis
干姜	*gān jiāng*	3 *liǎng*	Rhizoma Zingiberis
细辛	*xì xīn*	3 *liǎng*	Radix et Rhizoma Asari

Decoct the seven ingredients in 8 *shēng* of water to get 3 *shēng*. Remove the dregs and take 0.5 *shēng* when it is warm for each dose, 3 doses a day.

*****

[38] 咳满即止，而更复渴，冲气复发者，以细辛、干姜为热药也。服之当遂渴，而渴反止者，为支饮也。支饮者，法当冒，冒者必呕，呕者复内半夏以去其水。

桂苓五味甘草去桂加干姜细辛半夏汤[1]方：

茯苓四两甘草细辛干姜各二两五味子半夏各半升右六味，以水八升，煮取三升，去滓。温服半升，日三。

Annotations

[1] *Gui Ling Wu Wei Gan Cao Qu Gui Jia Gan Jiang Xi Xin Ban Xia Tang* (Cinnamon Twig, Poria, Schisandra, and Licorice Decoction minus Cinnamon Twig plus Dried Ginger, Asarum and Pinella): A modified *Ling Gan Wu Wei Jiang Xing Tang* (Poria, Licorice, and Schisandra Decoction plus Dried Ginger and Asarum) by decrasing the doses of *Xi Xin* (Radix et Rhizoma Asari) and *Gan Jiang* (Rhizoma Zingiberis) and adding *Ban Xia* (Rhizoma Pinelliae) to resolve fluid retention.

Interpretations

After taking the decoction, the cough and chest fullness alleviated; however, patients started to experience thirst and uprush of qi again due to the warm property of *Xi Xin* (Radix et Rhizoma Asari) and *Gan Jiang* (Rhizoma Zingiberis). Patients should normally feel thirsty but they don't because of internal fluid retention. Retained fluid may cause severe dizziness/vertigo or vomiting. In the case of vomiting, *Ban Xia* (Rhizoma Pinelliae) can be added to the previous formula to resolve water retention.

Fu Gan Wu Wei Jia Gan Jiang Xi Xin Ban Xia Tang

[Ingredients]

茯苓	*fú líng*	4 *liǎng*	Poria
甘草	*gān cǎo*	2 *liǎng*	Radix et Rhizoma Glycyrrhizae
五味子	*wǔ wèi zǐ*	0.5 *shēng*	Fructus Schisandrae Chinensis
干姜	*gān jiāng*	2 *liǎng*	Rhizoma Zingiberis
细辛	*xì xīn*	2 *liǎng*	Radix et Rhizoma Asari
半夏	*bàn xià*	0.5 *shēng*	Rhizoma Pinelliae

Decoct the six ingredients in 8 *shēng* of water to get 3 *shēng*. Remove the dregs and take 0.5 *shēng* when it is warm for each dose, 3 doses a day.

*****

[39] 水去呕止，其人形肿者，加杏仁主之。其证应内麻黄，以其人遂痹，故不内之。若逆而内之者，必厥。所以然者，以其人血虚，麻黄发其阳故也。

苓甘五味加姜辛半夏杏仁汤〔1〕方：

茯苓四两 甘草三两 五味子半升 干姜三两 细辛三两 半夏半升 杏仁半升，去皮、尖 右七味，以水一斗，煮取三升，去滓。温服半升，日三。

Annotations

[1] *Fu Gan Wu Wei Jia Jiang Xin Ban Xing Ren Tang* (Poria, Licorice, and Schisandra Decoction plus Dried Ginger, Asarum, Pinellia, and Apricot Kernel): A modified *Fu Gan Wu Wei Jia Jiang Tang* (Poria, Licorice, and Schisandra Decoction plus Dried Ginger and Asarum) plus *Ban Xia* (Rhizoma Pinelliae) and *Xing Ren* (Semen Armeniacae Amarum) to disperse lung qi and resolve fluid retention.

Interpretations

After taking the fluid-resolving decoction, patients stopped vomiting but developed general edema. In such case, *Xing Ren* (Semen Armeniacae Amarum) should be added to the formula. Normally *Ma Huang* (Herba Ephedrae) can be added to the formula; however, it cannot be combined in this case, because patients had kidney yang deficiency with Bi-impairment of hands/feet. The use of *Ma Huang* may cause cold limbs, as it disperses yang qi and consumes yin blood.

Fu Gan Wu Wei Jia Jiang Xin Ban Xing Da Huang Tang

[Ingredients]

茯苓	*fú líng*	4 *liǎng*	Poria
甘草	*gān cǎo*	3 *liǎng*	Radix et Rhizoma Glycyrrhizae
五味子	*wǔ wèi zǐ*	0.5 *shēng*	Fructus Schisandrae Chinensis
干姜	*gān jiāng*	3 *liǎng*	Rhizoma Zingiberis
细辛	*xì xīn*	3 *liǎng*	Radix et Rhizoma Asari
半夏	*bàn xià*	0.5 *shēng*	Rhizoma Pinelliae
杏仁	*xìng rén*	0.5 *shēng*	Semen Armeniacae Amarum (tip and skin removed)

Decoct the seven ingredients in 1 *dòu* of water to get 3 *shēng*. Remove the dregs and take 0.5 *shēng* when it is warm for each dose, 3 doses a day.

*****

[40] 若面热如醉，此为胃热上冲熏其面，加大黄以利之。

茯甘五味加姜辛半杏大黄汤[1]方：

茯苓四两 甘草三两五味子半升干姜三两细辛三两 半夏半升杏仁半升 大黄三两 右八味，以水一斗，煮取三升，去滓。温服半升，日三。

Annotations

[1] *Fu Gan Wu Wei Jia Jiang Xin Ban Xing Da Huang Tang* (Poria, Licorice, and Schisandra Decoction plus Dried Ginger, Asarum, Pinellia, Apricot Kernel and Rhubarb): A modified *Fu Gan Wu Wei Jia Jiang Xin Ban Xia Xing Ren Tang* (Poria, Licorice, and Schisandra Decoction plus Dried Ginger, Asarum, Pinellia, and Apricot Kernel) plus *Da Huang* (Radix et Rhizoma Rhei) to clear stomach heat.

Interpretations

(In addition to general edema), if patients feel hot in the face as if they were drunk, this is caused by uprush of stomach heat to the face. In such case, *Da Huang* (Radix et Rhizoma Rhei) should be added to the formula to promote bowel movements and clear stomach heat.

Fu Gan Wu Wei Jia Jiang Xin Ban Xing Da Huang Tang

[Ingredients]

茯苓	*fú líng*	4 *liǎng*	Poria
甘草	*gān cǎo*	3 *liǎng*	Radix et Rhizoma Glycyrrhizae
五味子	*wǔ wèi zǐ*	0.5 *shēng*	Fructus Schisandrae Chinensis
干姜	*gān jiāng*	3 *liǎng*	Rhizoma Zingiberis
细辛	*xì xīn*	3 *liǎng*	Radix et Rhizoma Asari
半夏	*bàn xià*	0.5 *shēng*	Rhizoma Pinelliae
杏仁	*xìng rén*	0.5 *shēng*	Semen Armeniacae Amarum
大黄	*dà huáng*	3 *liǎng*	Radix et Rhizoma Rhei

Decoct the eight ingredients in 1 *dòu* of water to get 3 *shēng*. Remove the dregs and take 0.5 *shēng* when it is warm for each dose, 3 doses a day.

*****

[41] 先渴后呕，为水停心下，此属饮家，小半夏茯苓汤主之〔1〕。方见上。

Annotations

[1] *Xiao Ban Xia Fu Ling Tang* (Minor Pinelliae Decoction plus Poria): A formula for vomiting due to phlegm fluid.

Interpretations

Patients (who had no vomiting) experience thirst, drink a large amount of water and vomit afterwards. This is caused by fluid retention below the heart and should be treated with *Xiao Ban Xia Fu Ling Tang* (Minor Pinelliae Decoction plus Poria) (to resolve water retention, harmonize the stomach, and down-regualte qi). The formula is discussed previous in this chapter (line 30).

消渴小便利淋病脉证并治第十三

Chapter 13 Wasting & Thirsting, Difficult Urination and Strangury—Pulses, Patterns and Treatment

Overview

This chapter discusses wasting and thirsting, difficult urination, and strangury. Wasting and thirsting is both a disease and syndrome. It refers to thirst with desire to drink and excessive urination afterwards. Difficult urination (a wrong spelling of "normal urination" in the original text) is a symptom in many external contracted conditions or internal dysfunctions. Strangury refers to painful, frequent urination in small volumes. The three conditions are discussed together because they share the same symptom of abnormal urination and are all associated with the kidney and urinary bladder.

*****

[01] 厥阴[1]之为病，消渴，气上冲心[2]，心中疼热，饥而不欲食，食即吐，下之不肯止。

Annotations

[1] *Jue Yin*: Jueyin disease, one of the six meridian diseases discussed in the *Shang Han Lun* (Treatise on Cold Damage).

[2] *Qi Shang Chong Xin*: Uprush of heat to the heart (referring to the stomach).

Interpretations

Jueyin disease may cause unusual thirst with a desire to drink water, uprush of heat to the stomach, a burning sensation and pain in the stomach, hunger but no desire to eat and vomiting after eating food (possibly vomiting up roundworms). The wrong use of draining downward method may cause persisten diarrhea.

*****

[02] 寸口脉浮而迟，浮即为虚，迟即为劳〔1〕，虚则卫气不足，劳则荣气竭〔2〕。

趺阳脉浮而数，浮则为气〔3〕，数即消谷而大坚〔4〕一作紧，气盛则溲数〔5〕，溲数即坚，坚数相搏，即为消渴〔6〕。

Annotations

[1] *Fu Ze Wei Xu, Chi Ze Wei Lao*: A superficial and slow pulse indicates general deficiency and exhaustion.

[2] *Xu Ze Wei Qi Bu Zu, Lao Ze Rong Qi Jie*: Deficiency mainly refers to deficiency of *Wei*-defensive qi; exhaustion mainly refers to exhaustion of *Ying*-nutrients qi. Deficiency of both *Ying*-nutrients and *Wei*-defense is the root cause of wasting and thirsting.

[3] *Fu Yang Mai Fu Er Shuo, Fu Ze Wei Qi*: The pulse felt at Chongyang (ST 42) tells the conditions of the spleen and stomach. A superficial pulse suggests excess stomach qi and heat.

[4] *Da Jian*: Hard stools.

[5] *Sou Shuo*: Frequent urination.

[6] *Xiao Ke*: Wasting and thirsting. The *Jin Gui Yao Lüè Xin Dian* (Personal Standards for the 'Essentials from the Golden Cabinet') states, "Stomach heat causes fast digestion and unusual thirst, which is later known as fast hunger after eating food. This is called wasting and thristing of the middle jiao". It is similar to diabetes mellitus in modern medicine.

Interpretations

A superficial and slow pulse felt at the *Cunkou* area indicates general deficiency and exhaustion, especially deficiency of the *Ying*-nutrients (blood) and *Wei*-defense (qi).

A superficial and rapid pulse felt at Chongyang (ST 42) indicates excess stomach qi and heat. Stomach heat may cause fast hunger after eating food and hard stools. Excess stomach qi may cause frequent urination. Frequent urination results in hard stools, while hard stools aggravate frequent urination. The two contend with each other and lead to wasting and thirsting disorder.

*****

[03] 男子〔1〕消渴〔2〕，小便反多，以饮一斗，小便一斗〔3〕，肾气丸主之。方见脚气中。

Annotations

[1] *Nan Zi:* Men; however, it also includes women.

[2] *Xiao Ke*: A condition characterized by increased thirst, increased hunger and increased urination. It is similar to diabetes mellitus or diabetes insipidus in modern medicine.

[3] *Yin Yi Dou, Xiao Bian Yi Dou*: Increase thirst and increased urination. This is more associated with the kidney and known as the wasting and thrist of the lower jiao.

Interpretations

Patients with wasting and thirsting experience increased urination and urinate the exact amount they drink. This should be treated with *Shen Qi Wan* (Kidney Qi Pill). For ingredients and usage of the formula, see chapter 5 (Cui's Eight Ingredients Pill).

*****

[04] 脉浮，小便不利，微热消渴〔1〕者，宜利小便、发汗，五苓散主之。

[05] 渴欲饮水，水入则吐〔2〕者，名曰水逆，五苓散主之。方见上。

Annotations

[1] *Mai Fu...Wei Re Xiao Ke:* A superficial pulse and mild fever indicate unresolved exterior syndrome; wasting and thirsting and difficult urination indicate interior heat.

[2] *Ke Yu Yin Shui, Shui Ru Ze Tu*: Thirst with a desire to drink water but vomit immediately after drinking water. This is caused by impaired qi transformation of the urinary bladder as well as disharmony of stomach qi. It is more severe than internal water retention.

Interpretations

A superficial pulse with difficult urination, mild fever, and thirst with a desire to drink water should be treated with *Wu Ling San* (Five Ingredients Powder with Poria) to promote urination and induce sweating.

Thirst with a desire to drink water but vomit immediately after drinking water is called upflow of water. This can also be treated with *Wu Ling San* (Five Ingredients Powder with Poria). For ingredients and usage of this formula, see chapter 12 (line 31).

*****

[06] 渴欲饮水不止者〔1〕，文蛤散〔2〕主之。

文蛤散方：文蛤〔3〕五两〔4〕右一味，杵为散，以沸汤五合，和服方寸匕。

Annotations

[1] *Ke Yu Yin Shui Bu Zhi Zhe*: Increased thirst that cannot be quenched due to insufficient body fluids. Thirst without fever indicates

that there is no exogenous pathogenic heat. Thirst without vomiting indicates that there is no retained fluid.

[2] *Wen Ge San* (Clamshell Powder): A formula to clear the lung, nourish yin and regenerate fluids.

[3] *Wen Ge*: There are different opinions regarding *Wen Ge*. One is clamshell, which acts to clear the lung, resolve phlegm, regenerate fluids and stop thirst. The other is *Wu Bei Zi* (Galla Chinensis).

[4] *Wu Liang: 5 liang*; 4 *liang* mentioned in YU's version.

Interpretations

Thirst with a desire to drink water and it seems the thirst cannot be quenched. This can be treated with *Wen Ge San* (Clamshell Powder).

Method: Grind 5 *liǎng* of clamshell into a fine powder and mix with 0.5 *shēng* of water. Take one square-inch spoon for each dose.

*****

[07] 淋〔1〕之为病，小便如粟状〔2〕，小腹弦急，痛引脐中。

Annotations

[1] *Lin*: Strangury that causes dribbling, hesitant or painful urination.

[2] *Xiao Bian Ru Su Zhuang*: Millet-like (dribbling) urine.

Interpretations

Strangury is a condition characterized by millet-like urine (dribbling, hesitant), along with lower abdominal tightness and pain that radiates to the umbilicus.

*****

[08] 趺阳脉数，胃中有热，即消谷引食，大便必坚，小便即数。

Interpretations

A rapid pulse felt at Chongyang (ST 42) indicates stomach heat, which is characterized by fast hunger after eating food, hard stools and increased urination.

*****

[09] 淋家不可发汗〔1〕，发汗则必便血。

Annotations

[1] *Lin Jia Bu Ke Fa Han*: Strangury is caused by heat in the lower jiao. Since heat consumes yin fluids, it cannot be treated by sweating even if the patient has a fever.

Interpretations

Strangury cannot be treated with sweating method, for it may result in bloody urine.

*****

[10] 小便不利者，有水气〔1〕，其人若渴，栝蒌瞿麦丸〔2〕主之。

栝蒌瞿麦丸方：

栝蒌根二两茯苓薯预各三两附子一枚，炮瞿麦一两　右五味，末之，炼蜜丸梧子大。饮服三丸，日三服。不知，增至七八丸，以小便利、腹中温为知。

Annotations

[1] *Xiao Bian Bu Li Zhe, You Shui Qi*: Difficult urination (without fever) indicates internal water qi retention due to kidney yang deficiency.

[2] *Gua Lou Qu Mai Wan* (Trichosanthes and Dianthus Pill): A formula to warm yang, transform qi, promote urination and moisten dryness. It is a modified formula of *Shen Qi Wan* (Kidney Qi Pill).

Interpretations

Difficult urination indicates internal retention of water qi. Increased thirst may also be present. This should be treated with *Gua Lou Qu Mai Wan* (Trichosanthes and Dianthus Pill).

Gua Lou Qu Mai Wan

[Ingredients]

栝蒌根	*guā lóu gēn*	2 *liǎng*	Radix Trichosanthis
茯苓	*fú líng*	3 *liǎng*	Poria
山药	*shān yào*	3 *liǎng*	Rhizoma Dioscoreae
附子	*huá shí*	1 piece	Radix Aconiti Lateralis Praeparata
瞿麦	*qú mài*	1 *liǎng*	Herba Dianthi

Grind the five ingredients into a fine powder and mix with the processed honey to make into pills the size of firmiana seeds. Take 3 pills with water for each dose, three doses a day. If no efficacy, increase the dose to 7 or 8 pills until the presence of normal urination and a warm sensation in the lower abdomen.

*****

[11] 小便不利〔1〕，蒲灰散〔2〕主之；滑石白鱼散〔3〕，茯苓戎盐汤〔4〕并主之。

蒲灰散方：蒲灰七分滑石三分右二味，杵为散。饮服方寸匕，日三服。

滑石白鱼散方：滑石二分乱发二分，烧 白鱼二分右三味，杵为散。饮服半钱匕，日三服。

茯苓戎盐汤方：茯苓半斤白术二两戎盐弹丸大一枚右三味。

Annotations

[1] *Xiao Bian Bu Li*: Dificult urination due to strangury.

[2] *Pu Hui San* (Typhae Pollen Powder): A formula to cool blood, resolve stasis and promote urination. It is indicated for strangury due to heat.

[3] *Hua Shi Bai Yu San* (Talcum and Silverfish Powder): A formula to stop bleeding, resolve stasis and promote urination. It is indicated for bloody strangury with blood-contained urine and lower abdominal pain.

[4] *Fu Ling Rong Yan Tang* (Poria and Halite Decoction): A formula to fortify the spleen, promote urination, benefit the kidney and reduce fire. It is indicated for turbid, milky or bloody urine.

Interpretations

There are three formulas for difficult urination— *Pu Hui San* (Typhae Pollen Powder) for dribbling, hesitant and painful urination; *Hua Shi Bai Yu San* (Talcum and Silverfish Powder) for bloody urine; and *Fu Ling Rong Yan Tang* (Poria and Halite Decoction) for turbid, milky or bloody urine.

Pu Hui San

[Ingredients]

蒲黄	*pú huáng*	7 *fēn*	Pollen Typhae
滑石	*huá shí*	3 *fēn*	Talcum

Grind the two ingredients into a fine powder. Drink 1 square-inch spoon for each dose, 3 doses a day.

Hua Shi Bai Yu San

[Ingredients]

滑石	huá shí	2 *fēn*	Talcum
乱发	*luàn fā*	2 *fēn*	Crinis (burnt)
白鱼	*bái yú*	2 *fēn*	Lepisma

Decoct the three ingredients into a fine powder. Drink 1 square-inch spoon for each dose, 3 doses a day.

Fu Ling Rong Yan Tang

[Ingredients]

茯苓	*fú líng*	0.5 *jīn*	Poria
白术	*bái zhú*	2 *liǎng*	Rhizoma Atractylodis Macrocephalae
戎盐	*róng yán*	1 piece (pellet-sized)	Halite

Decoct *Fu Ling* and *Bai Zhu* first and then add *Rong Yan*. Divide and take when it is warm in three times.

*****

[12] 渴欲饮水，口干舌燥者[1]，白虎加人参汤主之。方见中暍中。

Annotations

[1] *Ke Yu Yin Shui, Kou Gan She Zao Zhe*: Thirst with a desire to drink water and a dry mouth and tongue after drinking water. This indicates an unusual thirst due to excess heat in the lung and stomach, known as wasting and thirsting of the upper jiao. The *Jin Gui Yao Lüè Xin Dian* (Personal Standards for the 'Essentials from the Golden

Cabinet') states, "As this is caused by excess heat in the lung and stomach damaging fluids, *Bai Hu Tang* (White Tiger Decoction) is used to clear heat, *Ren Shen* (Radix et Rhizoma Ginseng) is combined to regenerate fluids and alleviate the thirst…". It is similar to type 1 diabetes in modern medicine.

Interpretations

Thirst with a desire to drink water and a dry mouth and tongue after drinking a large amount of water (in an externally contracted condition) should be treated with *Bai Hu Jia Ren Shen Tang* (White Tiger Decoction plus Ginseng). For ingredients and usage of the formula, see chapter 2 (line 26).

*****

[13] 脉浮发热，渴欲饮水，小便不利者〔1〕，猪苓汤〔2〕主之。

猪苓汤方：

猪苓去皮茯苓阿胶滑石泽泻各一两　右五味，以水四升，先煮四味，取二升，去滓，内胶烊消。温服七合，日三服。

Annotations

[1] *Mai Fu Fa Re, Ke Yu Yin Shui, Xiao Bian Bu Li Zhe*: These are similar symptoms indicated by *Wu Ling San* (Five Ingredients Powder with Poria)—a superficial pulse, fever, thirst and difficult urination in an externally contracted condition. However, the severity is different—mild fever versus fever, waisting and thirsting versus increased thirst with a desire to drink water. Apparently, there is severe heat and thirst here. Another difference lies in the sequence of symptoms –difficult urination, fever and thirst versus fever, thirst and difficult urination. To sum up, *Wu Ling San* (Five Ingredients Powder with Poria) is indicated for urination problem due to impaired qi transformation of the urinary bladder; *Zhu Ling Tang* (Polyporus Decoction) is indicated for micturition problem due to heat in the urinary bladder damaging yin.

[2] *Zhu Ling Tang* (Polyporus Decoction): A formula to nourish yin, clear heat and promote urination.

Interpretations

A superficial pulse, fever, thirst with a desire to drink water (due to heat accumulating in the urinary bladder) and difficult urination (in an externally contracted condition) should be treated with *Zhu Ling Tang* (Polyporus Decoction).

Zhu Ling Tang

[Ingredients]

猪苓	*zhū líng*	1 *liǎng*	Polyporus (skin removed)
茯苓	*fú líng*	1 *liǎng*	Poria
阿胶	*ē jiāo*	1 *liǎng*	Colla Corii Asini
滑石	*huá shí*	1 *liǎng*	Talcum
泽泻	*zé xiè*	1 *liǎng*	Rhizoma Alismatis

Decoct the four ingredients (except for *E Jiao*) in 4 *shēng* of water to get 3 *shēng*. Remove the dregs and add *E Jiao* to allow it to melt. Take 0.7 *shēng* when it is warm for each dose, 3 doses a day.

水气病脉证并治第十四
Chapter 14 Water Qi Retention—Pulses, Patterns and Treatment

Overview

This chapter discusses water qi retention, later known as body swelling or edema. It refers to internal retention of water fluids associated with dysfunctions of the lung, spleen and kidney. In this chapter, water qi is categorized into wind water, skin water, typical water, stone water and yellow sweats.

*****

[01] 师曰：病有风水，有皮水，有正水，有石水，有黄汗。风水〔1〕其脉自浮，外证骨节疼痛，恶风。皮水〔2〕其脉亦浮，外证胕肿，按之没指〔3〕，不恶风，其腹如鼓，不渴，当发其汗。正水〔4〕其脉沉迟，外证自喘。石水〔5〕其脉自沉，外证腹满不喘。黄汗〔6〕其脉沉迟，身发热，胸满，四肢头面肿，久不愈，必致痈脓。

Annotations

[1] *Feng Shui*: Wind water: A water qi disorder due to wind affecting the lung's function in regulating water metabolism. In addition to (exterior syndrome) symptoms including fever, chills, joint pain and a superficial, rapid pulse, it may cause facial puffiness and dysuria. It is characterized by a sudden onset of edema that starts from the face and eyes. It is similar to acute glomerulonephritis in modern medicine.

[2] *Pi Shui*: Skin water: A water qi disorder due to dysfunctions of the lung and spleen. It may cause generalized swelling, and in severe cases, ascites.

[3] *An Zhi Mo Zhi*: Pitting edema.

[4] *Zheng Shui*: Typical water: A water qi disorder due to yang deficiency of the spleen and kidney. It may cause shortness of breath or abdominal fullness.

[5] *Shi Shui*: Stone water: A water qi disorder due to kidney yang deficiency. It may cause lower abdominal hardness and fullness. The *Jin Gui Yao Lüè zhi Jie* (Direct Interpretation of the 'Essentials from the Golden Cabinet') states, "Typical water and stone water are both interior...the differene between the two is that typical water causes shortness of breath and the stone waterr does not.

[6] *Huang Han*: Yellow sweats: A condition that resembles water qi disorder due to water dampness transforming into heat. It is characterized by facial puffiness, limb swelling, yellowish sweats, dysuria, and over time, skin abscesses.

Interpretations

The Master said, "Water qi disorder is categorized into wind water, skin water, typical water, stone water and yellow sweats. For wind water, the pulse is superficial (water qi in the exterior); patients may present with joint pain and aversion to wind (fever), along with facial puffiness and dysuria. For skin water, the pulse is also superficial (water qi in the exterior); patients may present with generalized pitting edema, an absence of (exterior syndrome) symptoms such as aversion to wind, increased abdominal size like a drum, and absence of thirst. Wind water and skin water should both be treated by inducing sweating. For typical water, the pulse is deep and slow (water qi in the interior); patients may present with (abdominal fullness), shortness of breath and (dysuria). For stone water, the pulse is also deep; patients may present with lower abdominal fullness and distension but has no shortness of breath. For yellow sweats, the pulse is deep and slow; patients may present fever, yellowish sweats, chest fullness or distension, facial puffiness and limb swelling. Over time, patients may develop skin abscesses".

*****

[02] 脉浮而洪，浮则为风，洪则为气。风气相搏，风强则为隐疹[1]，身体为痒，痒为泄风[2]，久为痂癞。气强则为水，难以俛仰[3]，风气相击，身体洪肿，汗出乃愈。恶风则虚，此为风水[4]。不恶风者，小便通利，上焦有寒，其口多涎[5]，此为黄汗。

Annotations

[1] *Yin Zhen*: Literally means hidden rashes, similar to urticaria or hives. See chapter 5.

[2] *Xie Feng*: Literally means release of wind, referring to itchy skin rashes upon exposure to wind, which may, over time, form pus and scab.

[3] *Nan Yi Fu Yang*: Difficulty breathing.

[4] *Feng Qi Xiang Ji...Ci Wei Feng Shui*: Exposure to wind coupled with retained water qi may result in wind water

[5] *Shang Jiao You Han, Qi Kou Duo Xian*: Profuse saliva due to cold affecting the upper jiao (lung) (chapter 7). This seems irrelevant to "yellow sweats" in this context.

Interpretations

A superficial and surging pulse indicates combined exposure to wind and retained water qi, because a superficial pulse means wind and a surging pulse means excess water qi. Excess wind may cause itchy skin rashes. Over time, these rashes may form pus or scab. Excess water qi may cause water fluid retention and result in difficult breathing. Combined wind and water qi may cause severe edema, along with exterior-syndrome symptoms such as averstion to wind (fever). This is called wind water and can be treated with sweating method. An absence of aversion to wind, normal urination, and profuse saliva due to cold affecting the upper jiao indicate yellow sweats (*cold retained in the lung* makes more sense here).

*****

[03] 寸口脉沉滑者，中有水气，面目肿大，有热，名曰风水。视人之目裹上微拥，如蚕新卧起状[1]，其颈脉动，时时咳[2]，按其手足上，陷而不起者，风水。

Annotations

[1] *Mu Guo Shang Wei Yong, Ru Can Xin Wo Qi Fu*: Swollen eyelids with shiny, transparent skin that resembles silkworms before spinning the silk.

[2] *Jing Mai Dong, Shi Shi Ke*: Rapid pulsation of Renyin Pulse (ST 9 location: lateral to the Adam's apple, on the anterior border of m. sternocleidomastoideus, where the common carotid artery pulsates) (one of the eight ancient positions to feel the pulse) and frequent coughing.

Interpretations

A deep, slippery pulse at the *Cunkou* position indicates internal water retention. Facial puffiness coupled with fever (aversion to wind) is called wind water. Patients may present with mild eyelid swelling with shiny, transparent skin that resembles silkworms before spinning the silk. Rapid pulsations at Renyin (ST 9), frequent coughing and pitting edema on the feet when pressed with a finger. This is wind water.

*****

[04] 太阳病，脉浮而紧，法当骨节疼痛。反不疼，身体反重而酸，其人不渴，汗出即愈，此为风水[1]。恶寒者，此为极虚发汗得之。渴而不恶寒者，此为皮水，身肿而冷，状如周痹[2]。胸中室，不能食，反聚痛，暮躁不得眠，此为黄汗，痛在骨节[3]。

咳而喘，不渴者，此为脾胀。其状如肿〔4〕，发汗即愈。然诸病此者，渴而下利，小便数者，皆不可发汗。

Annotations

[1] *Tai Yang Bing...Ci Wei Feng Shui*: This is about the difference between Taiyang disease and wind water. Taiyang disease is characterized by fever, aversion to wind and joint pain. Wind water may also cause fever or aversion to cold but no joint pain, it is more characterized by body heaviness and swelling.

[2] *Ke Er Bu Wu Han Zhe...Zhaung Ru Zhou Bi*: This is about the difference between wind water and skin water. Wind water and skin water both have body swelling; however, wind water causes aversion to cold, whereas skin water does not. Skin water causes more severe body swelling than wind water. Just like generalized Bi-impediment (with migratory body pain due to cold-damp obstructing yang qi), skin water also causes aversion to cold because yang qi is obstructed.

[3] *Xiong Zhong Zhi...Tong Zai Gu Jie*: This is about the difference between wind water and yellow sweats. Yellow sweats may cause similar symptoms as wind water like body swelling, fever, sweating (see line 1 in this chapter) and joint pain; however, it also causes sweat stains in yellowish color that resembles phellodendron juice (see line 28 in this chapter), and in severe cases, chest tightness and pain, poor appetite, restlessness and insomnia.

[4] *Ke Er Chuan...Qi Zhuang Ru Zhong*: This is about the difference between wind water and lung distenstion (spleen distension is mentioned in the text). Wind water and lung distension can both cause edema and cough; however, lung distension is mainly characterized by cough and panting.

Interpretations

Presence of Taiyang disease symptoms (fever, chills, etc.) and a superficial, tight pulse; however, there is no joint pain but body heaviness (edema); and there is dysuria but no thirst (interior syndrome). All these symptoms can be treated with sweating method. This is called wind water. If patients experience averstion to cold, this is caused by deficieny plus sweating. Thirst without exterior-syndrome symptoms such as aversion to cold indicates skin water. It is characterized by body swelling, (dysuria) and a cold sensation on the skin as if yang qi is obstructed in generalized Bi-impediment. Presence of (fever, thirst, body swelling,) chest tightness and pain, poor appetite, restlessness at night and insomnia indicates yellow sweats. It also causes joint pain (and sweat stains in a yellowish color that resembles phellodendron juice). Presence of cough and panting without thirst indicates lung distension. It also causes body swelling, which can be treated by sweating method. Nonetheless, sweating method should not be used for thirst with diarrhea or frequent urination.

*****

[05] 里水〔1〕者，一身面目黄肿，其脉沉，小便不利，故令病水。假如小便自利，此亡津液，故令渴也。越婢加术汤〔2〕主之。方见下。

Annotations

[1] *Li Shui*: Interior water, i.e., skin water, as opposed to wind water (exterior).

[2] *Yue Bi Jia Zhu Tang* (Maidservant from Yue Decoction plus Atractylodes): A formula to induce sweating, promote urination and clear interior heat.

Interpretations

Patients with skin water may present with severe body swelling, a deep pulse, and dysuria, which in turn results in water retention. Thirst with normal urination is not water qi disorder but caused by insufficient body fluids. Water qi disorder should be treated with *Yue Bi Jia Zhu Tang* (Maidservant from Yue Decoction plus Atractylodes). For ingredients and usage of the formula, see chapter 5 (line 20).

*****

[06] 趺阳脉当伏，今反紧，本自有寒，疝瘕〔1〕，腹中痛，医反下之，下之即胸满短气。

[07] 趺阳脉当伏，今反数，本自有热，消谷〔2〕小便数，今反不利，此欲作水。

Annotations

[1] *Shan Jia*: Paiful abdominal masses due to cold retention and qi stagnation. The first word *Shan* suggests cold retention, where the second word *Jia* suggests qi stagnation. Here it refers to cold-related masses (see chapter 10).

[2] *Xiao Gu*: Fast hunger after eating food in wasting and thirsting disorder.

Interpretations

The pulse felt at Chongyang (ST 42) should be deep and hidden. When it is tight instead, it is caused by abdominal pain due to coagulated cold qi. The wrong use of draining downward method may cause chest fullness and shortness of breath.

The pulse felt at Chongyang (ST 42) should be deep and hidden. When it is rapid instead, it is caused by stomach heat. Patients may experience fast hunger after eating food and increased urination. Presence of dysuria is a sign indicative of water qi disorder (due to stomach heat).

*****

[08] 寸口脉浮而迟，浮脉则热，迟脉则潜，热潜相搏，名曰沉〔1〕。趺阳脉浮而数，浮脉即热，数脉即止，热止相搏，名曰

伏[2]。沉伏相搏，名曰水。沉则脉络虚，伏则小便难，虚难相搏，水走皮肤，即为水矣。

Annotations

[1] *Cun Kou Mai Fu Er Chi...Ming Yue Chen*: Stagnant heat in the upper jiao (lung).

[2] *Fu Yang Mai Fu Er Shuo...Ming Yue Fu*: Accumulated heat in the middle jiao (stomach).

Interpretations

A superficial and slow pulse felt at the *Cunkou* position indicates retained heat in the upper jiao (lung), and the heat lingers. A superficial and rapid pulse felt at Chongyang (ST 42) indicates accumulated heat in the middle jiao (stomach), and the heat persists. Retained heat in the lung and stomach may cause internal retention of water fluids. This, coupled with deficiency of collaterals, may result in difficult urination and cause water to flow over the skin, leading to water qi disorder.

*****

[09] 寸口脉弦而紧，弦则卫气不行，即恶寒，水不沾流，走于肠间[1]。

[10] 少阴脉紧而沉，紧则为痛，沉则为水[2]，小便即难。

Annotations

[1] *Cun Kou Mai Xian Er Jin...Zou Yu Chang Jian*: Cold affecting the lung may cause water retention in the abdomen.

[2] *Shao Yin Mai Jin Er Chen, Jin Ze Wei Tong, Chen Ze Wei Shui*: Cold in the kidney may cause water qi disorder.

Interpretations

A wiry and tight pulse felt at the *Cunkou* position indicates the *Wei*-defensive yang is blocked (by cold in the lung) and patients may experience aversion to cold. As cold impairs the lung's function in regulating the waterways, water fails to flow down to the urinary bladder but to the abdomen (causing ascites).

A tight and deep pulse felt at Taixi (KI 3) indicates body ache, edema and difficult urination.

*****

[11] 脉得诸沉〔1〕，当责有水，身体肿重。水病脉出〔2〕者，死。

Annotations

[1] *Mai De Zhu Chen*: The *Jin Gui Yao Lüè Shi Yi* (Interpretations of of the 'Essentials from the Golden Cabinet') states, "Water is a yin pathogen, so it often causes a deep pulse. Water flowing over the skin may obstruct the *Ying*-nutrients and *Wei*-defense and cause a deep pulse. Consequently, there is a saying goes that 'a deep pulse often indicates water'. However, internal yin cold also causes a deep pulse. A deep pulse coupled with body swelling and heaviness suggests water disorder".

[2] *Shui Bing Mai Chu*: A sudden change from a deep pulse into a superficial, rootless pulse is a life-threatening sign indicative of collapse of healthy qi and floating of deficiency yang.

Interpretations

A deep pulse might indicate water qi disorder; however, it's necessay to combine with body swelling and heaviness. A sudden change from a deep pulse into a superficial, rootless pulse with unresolved edema is a life-threatening sign.

*****

[12] 夫水病人，目下有卧蚕，面目鲜泽〔1〕，脉伏〔2〕，其人消渴〔3〕，病水腹大，小便不利，其脉沉绝〔4〕者，有水，可下之。

Annotations

[1] *Mian Mu Xian Ze*: Shiny, swollen face and eyes, especially the eyelids.

[2] *Mai Fu*: A severe deep pulse, indicating severe edema.

[3] *Xiao Ke*: Thirsting and wasting with increased thirst and excessive drinking.

[4] *Mai Chen Jue*: An extreme deep, hidden pulse, indicating excessive internal retention of water fluids.

Interpretations

Patients with water qi disorder first present with shiny, swollen eyelids like a sleeping silkworm and then have a deep, hidden pulse, along with increased thirst, excessive drinking, difficult urination, and increased abdominal size. Over time, they may have an extremely deep, hidden pulse due to excessive internal retention of water fluids. This can be treatd by drastic watwer-expelling method.

*****

[13] 问曰：病下利后，渴饮水，小便不利，腹满因肿者，何也？答曰：此法当病水。若小便自利及汗出者，自当愈。

Interpretations

Question: After diarrhea (due to spleen deficiency), patients drank a lot of water but developed difficult urination, abdominal fullness/distension and body swelling. Why is that?

Answer: This is water disorder. Patients can recover if they have normal urination (normal functioning of kidney qi in qi transformation) and sweats (normal functioning of lung qi in regulating waterways).

*****

[14] 心水者，其身重而少气，不得卧，烦而躁，其人阴肿〔1〕。

[15] 肝水者，其腹大，不能自转侧，胁下腹痛，时时津液〔2〕微生，小便续通。

[16] 肺水者，其身肿，小便难，时时鸭溏〔3〕。

[17] 脾水者，其腹大，四肢苦重，津液不生，但苦少气，小便难。

[18] 肾水者，其腹大，脐肿〔4〕腰痛，不得溺，阴下湿如牛鼻上汗〔5〕，其足逆冷，面反瘦。

Annotations

[1] *Yin Zhong*: Genital (labioscrotal) swelling.

[2] *Jin Ye*: It literally means body fluids; however, it refers to urine.

[3] *Ya Tang:* Loose stools like duck droppings.

[4] *Qi Zhong*: Outward bulging of the umbilicus. It is now known as umbilical hernia caused by increased intra-abdominal pressure.

[5] *Yin Xia Shi Ru Niu Bi Shang Han*: Wet scrotum like sweat on an ox's nose.

Interpretations

Water qi affecting the heart may cause generalized swelling, shortness of breath, an inability to lie flat, restlessness, and labioscrotal swelling.

Water qi affecting the liver may cause increased abdominal size (build-up fluid in the abdomen), abdominal fullness/distension, pain in the subcostal region, decreased urine volume, and intermittent urination (sometimes smooth, sometimes hesitant).

Water qi affecting the lung may cause generalized swelling, difficult urination, frequent loose stools like duck droppings.

Water qi affecting the spleen may cause increased abdominal size (build-up fluid in the abdomen), abdominal fullness, difficulty breathing, limb swelling and heaviness, and difficult urination.

Water qi affecting the kidney may cause increased abdominal size (build-up fluid in the abdomen), abdominal fullness/distension, outward bulging of the umbilicus, low back pain, urine retention, wet scrotum like sweat on an ox's nose, and cold, swollen limbs. In addition, patients appear emaciated.

*****

[19] 师曰：诸有水者，腰以下肿，当利小便；腰以上肿，当发汗乃愈。

Interpretations

The Master said, "For water qi disorders, noticeable swelling below the low back should be treated by inducing urination; noticeable swelling above the low back should be treated by inducing sweating".

*****

[20] 师曰：寸口脉沉而迟，沉则为水，迟则为寒，寒水相搏〔1〕。趺阳脉伏，水谷不化，脾气衰则鹜溏，胃气衰则身肿〔2〕。少阳脉卑，少阴脉细，男子则小便不利，妇人则经水不通〔3〕。经为血，血不利则为水，名曰血分。

Annotations

[1] *Cun Kou Mai Chen Er Chi...Han Shui Xiang Bo*: A pulse felt at the *Cunkou* position tells the condition of the upper jiao (lung): A ddep, slow pulse indicates cold water affecting the lung, i.e., water qi disorder

due to wind cold affecting the lung. It affects the qi phase, such as wind water.

[2] *Fu Yang Mai Fu...Wei Qi Shuai Ze Shen Zhong*: A pulse felt at Chongyang (ST 42) tells the condition of the middle jiao (spleen and stomach). A deep, hidden pulse indicates deficiency or water. Here it refers to water qi disorder caused by qi deficieny of the spleen and stomach. Patients may experience poor digestion, loose stools like duck droppings and body swelling like typical water.

[3] *Shao Yang Mai Bei...Fu Ren Ze Jing Shui Bu Tong*: A (Shaoyang) pulse felt at Qiuxu (GB 40) tells the conditions of the liver and gallbladder. A (Shaoyin) pulse felt at Taixi (KI 3) tells the condition of the kidney. A faint pulse at Qiuxu (GB 40) and a thready pulse at Taixi (KI 3) indicate water qi disorder due to deficiency of the liver and kidney. Women may experience absence of menstral period and men may experience difficult urination.

Interpretations

The Master said, "A deep and slow pulse felt at the *Cunkou* position indicates cold water affecting the upper jiao (lung) (water qi disorder in the qi phase). A hidden pulse felt at Chongyang (ST 42) indicates qi deficiency of the spleen and stomach. Patients may present with poor digestion, loose stools like duck droopings and body swelling (also water qi disorder in the qi phase). A faint, thready pulse at Qiuxu (GB 40) and Taixi (KI 3) indicates deficiency of the liver and kidney. Women experience absence of menstration and men experience difficult urination. Absence of menstruation may cause retention of water fluids. This is water qi disorder in the blood phase.

*****

[21] 问曰：病者苦水，面目身体四肢皆肿，小便不利。脉之，不言水，反言胸中痛，气上冲咽，状如炙肉〔1〕，当微咳喘，审如师言，其脉何类？

师曰：寸口脉沉而紧，沉为水，紧为寒，沉紧相搏，结在关元[2]。始时当微，年盛不觉。阳衰之后[3]，荣卫相干，阳损阴盛[4]，结寒微动。肾气上冲[5]，喉咽塞噎，胁下急痛。医以为留饮，而大下之[6]，气击不去，其病不除[7]。后重吐之，胃家虚烦[8]，咽燥欲饮水，小便不利，水谷不化，面目手足浮肿。又与葶苈丸下水，当时如小差，食饮过度，肿复如前，胸胁苦痛，象若奔[9]，其水扬溢，则浮咳喘逆[10]，当先攻击冲气，令止，乃治咳。咳止，其喘自差。先治新病，病当在后。

Annotations

[1] *Qi Shang Chong Yan, Zhuang Ru Zhi Rou*: Uprush of qi to the throat causes a sense of obstruction in the throat like a piece of roast meat stuck there.

[2] *Guan Yuan*: An acupuncture point on the Ren meridian (aka Conceptonal Vessel). Location: 3 cun below the umbilicus. Here it refers to the lower jiao.

[3] *Yang Shuai Zhi Hou*: Literally means after yang deficiency. Here it refers to after middle age.

[4] *Rong Wei Xiang Gan, Yang Sun Yin Shen*: Following the successive insufficiency of qi, blood, *Ying*-nutrients and *Wei*-defense, yang qi gradually declines and yin qi relatively prevails.

[5] *Jie Han Wei Dong, Shen Qi Shang Chong*: Cold water in the lower jiao (the kidney) starts to rush upward.

[6] *Yi Yi Wei Liu Yin, Er Da Xia Zhi*: Physicians may mistakenly assume this as internal retention of water fluids and treat it with water-expelling method.

[7] *Qi Ji Bu Qu, Qi Bing Bu Chu*: Cold qi was not removed, and healthy qi was impaired. As a result, there was no alleviation of the disease.

[8] *Hou Zhong Tu Zhi, Wei Jia Xu Fan*: Then physicians mistakenly use the method of inducing vomiting to treat the disease. This may impair stomach qi and cause deficiency heat symptoms.

[9] *Xiong Xie Ku Tong, Xiang Ruo Ben*: Intense pain in the subcostal region like a running piglet (see chapter 8).

[10] *Qi Shui Yang Yi, Ze Fu Ke Chuan Ni*: Water qi affecting the lung may cause cough and panting.

Interpretations

Question: A patient with severe water qi disorder experience difficult urination and swelling of the face, eyes and limbs. However, instead of water qi, the Master felt the pulse and said there was chest pain and uprush of qi into the throat causing a sensation of obstruction like a piece of roast meat stuck there, coupled with mild cough and panting. After talking to the patient, the Master is indeed correct. How do you analyze the pulse?

Answer: A deep, tight pulse was felt at the *Cunkou* position. Initially, cold water retained in the upper jiao and then gradually accumulated in the lower jiao. Young, strong patients were not aware of the condition because it was mild and asymptomatic. After middle age, along with the successive insufficiency of *Ying*-nutrients, *Wei*-defense, qi and blood, yang qi gradually declines and yin cold prevails. As a result, cold water retained in the lower jiao start to stir and rush upward, causing a sensation of obstruction in the throat and absence of contracture or pain in the subcostal region. The physician mistakenly assumed this is caused by internal retention of water fluids and treated with water-expelling method. However, the cold qi was not resolved and the healthy qi was damaged. Not surprisingly, the disease was not alleviated. Then the physician mistakenly treated with the method of inducing vomiting. This consumed stomach fluids and caused deficiency heat, a dry mouth and tongue, thirst with a desire to drink water, difficult urination, poor transformation of water and grains, and subsequently, swelling of the face, eyes and limbs. Then the physician prescribed *Ting Li Wan* (Lepidium Pill) to expel water. The swelling seems slightly alleviated, but returns after drinking water. In addition, the patient developed intense pain in the subcostal region like a running piglet. Over time, water qi continues to affect the lung and cause cough and panting. The correct treatment procedure should start with the uprush of cold qi, followed by cough and panting. In other words, the treatment should focus on the acute symptoms first and then the chronic condition (water qi).

*****

[22] 风水，脉浮，身重，汗出，恶风者，防己黄芪汤[1]主之。腹痛加芍药。

防己黄芪汤方：

防己一两黄芪一两一分白术三分甘草半两，炙 右锉。每服五钱匕，生姜四片、枣一枚，水盏半，煎取八分，去滓。温服，良久再服。

Annotations

[1] *Fang Ji Huang Qi Tang* (Stephania Root and Astragalus Decoction): A formula to supplement qi, secure the exterior, promote urination and drain dampness. It is discussed in chapter 2 for wind-dampness exterior deficiency syndrome. However, the dose of *Bai Zhu* (Rhizoma Atractylodis Macrocephalae) and aftercare methods are different.

Interpretations

Wind water with a superficial pulse, body heaviness (swelling), sweating, and aversion to wind should be treated with *Fang Ji Huang Qi Tang* (Stephania Root and Astragalus Decoction). Add *Shao Yao* (Radix Paeoniae) for abdominal pain.

Fang Ji Huang Qi Tang

[Ingredients]

防己	*fáng jǐ*	1 *liǎng*	Radix Stephaniae Tetrandrae
甘草	*gān cǎo*	0.5 *liǎng*	Radix et Rhizoma Glycyrrhizae (stir-fried)
白术	*bái zhú*	3 *fēn*	Rhizoma Atractylodis Macrocephalae
黄芪	*huáng qí*	11 *fēn*	Radix Astragali

Grind the above ingredients into a powder. Take five coin-spoonfuls for each dose and add four slices of fresh ginger and one jujube fruit to one and a half cups of water to get eight *fen*. Remove the dregs and take the decoction when it is warm. Take the second dose after a couple of hours.

*****

[23] 风水，恶风，一身悉肿，脉浮，不渴，续自汗出，无大热〔1〕，越婢汤〔2〕主之。

越婢汤方：

麻黄六两石膏半斤生姜三两大枣十五枚甘草二两　右五味，以水六升，先煮麻黄，去上沫，内诸药，煮取三升。分温三服。恶风〔3〕者加附子一枚炮。风水〔4〕加术四两《古今录验》。

Annotations

[1] *Bu Ke, Xu Zi Han Chu, Wu Da Re*: *Bu Ke* here literally means absence of thirst; however, it actually means thirst. Thirst with persistent sweating is caused by interior excess heat. *Wu Da Re* means there is no noticeable fever (due to sweating).

[2] *Yue Bi Tang* (Maidservant from Yue Decoction): A formula to resolve water qi and clear interior heat. For yang deficiency with aversion to cold, add *Fu Zi* (Radix Aconiti Lateralis Praeparata) to warm meridians and secure the exterior; for skin water, add *Bai Zhu* (Rhizoma Atractylodis Macrocephalae) to enhance the effect of draining dampness.

[3] *Wu Feng*: Literally means aversion to wind; actually it refers to aversion to cold.

[4] *Feng Shui*: Literally means wind water; actually it refers to skin water.

Interpretations

Wind (skin) water with aversion to wind (cold), body swelling, a superficial pulse, thirst, persistent sweating and absence of high-grade fever (but intense interior heat) should be treated with *Yue Bi Tang* (Maidservant from Yue Decoction).

Yue Bi Tang

[Ingredients]

麻黄	*má huáng*	6 *liǎng*	Herba Ephedrae
石膏	*shí gāo*	0.5 *jīn*	Gypsum Fibrosum
生姜	*shēng jiāng*	3 *liǎng*	Rhizoma Zingiberis Recens
大枣	*dà zǎo*	15 pieces	Fructus Jujubae
甘草	*gān cǎo*	2 *liǎng*	Radix et Rhizoma Glycyrrhizae

Decoct *Ma Huang* (Herba Ephedrae) first in 6 *shēng* of water, skim off the foam and add the rest of the ingredients to get 3 *shēng*. Divide into three doses and take when it is warm. For aversion to cold, add 1 piece of *Fu Zi* (Radix Aconiti Lateralis Praeparata). For skin water, add 4 *liǎng* of *Bai Zhu* (Rhizoma Atractylodis Macrocephalae) [the *Gu Jin Lu Yan* (Ancient and Modern Records of Proven Formulas)].

*****

[24] 皮水为病，四肢肿，水气在皮肤中，四肢聂聂动〔1〕者防己茯苓汤〔2〕主之。

防己茯苓汤方：

防己三两黄芪三两桂枝三两茯苓六两甘草二两　右五味，以水六升，煮取二升。分温三服。

Annotations

[1] *Si Zhi Nie Nie Dong*: Involuntary twitching of the limbs. It is caused by limb swelling and retained water obstructing yang qi.

[2] *Fang Ji Fu Ling Tang* (Stephania Root and Poria Decoction): A formula to supplement qi, promote urination, unblock yang, and eliminate the impediment. It shares similar ingredients with *Fang Ji Huang Qi Tang* (Stephania Root and Astragalus Decoction), but use a larger dose of *Fang Ji* (Radix Stephaniae Tetrandrae), *Huang Qi* (Radix Astragali) and *Fu Ling* (Poria) to resolve the severe swelling.

Interpretations

Skin water with noticeable limb swelling, retained water qi in the skin and involuntary twitching of the hands and feet should be treated with *Fang Ji Fu Ling Tang* (Stephania Root and Poria Decoction).

Fang Ji Fu Ling Tang

[Ingredients]

防己	*fáng jǐ*	3 *liǎng*	Radix Stephaniae Tetrandrae
黄芪	*huáng qí*	3 *liǎng*	Radix Astragali
桂枝	*guì zhī*	3 *liǎng*	Ramulus Cinnamomi
茯苓	*fú líng*	6 *liǎng*	Poria
甘草	*gān cǎo*	2 *liǎng*	Radix et Rhizoma Glycyrrhizae (stir-fried)

Decoct the five ingredients in 6 *shēng* of water and get 2 *shēng*. Divide into three doses and take when it is warm.

*****

[25] 里水，越婢加术汤〔1〕主之；甘草麻黄汤〔2〕亦主之。

越婢加术汤方见上，于内加白术四两，又见脚气中。

甘草麻黄汤方：

甘草二两麻黄四两　右二味。以水五升，先煮麻黄，去上沫，内甘草，煮取三升。温服一升，重复汗出。不汗，再服，慎风寒。

Annotations

[1] *Yue Bi Jia Zhu Tang* (Maidservant from Yue Decoction plus Atractylodis Macrocephalae): A formula for skin water with interior heat (see line 23).

[2] *Gan Cao Ma Huang Tang* (Licorice and Ephedra Decoction): A formula to induce sweating and promote urination. It is used for mild skin water without interior heat.

Interpretations

Skin water with interior heat can be treated with *Yue Bi Jia Zhu Tang* (Maidservant from Yue Decoction plus Atractylodis Macrocephalae); skin water without interior heat (patients may present with mild edema, difficult urination and absence of sweating) can be treated with *Gan Cao Ma Huang Tang* (Licorice and Ephedra Decoction).

For ingredients and usage of *Yue Bi Jia Zhu Tang* (Maidservant from Yue Decoction plus Atractylodis Macrocephalae), see *Yue Bi Tang* (Maidservant from Yue Decoction) (line 23 in this chapter) plus 4 *liǎng* of *Bai Zhu* (Rhizoma Atractylodis Macrocephalae) (the formula is also mentionedin chapter 5).

Gan Cao Ma Huang Tang

[Ingredients]

甘草	*gān cǎo*	2 *liǎng*	Radix et Rhizoma Glycyrrhizae
麻黄	*má huáng*	4 *liǎng*	Herba Ephedrae

Decoct *Ma Huang* (Herba Ephedrae) first in 5 *shēng* of water, skim off the foam and add *Gan Cao* (Radix et Rhizoma Glycyrrhizae) to get 3 *shēng*. Take 1 *shēng* for each dose when it is warm. Sweating is good for the recovery. If no sweating, take another dose and stay away from wind cold.

*****

[26] 水之为病〔1〕，其脉沉小，属少阴〔2〕；浮者为风〔3〕。无水虚胀者为气〔4〕。水，发其汗即已〔5〕。脉沉者宜麻黄附子汤〔6〕；浮者宜杏子汤〔7〕。

麻黄附子汤方：

麻黄三两甘草二两附子一枚，炮右三味，以水七升，先煮麻黄，去上沫，内诸药，煮取二升半。温服八分〔8〕，日三服。杏子汤方未见，恐是麻黄杏仁甘草石膏汤。

Annotations

[1] *Shui Zhi Wei Bing*: Typical water and wind water.

[2] *Mai Chen Xiao, Shu Shao Yin*: A deep, small pulse indicates interior. *Shao Yin* here refers to the kidney. Here it refers to typical water due to kidney yang deficiency.

[3] *Fu Zhe Wei Feng*: A superficial pulse indicates exterior. Here it refers to wind water upon exposure to wind.

[4] *Wu Shui Xu Zhang Zhe Wei Qi*: Abdominal fullness due to qi stagnation instead of the build-up of water.

[5] *Shui, Fa Qi Han Ji Yi*: Wind water and typical water can both be treated by sweating. This suggests that abdominal fullness due to qi stagnation cannot be treated by inducing sweating.

[6] *Ma Huang Fu Zi Tang* (Ephedra and Aconite Decoction): A formula to warm meridians and induce sweating. It is also used for typical water.

[7] *Xing Zi Tang* (Apricot Kernel Decoction): No detailed information. It could be *Ma Huang Xing Ren Gan Cao Shi Gao Tang* (Ephedra, Apricot Kernel, Gypsum and Licorice Decoction).

[8] *Ba Fen*: It should be *Ba Ge* (=0.8 *shēng*).

Interpretations

Water qi disorder with a deep, small pulse indicates typical water due to kidney yang deficiency. Water qi disorder with a superficial pulse indicates wind water upon exposure to wind. Abdominal fullness without build-up fluids is caused by qi stagnation (and cannot be treated by inducing sweating). Typical water and wind water can both be treated by inducing sweating. A deep pulse indicates typical water and should be treated with *Ma Huang Fu Zi Tang* (Ephedra and Aconite Decoction). A superficial pulse indicates wind water and should be treated with *Xing Zi Tang* (Apricot Kernel Decoction).

Ma Huang Fu Zi Tang

[Ingredients]

麻黄	*má huáng*	3 *liǎng*	Herba Ephedrae
甘草	*gān cǎo*	2 *liǎng*	Radix et Rhizoma Glycyrrhizae
附子	*fù zǐ*	1 piece	Radix Aconiti Lateralis Praeparata

Decoct *Ma Huang* (Herba Ephedrae) first in 7 *shēng* of water, skim off the foam and add the rest of the ingredients to get 2.5 *shēng*. Take 0.8 *shēng* for each dose when it is warm, 3 doses a day.

There was no detailed information of *Xing Zi Tang* (Apricot Kernel Decoction). It could be *Ma Huang Xing Ren Gan Cao Shi Gao Tang* (Ephedra, Apricot Kernel, Gypsum and Licorice Decoction).

*****

[27] 厥而皮水〔1〕者，蒲灰散〔2〕主之。方见消渴中。

Annotations

[1] *Jue Er Pi Shui*: Skin water with cold limbs due to water obstructing yang qi.

[2] *Pu Hui San* (Typhae Pollen Powder): A formula to promote urination and unblock yang. For more information, see chapter 13 (line 11).

Interpretations

Skin water (generalized edema, difficult urination and a deep pulse) with cold limbs should be treated with *Pu Hui San* (Typhae Pollen Powder). The formula is discussed in chapter 13 (line 11).

*****

[28] 问曰：黄汗〔1〕之为病，身体肿一作重，发热，汗出而渴，状如风水，汗沾衣，色正黄如蘗汁〔2〕，脉自沉，何从得之？师曰：以汗出入水中浴，水从汗孔入〔3〕得之，宜芪芍桂酒汤〔4〕主之。

黄芪芍药桂枝苦酒汤方：

黄芪五两芍药三两桂枝三两　　右三味，以苦酒〔5〕一升，水七升，相和，煮取三升。温服一升，当心烦，服至六七日乃解。若心烦不止者，以苦酒阻故也。一方用美酒醯〔6〕代苦酒。

Annotations

[1] *Huang Han*: Yellow sweats due to damp heat accumulating in the surface of the body (see line 1 in this chapter).

[2] *Nie Zhi*: Here it refers to phellodendron juice.

[3] *Han Chu Ru Shui Zhong Yu, Shui Cong Han Kong Ru*: Yellow sweats occurs as a result of taking cold showers upon sweating and the water dampness enters the body through the pores in the skin.

[4] *Qi Shao Gui Jiu Tang* (Astragalus, Peony, Cinnamon Twig, and Vinegar Decoction): A formula to supplement qi, resolve dampness and harmonize the *Ying*-nutrients and *Wei*-defense.

[5] *Ku Jiu*: Rice vinegar

[6] *Mei Jiu Xi*: Red vinegar.

Interpretations

Question: Yellow sweats may cause body swelling (body heaviness in other texts), fever, sweating, and thirst. These symptoms are similar to wind water. The sweat stains appear yellowish like phellodendron juice. The pulse is deep in patients with yellow sweats. How did this condition happen?

Answer: It occurs as a result of taking cold showers upon sweating and the water dampness enters the body through the pores in the skin. It should be treated with *Qi Shao Gui Jiu Tang* (Astragalus, Peony, Cinnamon Twig, and Vinegar Decoction).

Qi Shao Gui Jiu Tang

[Ingredients]

黄芪	*huáng qí*	5 *liǎng*	Radix Astragali
芍药	*sháo yào*	3 *liǎng*	Radix Paeoniae
桂枝	*guì zhī*	3 *liǎng*	Ramulus Cinnamomi

Decoct the three ingredients in 1 *shēng* of rice vinegar and 7 *shēng* of water to get 3 *shēng*. Take 1 *shēng* a day when it is warm. Patients may feel a hot sensation in the stomach. The sensation normally resolves in 6 or 7 days; however, it may persist because of the use of rice vinegar (the red vinegar was used in another formula).

*****

[29] 黄汗之病，两胫自冷；假令发热，此属历节[1]。食已汗出，又身常暮盗汗出者，此劳气也。若汗出已，反发热者，久久其身必甲错。发热不止者，必生恶疮[2]。

若身重，汗出已，辄轻者，久久必身，即胸中痛，又从腰以上必汗出，下无汗，腰髋弛痛，如有物在皮中状。剧者不能食，身疼重，烦躁，小便不利，此为黄汗。桂枝加黄芪汤[3]主之。

桂枝加黄芪汤方：

桂枝芍药各三两甘草二两生姜三两大枣十二枚黄芪二两　右六味，以水八升，煮取三升。温服一升。须臾，饮热稀粥一升余，以助药力，温服，取微汗。若不汗，更服。

Annotations

[1] *Huang Han Zhi Bing…Ci Shu Li Jie*: Yellow sweats may cause joint pain (see line 4 in this chapter). Joint disorders are characterized by pain, warmth and impaired flexion and extension of the joints. The difference between the two lies in the "warmth" in joint disorders and "leg coldness" in yellow sweats.

[2] *Shi Yi Han Chu…Bi Sheng E Chuang*: Yellow sweats is characterized by yellowish sweats and fever. Deficiency exhaustion is characterized by night sweats and low-grade fever. The difference between the two lies in "rough, scaly skin" in deficiency exhaustion and "skin boils" in yellow sweats (see line 1 in this chapter).

[3] *Gui Zhi Jia Huang Qi Tang* (Cinnamon Twig Decoction plus Astragalus): A formula to harmonize the *Ying*-nutrients and *Wei*-defense, unblock yang and drain dampness. This formula and *Qi Shao Gui Jiu Tang* (Astragalus, Peony, Cinnamon Twig, and Vinegar Decoction) are both indicated for yellow sweats; however, this formula uses *Gui Zhi* (Ramulus Cinnamomi) as the monarch ingredient to release the exterior, drain dampness and unblock yang, whereas *Qi Shao Gui Jiu Tang* used *Huang Qi* (Radix Astragali) as the monarch ingredient to tonify qi.

Interpretations

Although yellow sweats may cause joint pain, patients have leg coldness. A warm sensation around the joint indicates a joint problem. Sweating after meals, especially night sweats, fever that cannot be resolved by sweats, and rough, scaly skin are manifestations indicative of deficiency exhaustion. Yellow sweats may cause persistent fever and skin sores or boils. In addition, yellow sweats also cause body swelling and heaviness that slightly alleviate after sweating. Over time, patients may experience muscle cramps, and chest tightness or pain. Other symptoms of yellow sweats include sweats on the upper body only, and a dull pain in the low back and hip as if there is something stuck in the skin. In severe cases, body ache, poor appetite, restlessness and difficult urination may be present. Yellow sweats should be treated with *Gui Zhi Jia Huang Qi Tang* (Cinnamon Twig Decoction plus Astragalus).

Gui Zhi Jia Huang Qi Tang

[Ingredients]

桂枝	*guì zhī*	3 *liǎng*	Ramulus Cinnamomi
芍药	*sháo yào*	3 *liǎng*	Radix Paeoniae
甘草	*gān cǎo*	2 *liǎng*	Radix et Rhizoma Glycyrrhizae
生姜	*shēng jiāng*	3 *liǎng*	Rhizoma Zingiberis Recens
大枣	*dà zǎo*	12 pieces	Fructus Jujubae
黄芪	*huáng qí*	2 *liǎng*	Radix Astragali

Decoct the six ingredients in 8 *shēng* of water to get 3 *shēng*. Take 1 *shēng* when it is warm, and after a while, eat more than 1 *shēng* of warm congree to help with the efficacy. Sweating is good for the recovery. If no sweating, take another dose.

*****

[30] 师曰：寸口脉迟而涩，迟则为寒，涩为血不足。趺阳脉微而迟，微则为气，迟则为寒〔1〕。寒气不足，则手足逆冷。手足逆冷，则荣卫不利。荣卫不利，则腹满胁鸣相逐。气转膀胱，荣卫俱劳。阳气不通即身冷，阴气不通即骨疼。阳前通则恶寒，阴前通则痹不仁〔2〕。阴阳相得，其气乃行，大气一转，其气乃散。实则失气，虚则遗尿〔3〕，名曰气分。

Annotations

[1] *Cun Kou Mai Chi Er Se...Chi Ze Wei Han*: Pathogenesis of qi phase disorder—a deep pulse indicates cold qi; a hesitant pulse indicates deficiency of qi and blood.

[2] *Han Qi Bu Zu...Ze Bi Bu Ren*: Symptoms of qi phase disorder—yang qi deficiency causes cold hands and feet. Obstruction of *Ying*-nutrients and *Wei*-defense causes abdominal fullness and bowel sounds. Obstruction of yin and yang causes aversion to cold and numbness.

[3] *Yin Yang Xiang De...Xu Ze Yi Niao*: Treatment strategy of qi phase disorder: harmonizes yin and yang to unblock qi. Normal functioning of zong-pectoral qi helps to resolve water qi. Abdominal fullness can be treated by promoting bowel movements; and water fluid can be treated by promoting urination.

Interpretations

The Master said, "The pulse is deep and hesitant at the *Cunkou* position—a deep pulse indicates cold qi, and a hesitant pulse indicates deficiency of qi and blood. The pulse is faint and slow at Chongyang (ST 42)—a faint pulse indicates qi deficiency and a slow pulse indicates cold qi. Yang qi deficiency and obstruction of *Ying*-nutrients and *Wei*-defense may cause cold hands and feet, abdominal fullness and bowel sounds. Pathogenic qi entering the urinary bladder may impair its qi transformation and affect both the *Ying*-nutrients and *Wei*-defense. Obstruction of yin and yang may cause chills and bone pain, followed by aversion to cold and numbness. The treatment strategy is to harmonize yin and yang and move qi. Normal functioning of the zong-pectoral qi helps to resolve water qi. The efficacy can be achieved by promoting bowel and bladder movements. This is called qi phase disorder.

*****

[31] 气分，心下坚，大如盘，边如旋杯〔1〕，水饮所作〔2〕，桂枝去芍加麻辛附子汤〔3〕主之。

桂枝去芍药加麻黄细辛附子汤方：

桂枝三两生姜三两甘草二两大枣十二枚 麻黄细辛各二两附子一枚，炮 右七味，以水七升，煮麻黄，去上沫，内诸药，煮取二升。分温三服。当汗出，如虫行皮中，即愈。

Annotations

[1] *Xin Xia Jian, Da Ru Pan, Bian Ru Xuan Bei*: Hardness below the heart: the hard area is as big as a plate with edges like an inverted cup.

[2] *Shui Yin Suo Zuo*: It is caused by build-up of water fluid.

[3] *Gui Zhi Qu Shao Yao Jia Ma Huang Xi Xin Fu Zi Tang* (Cinnamon Twig Decoction Minus Peony plus Ephedra, Asarum ad Aconite): A formula to warm yang and promote urination.

Interpretations

In addition to common symptoms, water fluid in the qi phase may cause hardness below the heart and the hard area is as big as a plate with edges like an inverted cup. This is caused by the build-up of water fluid and should be treated with *Gui Zhi Qu Shao Yao Jia Ma Huang Xi Xin Fu Zi Tang* (Cinnamon Twig Decoction minus Peony plus Ephedra, Asarum ad Aconite).

Gui Zhi Qu Shao Yao Jia Ma Huang Xi Xin Fu Zi Tang

[Ingredients]

桂枝	*guì zhī*	3 *liǎng*	Ramulus Cinnamomi
生姜	*shēng jiāng*	3 *liǎng*	Rhizoma Zingiberis Recens
甘草	*gān cǎo*	2 *liǎng*	Radix et Rhizoma Glycyrrhizae
麻黄	*má huáng*	2 *liǎng*	Herba Ephedrae
细辛	*xì xīn*	2 *liǎng*	Radix et Rhizoma Asari
大枣	*dà zǎo*	12 pieces	Fructus Jujubae
附子	*fù zǐ*	1 piece	Radix Aconiti Lateralis Praeparata

Decoct *Ma Huang* (Herba Ephedrae) first in 7 *shēng* of water, skim off the foam and add the rest of the ingredients to get 2 *shēng*. Divide into three doses and take when it is warm. Sweating is good for the recovery. A sensation that resembles that of small insects crawling on or under the skin indicates a full recovery.

*****

[32] 心下坚，大如盘，边如旋盘〔1〕，水饮所作，枳术汤〔2〕主之。

枳术汤方：

枳实七枚白术二两　右二味，以水五升，煮取三升。分温三服。腹中软即当散也。

Annotations

[1] *Xin Xia Jian, Da Ru Pan, Bian Ru Xuan pan*: Hardness below the heart: the hard area is as big as plate with edges like an inverted plate.

[2] *Zhi Zhu Tang* (Immature Bitter Orange and Atractylodes Macrocephala Decoction): A formula to move qi, resolve masses, fortify the spleen, and promote urination.

Interpretations

Water fluid in the qi phase may cause hardness below the heart and the hard area is as big as a plate with edges like an inverted plate. This is caused by the build-up of water fluid and should be treated with *Zhi Zhu Tang* (Immature Bitter Orange and Atractylodes Macrocephala Decoction).

Zhi Zhu Tang

[Ingredients]

枳实	*zhǐ shí*	7 pieces	Fructus Aurantii Immaturus
白术	*bái zhú*	2 *liǎng*	Rhizoma Atractylodis Macrocephalae

Decoct the two ingredients in 5 *shēng* of water to get 3 *shēng*. Divide into three doses and take when it is warm. The sensation of hardness turning into softness indicates resolved water qi.

*****

Annex formula *Wai Tai Fang Ji Huang Qi Tang* (Stephania Root and Astragalus Decoction)

附方

《外台》防己黄芪汤，治风水，脉浮为在表，其人或头汗出，表无他病[1]。病者但下重[2]，从腰以上为和，腰以下当肿及阴[3]，难以屈伸。方见风湿中。

Annotations

[1] *Biao Wu Ta Bing*: No exterior-syndrome symptoms such as fever or chills.

[2] *Dan Xia Zhong*: Edema and heaviness below the low back.

[3] *Zhong Ji Yin*: Genital swelling.

Interpretations

The *Fang Ji Huang Qi Tang* (Stephania Root and Astragalus Decoction) in the *Wai Tai Mi Yao* (Arcane Essentials from the Imperial Library) can be used to treat wind water (exterior deficiency syndrome) with a superficial pulse and water qi in the exterior. Some patients may have sweats on the head but no exterior-syndrome symptoms (like fever). Patients may present with edema and heaviness below the low back with impaired flexion and extension. Some may even have genital swelling but no swelling above the low back (the formula is discussed in chapter 2).

黄疸病脉证并治第十五
Chapter 15 Jaundice—Pulses, Patterns and Treatment

Overview

This chapter discusses jaundice—a condition characterized by a yellowish discoloration of the eyes, skin and urine. In this chapter, jaundice is categorized into four types—grain jaundice, alcohol jaundice, female deficiency jaundice and black jaundice.

*****

[01] 寸口脉浮而缓，浮则为风，缓则为痹。痹非中风，四肢苦烦〔1〕，脾色必黄，瘀热以行。

Annotations

[1] *Bi Fei Zhong Feng, Si Zhi Ku Fan*: Jaundice results from exposure to wind and internal build-up of damp heat. It is different from Bi-impediment with joint pain.

Interpretations

The pulse is superficial and delayed at the *Cunkou* position. A superifical pulse indicates exposure to wind and a delayed pulse indicates dampness. However, combined wind and dampness do not cause bone or joint pain. Damp heat retained in the spleen causes yellowish discoloration of the skin and affects all over the body through blood circulation (leading to jaundice).

*****

[02] 趺阳脉紧而数，数则为热，热则消谷，紧则为寒，食即为满。尺脉浮为伤肾，趺阳脉紧为伤脾〔1〕。风寒相搏，食谷即眩，谷气不消，胃中苦浊，浊气下流，小便不通，阴被其寒，热流膀胱，身体尽黄〔2〕，名曰谷疸〔3〕。额上黑〔4〕，微汗出，手足中热，薄暮即发，膀胱急〔5〕，小便自利，名曰女劳疸〔6〕；腹如水状不治〔7〕。心中懊而热〔8〕，不能食，时欲吐，名曰酒疸〔9〕。

Annotations

[1] *Chi Mai Fu Wei Shang Shen, Fu Yang Mai Jin Wei Shang Pi*: A superficial pulse at the *Chi* position indicates kidney deficiency, the cause of female deficiency jaundice. A tight pulse at Chongyang (ST 42) indicates dampness due to spleen deficiency, the cause of grain jaundice. This tells the difference between female deficiency jaundice and grain jaundice in causative factor and location.

[2] *Yin Bei Qi Han…Shen Ti Jin Huang*: Retained cold dampness in the spleen may, over time, transform into heat. Then the damp heat flows down to the urinary bladder and impair the qi transformation of the urinary bladder, leading to difficult urination and yellowish discoloration of the skin. The first word *Yin* here fers to the spleen.

[3] *Gu Dan*: Grain jaundice due to damp heat in the spleen and stomach. It is characterized by poor digestion, difficult urination and yellowish discoloration of the skin. It is similar to hepatocellular jaundice in modern medicine.

[4] *E Shang Hei*: A dark complexion.

[5] *Pang Guang Ji*: Lower abdominal contracture.

[6] *Nǚ Lao Dou*: Female deficiency jaundice due to kidney deficiency. It is characterized by a dark complexion, mild sweating, feverish sensations in the palms, soles and chest, aftertoon fever, and lower abdominal contracture with normal urination.

[7] *Fu Ru Shui Zhuang Bu Zhi*: Build-up of water fluids in the abdomen in late stage of female deficiency jaundice. Difficult urination in this stage is difficult to treat.

[8] *Xin Zhong Ao Er Re*: A burning sensation in the stomach.

[9] *Jiu Dan*: Alcohol jaundice due to long-term intake of alcohol. It is characterized by a burning sensation in the stomach, poor appetite, nausea, vomiting, yellowish discoloration of the skin and difficult urination.

Interpretations

A tight, rapid pulse at Chongyang (ST 42) indicates heat in the spleen and stomach. Stomach heat increases digestion; however, cold dampness retains in the spleen and causes poor digestion, resulting in abdominal fullness and distension. A superficial pulse at the *Chi* position indicates kidney deficiency (female deficiency jaundice). A tight pulse at Chongyang (ST 42) indicates damp heat in the spleen and stomach (grain jaundice). Exposure to wind, coupled with heat transformed from dampness in the spleen may cause poor digestion and obstruct clear yang, leading to dizziness. Damp heat may flow down to the urinary bladder and impair its qi transformation, leading to difficult urination and yellowish discoloration of the skin. This is grain jaundice. A dark complexion, mild sweating, feverish sensations in the palms, soles and chest, afternoon fever, lower abdominal contracture and a normal urination are symptoms indicative of female deficiency jaundice. The presence of build-up the water fluids in the abdomen (late stage) is difficult to treat. A burning sensation in the stomach (due to long-term intake of alcohol), poor appetite and frequent nausea and vomiting (with yellowish discoloration of the skin) are symptoms indicative of alcohol jaundice.

*****

[03] 阳明病，脉迟者，食难用饱。饱则发烦头眩，小便必难，此欲作谷疸。虽下之，腹满如故。所以然者，脉迟故也。

Interpretations

Patients with yangming disease (excess heat in the stomach) but a slow pulse (due to cold dampness impairing the spleen's function in transformation and transportation of water and grain) may experience an inability to eat a full meal; otherwise they feel abdominal discomfort (damp retained in the middle jiao), dizziness (due to ascending of dampness to obstruct clear yang), difficult urination (due to dampness flowing downward to the urinary bladder). These are the signs indicative of grain jaundice. Abdominal fullness and distension cannot be resolved by draining downward method, because a slow pulse indicates cold dampness in the spleen.

*****

[04] 夫病酒黄疸，必小便不利，其候心中热[1]，足下热[2]是其证也。

Annotations

[1] *Xin Zhong Re*: A burning sensation in the heart.
[2] *Zu Xia Re*: Feverish sensations in the palms, soles and chest.

Interpretations

Alcohol jaundice (yellowish discoloration of the skin) may cause difficult urination. Other distinctive symptoms include a burning sensation in the heart and feverish sensations in the palms, soles and chest.

*****

[05] 酒黄疸者，或无热，请言了，腹满欲吐，鼻燥。其脉浮者先吐之；沉弦者先下之。

Interpretations

Some patients with alcohol jaundice may have a calm mind and clear speech with a burning sensation in the stomach; however, they experience abdominal fullness, nausea and dry nose. A superficial pulse with nausea and a dry nose should first be treated by inducing vomiting. A deep, wiry pulse with abdominal fullness should first be treated by draining downward method.

*****

[06] 酒疸，心中热，欲呕者，吐之愈。

Interpretations

In addition to yellow discoloration of the skin and difficult urination, alchol jaundice may also cause a burning sensation in the stomach and nausea. This can be treated by inducing vomiting.

*****

[07] 酒疸下之，久久为黑疸[1]，目青面黑，心中如啖蒜齑状[2]，大便正黑，皮肤爪之不仁[3]，其脉浮弱，虽黑微黄，故知之。

Annotations

[1] *Hei Dan*: Further development of alcohol jaundice. It is characterized by a dark bluish complexion, a burning sensation in the stomach, black stools and skin numbness.

[2] *Xin Zhong Ru Dan Suan Ji Zhuang*: A severe burning sensation in the stomach like eating mashed garlic.

[3] *Pi Fu Zhua Zhi Bu Ren*: Skin numbness when scratched.

Interpretations

When alcohol jaundice was mistakenly treated by draining downward method, it may gradually develop into black jaundice. Patients may present with a dark bluish complexion, a severe burning sensation in the stomach like eating mashed garlic, skin numbness when scratched, and a superficial, weak pulse. The presence of yellowness in the dark complexion indicates this condition develops from (alcohol) jaundice.

*****

[08] 师曰：病黄疸，发热烦喘，胸满口燥[1]者，以病发时火劫其汗，两热所得[2]。然黄家所得，从湿得之。一身尽发热而黄，肚热[3]。热在里，当下之。

Annotations

[1] *Fa Re Fan Chuan, Xiong Man Kou Zao*: Fever is a common symptom of jaundice; severe panting, chest tightness and a dry mouth and tongue are caused by the wrong use of inducing sweating with fire (warming needling, fumination, hot compression, etc).

[2] *Huo Jie Qi Han, Liang Re Suo De*: To induce sweating with fire is to add heat to the pre-existing damp heat.

[3] *Du Re:* Heat in the interior, highlighting that there is more interior heat than exterior heat.

Interpretations

The Master said, "In addition to fever, presence of severe panting, chest tightness and a dry mouth and tongue in jaundice are caused by the wrong use of inducing sweating with fire (such as warming needle, fumigation, hot compression, etc.) at its onset. The fire (that induces sweating) combined with the pre-existing heat aggravated the condition. Associated with damp heat, jaundice causes fever and yellowish discoloration of the skin. The interior excess heat in jaundice should be treated with the draining downward method.

*****

[09] 脉沉，渴欲饮水，小便不利者，皆发黄。

Interpretations

A deep pulse (indicates an interior syndrome), thirst with a desire to drink water (due to interior heat), difficult urination (due to dampness retention) and yellowish discoloration of the skin (retained damp heat).

*****

[10] 腹满〔1〕，舌痿黄〔2〕，燥不得睡〔3〕，属黄家。舌痿疑作身痿。

Annotations

[1] *Fu Man*: Abdominal fullness and distension (due to build-up of water fluids).

[2] *She Wei Huang*: A small tongue with yellow, greasy coating.

[3] *Zao Bu De Shui:* Restlessness or delirium. This is later known as acute aggravation of jaundice, similar to severe hepatitis (necrotizing hepatitis).

Interpretations

Abdominal fullness due to build-up of water fluids, a smaller tongue with yellow, greasy coating (dark, ginger-like yellowish skin in other texts), restlessless, and sleeplessness are symptoms indicative of severe jaundice.

*****

[11] 黄疸之病，当以十八日为期。治之十日以上瘥。反极为难治。

Interpretations

Normally jaundice lasts approximately 18 days. It should respond to treatment after 10 days. It is hard to treat if jaundice aggravates after 10 days.

*****

[12] 疸而渴〔1〕者，其疸难治；疸而不渴〔2〕者，其疸可治。发于阴部〔3〕，其人必呕；阳部〔4〕，其人振寒而发热也。

Annotations

[1] *Dan Er Ke*: Severe interior heat in jaundice.

[2] *Dan Er Bu Ke*: Mild interior heat in jaundice.

[3] *Fa Yu Yin Bu: Yin Bu* refers to the interior. Patients may experience nausea or vomiting.

[4] *(Fa Yu) Yang Bu*: *Yang Bu* refers to the exterior. Patients may experience fever and chills.

Interpretations

Jaundice with severe interior heat and thirst is hard to treat. Jaundice with mild interior heat and absence of thirst is easier to treat. Jaundice affecting the interior may cause nausea or vomiting. Jaundice affecting the exterior may cause chills and fever.

*****

[13] 谷疸之为病，寒热不食，食即头眩，心胸不安，久久发黄为谷疸。茵陈蒿汤〔1〕主之。

茵陈蒿汤方：

茵陈蒿六两栀子十四枚大黄二两右三味，以水一斗，先煮茵陈，减六升，内二味，煮取三升，去滓。分温三服。小便当利，尿如皂角汁状，色正赤。一宿腹减，黄从小便去也。

Annotations

[1] *Yin Chen Hao Tang* (Virgate Wormwood Decoction): A formula to resolve dampness and clear heat. Of the three ingredients, *Yin Chen* (Herba Artemisiae Scopariae) and *Shan Zhi* (Fructus Gardeniae) clear heat and resolve dampness; and *Da Huang* (Radix et Rhizoma Rhei) promotes bowel movements and clear fire.

Interpretations

Patients with early stage grain jaundice may experience chills, fever, poor appetite, dizziness after eating food, and abdominal discomfort (distenion and pain in the right subcostal region). Over time, they may present with yellowish discoloration of the skin (along with difficult urination, abdominal fullness, constipation, etc.). This should be treated with *Yin Chen Hao Tang* (Virgate Wormwood Decoction).

Yin Chen Hao Tang

[Ingredients]

茵陈蒿	*yīn chén hāo*	6 *liǎng*	Herba Artemisiae Scopariae
山栀	*shān zhī*	14 pieces	Fructus Gardeniae
大黄	*dà huáng*	2 *liǎng*	Radix et Rhizoma Rhei

Decoct *Yin Chen Hao* (Herba Artemisiae Scopariae) in 1 *dòu* of water to get 6 *shēng*, and then add the other two ingredients to get 3 *shēng*. Remove the dregs, divide into three doses and take when it is warm. After taking the formula, patients shall have normal urination with urine that resembles (red) gleditsia juice. Abdominal distension alleviated the next day, so did the yellowish discoloration.

*****

[14] 黄家日晡所发热〔1〕，而反恶寒，此为女劳得之。膀胱急，少腹满〔2〕，身尽黄，额上黑，足下热，因作黑疸。其腹胀如水状，大便必黑，时溏〔3〕，此女劳之病，非水也〔4〕。腹满者难治〔5〕。消石矾石散〔6〕主之。

消石矾石散方：

消石矾石烧，等分右二味，为散，以大麦粥汁〔7〕和服方寸匕，日三服。病随大小便去，小便正黄，大便正黑〔8〕，是候也。

Annotations

[1] *Ri Bu Suo Fa Re*: Fever between 3 pm and 5 pm.

[2] *Pang Guang Ji, Shao Fu Man*: Lower abdominal contracture, fullness and distension.

[3] *Da Bian Bi Hei, Shi Tang*: Black, loose stools (indicating gastrointestinal bleeding).

[4] *Ci Nǚ Lao Zhi Bing, Fei Shui Ye*: This results from female deficiency jaundice instead of water qi disorder.

[5] *Fu Man Zhe Nan Zhi*: Jaundice with abdominal fullness with build-up of water fluids is hard to treat.

[6] *Xiao Shi Fan Shi San* (Niter and Alum Powder): A formula to break stasis and expel dampness. It is a major formula for female deficiency jaundice, not for build-up of water in the abdomen or black stools.

[7] *Da Mai Zhou Zhi*: Barley congree. It acts to harmonize the middle jiao and nourish the stomach. Here it is used to protect

stomach qi from being damaged by *Xiao Shi* (Natrii Sulfas) and *Fan Shi* (Alumen).

[8] *Da Bian Zheng Hei*: Black stools after taking the formula.

Interpretations

For patients with chronic jaundice, afternoon fever with aversion to cold indicates female deficiency jaundice. Lower abdominal contracture, fullness and distension, yellowish discoloration of the skin, a dark gray complexion and feverish sensations in palms, soles and chest indicate a progression into black jaundice. In such case, abdominal fullness and distension due to build-up of water fluids and black, loose stools are developed from female deficiency jaundice instead of water qi disorder. Black jaundice with abdominal fullness and distension due to build-up of water is hard to treat. *Xiao Shi Fan Shi San* (Niter and Alum Powder) is recommended.

Xiao Shi Fan Shi San

[Ingredients]

消石	*xiāo shí*	Natrii Sulfas
矾石	*fán shí*	Alumen (burnt)

Grind equal parts of the two ingredients into a powder. Take one square inch-sponn of the powder with barley congree, 3 times a day. It's normal to have yellow urine and black stools after taking the formula.

*****

[15] 酒黄疸，心中懊或热痛，栀子大黄汤[1]主之。

栀子大黄汤方：

栀子十四枚大黄一两枳实五枚豉一升 右四味，以水六升，煮取二升。分温三服。

Annotations

[1] *Zhi Zi Da Huang Tang* (Gardenia and Rhubarb Decoction): A formula to clear excess heat. This formula and *Yin Chen Hao Tang* (Virgate Wormwood Decoction) are both indicated for jaundice due to damp heat. The difference between the two is that *Yin Chen Hao Tang* uses *Yin Chen* (Herba Artemisiae Scopariae) as the monarch ingredient and focuses on clearing damp heat, whereas this one uses *Shan Zhi* (Fructus Gardeniae) as the monarch ingredient and focuses on clearing excess heat. In addition, this formula is not only indicated for alcohol jaundice but for all types of jaundice with more heat than dampness.

Interpretations

Alcohol jaundice with stomach discomfort or burning pain (yellowish discoloration of the skin, difficult urination, abdominal fullness and constipation) should be treated with *Zhi Zi Da Huang Tang* (Gardenia and Rhubarb Decoction).

Zhi Zi Da Huang Tang

[Ingredients]

山栀	*shān zhī*	14 pieces	Fructus Gardeniae
大黄	*dà huáng*	1 *liǎng*	Radix et Rhizoma Rhei
枳实	*zhǐ shí*	5 pieces	Fructus Aurantii Immaturus
豆豉	*dòu chǐ*	1 *shēng*	Semen Sojae Praeparatum

Decoct the four ingredients in 6 *shēng* of water and get 2 *shēng*. Divide into three doses and drink when it is warm.

*****

[16] 诸病黄家，但利其小便〔1〕。假令脉浮〔2〕，当以汗解之，宜桂枝加黄芪汤〔3〕主之。方见水病中。

Annotations

[1] *Zhu Bing Huang Jia, Dan Li Qi Xiao Bian*: A standard treatment strategy for all types of jaundice is to resolve dampness and clear heat through urination.

[2] *Jia Ling Mai Fu*: If exterior-syndrome symptoms occur, such as fever, aversion to wind or spontaneous sweating, etc.

[3] *Gui Zhi Jia Huang Qi Tang* (Cinnamon Twig Decoction plus Astragalus): See chapter 14 (line 29). A formula originally for yellow sweats.

Interpretations

Normally all types of jaundice can be treated by inducing urination (to clear damp heat). In case a superficial pulse (fever, aversion to wind or spontaneous sweating) is present, *Gui Zh Jia Huang Qi Tang* (Cinnamon Twig Decoction plus Astragalus) can be used to induce sweating and release the exterior (For ingredients and usage of the formula, see chapter 14).

*****

[17] 诸黄〔1〕，猪膏发煎〔2〕主之。

猪膏发煎方：

猪膏半斤乱发如鸡子大三枚 二味，和膏中煎之，发消药成。分再服。病从小便出〔3〕。

Annotations

[1] *Zhu Huang*: Here it refers to jaundice with intestinal dryness and constipation.

[2] *Zhu Gao Fa Jian* (Lard and Human Hair Decoction): A formula to moisten drynesss and resolve stasis. It is often used for dry stools.

[3] *Bing Cong Xiao Bian Chu*: The disease is flushed out through bladder movements (a wrong spelling of bowel movements).

Interpretations

All types of jaundice in remissive stage (intestinal dryness and constipation) can be treated with *Zhu Gao Fa Jian* (Lard and Human Hair Decoction).

Zhu Gao Fa Jian

[Ingredients]

猪膏	*zhū gāo*	0.5 *jīn*	Adeps Suis
乱发	*luàn fā*	3 lumps (egg-sized)	Crinis

Decoct the two ingredients until the hair is completely dissolved. Divide into two doses. The condition alleviates upon the passing of dry stools.

*****

[18] 黄疸病〔1〕，茵陈五苓散〔2〕主之。一本云茵陈汤及五苓散并主之。

茵陈五苓散方：

茵陈蒿末十分五苓散五分。方见痰饮中。右二物和。先食饮方寸匕，日三服。

Annotations

[1] *Huang Dan Bing*: Here it refers to jaundice with more dampness than heat. Symptoms may include yellowish discoloration of the skin, fatigue, chest tightness, a poor appetite, thirst but no desire to drink water, difficult urination or loose stools.

[2] *Yin Chen Wu Ling San* (Five ingredients Powder with Poria plus Virgate Wormwood): A formula to clear heat and resolve dampness. Of the ingredients, *Yin Chen* (Herba Artemisiae Scopariae) clears damp heat and *Wu Ling San* (Five Ingredients Powder with Poria) promotes urination.

Interpretations

Jaundice (with more dampness than heat, characterized by yellowish discoloration of the skin, fatigue, poor appetite, thirst but no desire to drink water, difficult urination or loose stools) can be treated with *Yin Chen Wu Ling San* (Five ingredients Powder with Poria plus Virgate Wormwood) (*Yin Chen Hao Tang* and *Wu Ling San* in other texts).

Yin Chen Wu Ling San

[Ingredients]

茵陈蒿	*yīn chén hāo*	10 *fēn*	Herba Artemisiae Scopariae
五苓散	*wǔ líng sǎn*	5 *fēn*	Five ingredients Powder with Poria (see chapter 12)

Mix the two powders and take 1 square inch-spoon before meals, three times a day.

*****

[19] 黄疸，腹满，小便不利而赤，自汗出，此为表和里实〔1〕。当下之，宜大黄消石汤〔2〕。

大黄消石汤方：

大黄黄柏消石各四两栀子十五枚　　右四味，以水六升，煮取二升，去滓，内消，更煮取一升。顿服。

Annotations

[1] *Biao He Li Shi*: No noticeable exterior-syndrome symptoms but excess interior heat. Patients may experience yellowish discoloration of the skin, difficult urination and yellow urine, along with abdominal fullness and constipation.

[2] *Da Huang Xiao Shi Tang* (Rhubarb and Niter Decoction): A formula to unblock fu-organs and clear heat. Of the ingredients, *Da*

Huang (Radix et Rhizoma Rhei) and *Xiao Shi* (Natrii Sulfas) promote bowel movements; *Huang Bai* (Cortex Phellodendri Chinensis) and *Shan Zhi* (Fructus Gardeniae) clear damp heat. The *Jin Gui Yao Lüè Jin Shi* (Modern Interpretation of the 'Essentials from the Golden Cabinet') states, "this formula is indicated for stagnant jaundice and gall stones".

Interpretations

Presence of abdominal fullness, difficult urination with yellow urine, spontaneous sweating (and constipation) in jaundice indicates absence of exterior syndrome but interior excess heat. This should be treated with *Da Huang Xiao Shi Tang* (Rhubarb and Niter Decoction) to drain downward.

Da Huang Xiao Shi Tang

[Ingredients]

大黄	*dà huáng*	4 *liǎng*	Radix et Rhizoma Rhei
黄柏	*huáng bǎi*	4 *liǎng*	Cortex Phellodendri Chinensis
消石	*xiāo shí*	4 *liǎng*	Natrii Sulfas
山栀	*shān zhī*	15 pieces	Fructus Gardeniae

Decoct *Da Huang* (Radix et Rhizoma Rhei), *Huang Bai* (Cortex Phellodendri Chinensis) and *Shan Zhi* (Fructus Gardeniae) in 6 *shēng* of water and get 2 *shēng*. Then add *Xiao Shi* (Natrii Sulfas) and decoct to get 1 *shēng*. Drink up the decoction at a draught.

*****

[20] 黄疸病，小便色不变，欲自利〔1〕，腹满而喘，不可除热，热除必哕。哕者，小半夏汤〔2〕主之。方见消渴中。

Annotations

[1] *Xiao Bian Se Bu Bian, Yu Zi Li*: Normal bladder movements with normal urine color. This indicates deficiency cold of the spleen and stomach instead of damp heat.

[2] *Xiao Ban Xia Tang* (Minor Pinellia Decoction): A formula to warm the stomach and down-regulate qi.

Interpretations

For patients with jaundice, normal bladder movements with normal urine color, abdominal distension and panting (due to deficiency cold of the spleen and stomach) cannot be treated with draining downward method (to clear heat), otherwise patients may experience hiccups. This should be treated with *Xiao Ban Xia Tang* (Minor Pinellia Decoction) (for the ingredients and usage of the formula, see chapter 12).

*****

[21] 诸黄，腹痛而呕〔1〕者，宜柴胡汤〔2〕。必小柴胡汤，方见呕吐中。

Annotations

[1] *Fu Tong Er Ou*: Abdominal pain, pain or hardness in the subcostal region, fever (or alternating fever and chills), and vomiting with no appetite to eat. Despite the yellowish discoloration of the skin, this is not jaundice but similar to acute cholecystitis or gall stones.

[2] *Chai Hu Tang* (Bupleurum Decoction): A formula to clear interior heat. Normally it refers to *Xiao Chai Hu Tang* (Minor Bupleurum Decoction). Use *Da Chai Hu Tang* (Major Bupleurum Decoction) for abdominal fullness and constipation (see chapter 10).

Interpretations

Yellow discoloration of the skin, severe abdominal pain or pain in the right upper abdomen and vomiting should be treated with *Chai Hu Tang* (Bupleurum Decoction) (for ingredients and usage of *Xiao Chai Hu Tang*, see chapter 17).

*****

[22] 男子黄，小便自利〔1〕，当与虚劳小建中汤〔2〕。方见虚劳中。

Annotations

[1] *Xiao Bian Zi Li*: Normal urination, indicating deficiency jaundice instead of damp-heat jaundice. It is similar to autoimmune hemolytic anemia in modern medicine.

[2] *Xiao Jian Zhong Tang* (Minor Middle Jiao-Fortifying Decoction): see chapter 6 (line 14).

Interpretations

Patients with yellow discoloration of the skin and normal urination should be treated with *Xiao Jian Zhong* (Minor Middle Jiao-Fortifying Decoction) to reinforce the body (for ingredients and usage of the formula, see chapter 6).

*****

Annex formula # 1 *Gua Di Tang* (Melon Stalk Decoction)

瓜蒂汤治诸黄。方见暍病中。

Interpretations

Gua Di Tang (Melon Stalk Decoction) can be used to treat all types of jaundice (for ingredients and usage of the formula, see chapter 2).

*****

Annex formula # 2 *Qian Jin Ma Huang Chun Jiu Tang* (Ephedra and Pure Liquor Decoction)

《千金》麻黄醇酒汤[1]治黄疸。

麻黄三两右一味，以美清酒五升，煮取二升半。顿服尽。冬月用酒，春月用水煮之。

Annotations

[1] *Ma Huang Chun Jiu Tang* (Ephedra and Pure Liquor Decoction): A formula to induce sweating, release the exterior, remove wind and resolve water retention.

Interpretations

The *Ma Huang Chun Jiu Tang* (Ephedra and Pure Liquor Decoction) recorded in the *Qian Jin Yao Fang* (Important Formulas Worth a Thousand Gold Pieces) is indicated for jaundice (with fever, chills and absence of sweats, etc.).

Method: Decoct 3 *liǎng* of *Ma Huang* (Herba Ephedra) in 5 *shēng* of high-quality liquor to get 2.5 *shēng* (1.5 *shēng* in other texts). Drink up at a draught. It's advisable to decoct with liquor in winter but with water in spring.

惊悸吐衄下血胸满瘀血病脉证治第十六

Chapter 16 Fright, Palpitations, Bleeding, Chest Fullness and Stagnant Blood—Pulses, Patterns and Treatment

Overview

This chapter discusses fright, palpitations, bleeding and stagnant blood. Fright is a sudden feeling of fear and restlessness. It is often seen in acute febrile diseases. Palpitations are the feelings of having faster heart beats. They are often seen in phlegm fluid retention. Bleeding includes coughing up blood, vomiting of blood, nosebleed, and blood in stools. Stagnant blood includes blood that flows out of the vessels. Chest fullness is a symptom of blood stasis. As fright and palpitations often occur in combination with bleeding in febrile diseases, these conditions are discussed together in this chapter.

*****

[01] 寸口脉动而弱[1]，动即为惊，弱则为悸。

Annotations

[1] *Mai Dong Er Ruo*: A rapid pulse felt at the *Guan* position. A weak pulse is soft, deep and thready.

Interpretations

The pulse is rapid and weak at the *Cunkou* position. A rapid pulse is felt in patients with fright; and a weak pulse in patients with palpitations.

*****

[02] 师曰：尺脉浮〔1〕，目睛晕黄〔2〕，衄未止。晕黄去，目睛慧了〔3〕，知衄今止。

Annotations

[1] *Chi Mai Fu*: A superficial pulse at the *Chi* position, indicating ascending of deficiency fire (in the kidney).

[2] *Mu Jing Yun Huang*: Blurred vision.

[3] *Mu Jing Hui Liao*: Clear vision.

Interpretations

The Master said, "With a superficial pulse at the *Chi* position and blurred vision, the nosebleed is not yet stopped. The nosebleed stops upon the restoration of a clear vision".

*****

[03] 又曰：从春至夏衄者太阳〔1〕，从秋至冬衄者阳明〔2〕。

Annotations

[1] *Cong Chun Zhi Xia Nǜ Zhe Tai Yang*: Nosebleed in spring and summer is often associated with Taiyang exterior syndrome.

[2] *Cong Qiu Zhi Dong Nǜ Zhe Tai Yang*: Nosebleed in autumn and winter is often associated with interior Yangming heat.

Interpretations

The Master also said, "Nosebleed in spring and summer is often caused by Taiyang exterior syndrome, whereas nosebleed in autumn and winter is often caused by interior Yangming heat".

*****

[04] 衄家〔1〕不可汗。汗出必额上陷脉〔2〕紧急，直视不能眴〔3〕，不得眠。

Annotations

[1] *Nǜ Jia*: It originally means nosebleed; however, it here refers to vomiting of blood and nosebleed.

[2] *Xian Mai*: Here it refers to face (forehead) along the pathways of meridians.

[3] *Zhi Shi Bu Neng Shun*: Stare straight ahead with an inability to move the eyeballs.

Interpretations

Vomiting of blood and nosebleed cannot be treated by inducing sweating, because sweating may cause the forehead along the pathways of meridians to become tense and spasmodic, leading to staring straight ahead with an inability to move the eyeballs. In such case, patients cannot close the eyes to sleep.

*****

[05] 病人面无色，无寒热〔1〕。脉沉弦者，衄；浮弱，手按之绝者〔2〕，下血〔3〕；烦咳〔4〕者，必吐血。

Annotations

[1] *Mian Wu Se, Wu Han Re*: A pale, lusterless complexion with no fever or chills (no external contraction of pathogenic factors).

[2] *Fu Ruo, Shou An Zhi Jue Zhe*: A weak pulse with light pressure and faint (can hardly be felt) with heavy pressure.

[3] *Xia Xue*: Bloody stools.

[4] *Fan Ke*: Severe coughing.

Interpretations

When a patient presents with a pale, lusterless complexion with no fever or chills (it might suggest bleeding but needs also to feel the pulse), a deep, wiry pulse indicates nosebleed, a weak pulse with light pressure but faint with heavy pressure often indicates bloody stools. In addition, concurrent severe cough may cause coughing up blood.

*****

[06] 夫吐血〔1〕，咳逆上气，其脉数而有热，不得卧〔2〕者死。

Annotations

[1] *Tu Xue*: Here it refers to coughing up blood.

[2] *Mai Shuo Er You Re, Bu De Wo*: A rapid pulse indicates heat. Patients experience shortness of breath with an inability to lie flat.

Interpretations

In patients with coughing up blood, panting, a rapid pulse, feverish sensations and an inability to lie flat are life-threatening signs indicative of an unfavorable prognosis.

*****

[07] 夫酒客[1]咳者，必致吐血，此因极饮过度所致也。

Annotations

[1] *Jiu Ke*: Long-term alcohol drinkers.

Interpretations

Cough and vomiting of blood in long-term drinkers are caused by excessive consumption of alcohol.

*****

[08] 寸口脉弦而大，弦则为减，大则为芤，减则为寒，芤则为虚，寒虚相击，此名曰革，妇人则半产漏下，男人则亡血。

Interpretations

See chapter 6 (line 13)

*****

[09] 亡血[1]不可发其表[2]。汗出即寒栗[3]而振。

Annotations

[1] *Wang Xue*: Loss of blood.

[2] *Fa Qi Biao*: Release the exterior (induce sweating in *Shang Han Lun*).

[3] *Han Li*: Chills (shivering).

Interpretations

Patients with loss of blood cannot be treated by inducing sweating to release the exterior; otherwise they may experience chills (shivering) due to sudden collapse of yang qi.

*****

[10] 病人胸满，唇痿舌青〔1〕，口燥，但欲嗽水不欲咽，无寒热，脉微大来迟〔2〕，腹不满，其人言我满〔3〕，为有瘀血。

Annotations

[1] *Chun Wei She Qing*: Dry, bluish tongue and lips, indicating blood stasis.

[2] *Mai Wei Da Lai Chi*: A hesitant pulse, indicating stagnation of blood.

[3] *Fu Bu Man, Qi Ren Yan Wo Man*: Complaints of abdominal fullness and distension but no increase in abdominal size.

Interpretations

Chest tightness, dry, bluish lips and tongue, a dry mouth with desire to drink water but no desire to swallow, absence of chills or fever, a subjective feeling of abdominal fullness but no increase in abdominal size. All these symptoms indicate internal obstruction of stagnant blood.

*****

[11] 病者如热状，烦满，口干燥而渴，其脉反无热〔1〕，此为阴状〔2〕，是瘀血也。当下之。

Annotations

[1] *Bing Zhe Ru Re Zhuang...Qi Mai Fa Wu Re*: Despite the heat symptoms, the pulse does not indicate heat.

[2] *Yin Zhuang*: Here it refers to yin pathogen – blood stasis.

Interpretations

Patients present with symptoms that indicate internal heat such as restlessness, a dry mouth, and thirst; however, the pulse does not indicate there is internal heat. Actually, it is caused by blood stasis and should be treated by resolving blood.

*****

[12] 火邪〔1〕者，桂枝去芍药加蜀漆牡蛎龙骨救逆汤〔2〕主之。

桂枝救逆汤方：

桂枝三两，去皮甘草二两，炙 生姜三两牡蛎五两，熬龙骨四两大枣十二枚蜀漆三两，洗去腥

右为末，以水一斗二升，先煮蜀漆，减二升，内诸药，煮取三升，去滓，温服一升。

Annotations

[1] *Huo Xie*: Here it refers to aggravated condition after inducing sweating with fire (warming needle, fumigation, hot compression, etc.), which may damage heart yang.

[2] *Gui Zhi Qu Shao Yao Jia Shu Qi Mu Li Long Gu Jiu Ni Tang* (Cinnamon Twig Rescue Decoction minus Peony plus Dichroa Leaf, Oyster Shell and Dragon Bone): A modified formula of *Gui Zhi Tang* (Cinnamon Twig Decoction). It acts to release the exterior, remove pathogenic factors, restore yang and prevent collapse.

Interpretations

Aggravated condition (retained fever and chills with fright and restlessness) due to the wrong use of inducing sweating with fire can be treated with *Gui Zhi Qu Shao Yao Jia Shu Qi Mu Li Long Gu Jiu Ni Tang* (Cinnamon Twig Rescue Decoction minus Peony plus Dichroa Leaf, Oyster Shell and Dragon Bone).

Gui Zhi Qu Shao Yao Jia Shu Qi Mu Li Long Gu Jiu Ni Tang

[Ingredients]

桂枝	*guì zhī*	3 *liǎng*	Ramulus Cinnamomi (skin removed) (2 *liǎng* in other text)
生姜	*shēng jiāng*	3 *liǎng*	Rhizoma Zingiberis Recens (6 *liǎng* in other text)
甘草	*gān cǎo*	2 *liǎng*	Radix et Rhizoma Glycyrrhizae Preparata(3 *liǎng* in other text)
牡蛎	*mǔ lì*	5 *liǎng*	Concha Ostreae (boiled)
龙骨	*lóng gǔ*	4 *liǎng*	Os Draconis
大枣	*dà zǎo*	12 pieces	Fructus Jujubae
蜀漆	*shǔ qī*	3 *liǎng*	Folium Dichroae (wash to remove the fishy smell)

Grind the above ingredients into a powder. First decoct *Shu Qi* (Folium Dichroae) in 1 *dòu* and 2 *shēng* of water to get 10 *shēng*, and then add the rest of the ingredients to get 3 *shēng*. Remove the dregs and take 1 *shēng* for each dose when it is warm.

*****

[13] 心下悸[1]者，半夏麻黄丸[2]主之。

半夏麻黄丸方：

半夏麻黄等分右二味，末之，炼蜜和丸，小豆大。饮服三丸，日三服。

Annotations

[1] *Xin Xia Ji*: Palpitations due to retained water fluid obstructing yang (see chapter 12, line 11).

[2] *Ban Xia Ma Huang Wan* (Pinellia and Ephedra Pill): A formula to resolve water retention. Of the two ingredients, *Ban Xia* (Rhizoma Pinelliae) resolves water fluid and *Ma Huang* (Herba Ephedrae) disperses yang.

Interpretations

Palpitations due to water fluid retention can be treated with *Ban Xia Ma Huang Wan* (Pinellia and Ephedra Pill).

Ban Xia Ma Huang Wan

[Ingredients]

半夏	*bàn xià*	Rhizoma Pinelliae
麻黄	*má huáng*	Herba Ephedrae

Grind the two ingredients into a powder. Mix with the prepared white honey to make into pills the size of a small bean. Take 3 pills for each dose with water, 3 doses a day.

*****

[14] 吐血不止[1]者，柏叶汤[2]主之。

柏叶汤方：

柏叶干姜各三两 艾三把 右三味，以水五升，取马通汁[3]一升合煮，取一升。分温再服。

Annotations

[1] *Tu Xue Bu Zhi*: Here it refers to persistent coughing up blood.

[2] *Bai Ye Tang* (Arborvitae Leaf Decoction): A formula to warm the middle jiao and stop bleeding.

[3] *Ma Tong Zhi*: Mixed horse manure and water. In ancient times, this was believed to stop bleeding but no longer used now.

Interpretations

Chronic coughing up blood can be treated with *Bai Ye Tang* (Arborvitae Leaf Decoction).

Ban Xia Ma Huang Wan

[Ingredients]

柏叶	*bǎi yè*	3 *liǎng*	Cacumen Platycladi
干姜	*gān jiāng*	3 *liǎng*	Rhizoma Zingiberis
艾叶	*ài yè*	3 handfuls	Folium Artemisiae Argyi

Decoct the three ingredients in 5 *shēng* of water and 1 *shēng* of horse manure juice to get 1 *shēng*. Divide into two doses and take when it is warm.

*****

[15] 下血，先便后血〔1〕，此远血〔2〕也，黄土汤〔3〕主之。

黄土汤方亦主吐血、衄血：

甘草干地黄白术附子炮阿胶黄芩各三两灶中黄土半斤右七味，以水八升，煮取三升。分温二服。

Annotations

[1] *Xian Bian Hou Xue*: Bleeding after defecation.

[2] *Yuan Xue:* Distal (upper gastrointestinal tract, away from the anus) bleeding.

[3] *Huang Tu Tang* (Yellow Earth Decoction): A well-known formula to warm the spleen and stop bleeding.

Interpretations

Bleeding after defecation is distal bleeding and can be treated with *Huang Tu Tang* (Yellow Earth Decoction).

Huang Tu Tang

[Ingredients]

甘草	*gān cǎo*	3 *liǎng*	Radix et Rhizoma Glycyrrhizae
干地黄	*gān dì huáng*	3 *liǎng*	Radix Rehmanniae
白术	*bái zhú*	3 *liǎng*	Rhizoma Atractylodis Macrocephalae
附子	*fù zǐ*	3 *liǎng*	Radix Aconiti Lateralis Praeparata
阿胶	*ē jiāo*	3 *liǎng*	Colla Corii Asini
黄芩	*huáng qín*	3 *liǎng*	Radix Scutellariae
灶心土	*zào xīn tǔ*	0.5 *jīn*	Terra Flava Usta

Decoct the seven ingredients in 8 *shēng* of water to get 3 *shēng*. Divide into two doses and take when it is warm.

*****

[16] 下血，先血后便〔1〕，此近血〔2〕也，赤小豆当归散〔3〕主之。方见狐惑中。

Annotations

[1] *Xian Xue Hou Bian*: Bleeding before defecation.

[2] *Jin Xue:* Local (to the anus, lower gastrointestinal tract) bleeding.

[3] *Chi Xiao Dou Dang Gui San* (Rice Bean and Chinese Angelica Powder): see chapter 2 (line 13).

Interpretations

Bleeding before defecation is local bleeding and can be treated with *Chi Xiao Dou Dang Gui San* (Rice Bean and Chinese Angelica Powder) (for the ingredients and usage of the formula, see chapter 2).

*****

[17] 心气不足〔1〕，吐血、衄血，泻心汤〔2〕主之。

泻心汤方亦治霍乱：

大黄二两黄连黄芩各一两右三味，以水三升，煮取一升。顿服之。

Annotations

[1] *Xin Qi Bu Zu*: Heart qi deficiency may cause hyperactivity of heart fire to cause the blood to flow recklessly and result in vomiting of blood and nosebleed.

[2] *Xie Xin Tang* (Heart-Draining Decoction): A formula to reduce fire and stop bleeding. Of the ingredients, *Da Huang* (Radix et Rhizoma Rhei) and *Huang Lian* (Rhizoma Coptidis) are bitter in taste and cold in property and act to reduce heart fire.

Interpretations

Vomiting of blood and nosebleed due to heart qi deficiency (causing hyperactivity of heart fire) can be treated with *Xie Xin Tang* (Heart-Draining Decoction).

Xie Xin Tang (can also be used for cholera)

[Ingredients]

大黄	*dà huáng*	2 *liǎng*	Radix et Rhizoma Rhei
黄连	*huáng lián*	1 *liǎng*	Rhizoma Coptidis
黄芩	*huáng qín*	1 *liǎng*	Radix Scutellariae

Decoct the three ingredients in 3 *shēng* of water to get 1 *shēng*. Drink up at a draught.

呕吐哕下利病脉证治第十七
Chapter 17 Retching, Vomiting, Hiccups and Diarrhea—Pulses, Patterns and Treatment

Overview

This chapter discusses retching/vomiting, hiccups and diarrhea. The three conditions are discussed together because they are all associated with the stomach and intestines.

*****

[01] 夫呕家有痈脓[1]，不可治呕，脓尽自愈。

Annotations

[1] *Fu Ou Jia You Yong Nong*: Patients with frequent vomiting of pus.

Interpretations

For patients with frequent vomiting of pus, the treatment should focus on the pus instead of vomiting. The vomiting stops upon the removal of pus.

*****

[02] 先呕却渴者，此为欲解[1]。先渴却呕者，为水停心下，此属饮家[2]。呕家本渴，今反不渴者，以心下有支饮故也，此属支饮。

Annotations

[1] *Xian Ou Que Ke Zhe, Ci Wei Yu Jie*: Thirst after vomiting indicates a high chance that vomiting will stop.

[2] *Xian Ke Que Ou Zhe...Ci Shu Yin Jia*: Thirst with excessive drinking before vomiting indicates water fluid retention (see chapter 12, line 28 for reference).

Interpretations

Thirst after vomiting predicts a high chance that vomiting will stop. Thirst with excessive drinking before vomiting is caused by retained water fluid in the stomach. Normally patients should feel thirsty after vomiting. Absence of thirst indicates water fluid in the stomach.

*****

[03] 问曰：病人脉数，数为热，当消谷引食，而反吐者，何也？师曰：以发其汗，令阳微，膈气虚〔1〕，脉乃数，数为客热〔2〕，不能消谷，胃中虚冷故也。脉弦者，虚也。胃气无余，朝食暮吐〔3〕，变为胃反〔4〕。寒在于上，医反下之，今脉反弦，故名曰虚。

Annotations

[1] *Ge Qi Xu*: It literally means deficiency of the zong-pectoral qi; however, here it refers to qi deficiency of the spleen and stomach.

[2] *Ke Re*: False heat.

[3] *Zhao Shi Mu Tu*: Eating in the morning but vomiting in the evening, indicating a longer period of food retention in the stomach.

[4] *Wei Fan*: Nausea and vomiting due to deficiency cold of the stomach.

Interpretations

Question: A patient has a rapid pulse. A rapid pulse indicates heat and stomach heat increases the digestion of food, but the patient vomits. Why is that?

Answer: The wrong use of medicinals that induce sweating may impair spleen yang and cause a rapid pulse. However, this is false heat (due to yang deficiency) and cannot digest grains because of deficiency cold in the stomach. A wiry pulse is also caused by stomach qi deficiency. When stomach qi fails to descend, the patient eats food in the morning but vomits in the evening. This is nausea and vomiting due to deficiency cold. The wrong use of sweating method aggravates the pre-existing deficiency cold and causes a wiry pulse.

*****

[04] 寸口脉微而数，微则无气〔1〕，无气则营虚〔2〕，营虚则血不足，血不足则胸中冷〔3〕。

Annotations

[1] *Wu Qi*: Deficiency of *Wei*-defensive qi.

[2] *Ying Xu*: Deficiency of *Ying*-nutrients qi.

[3] *Xiong Zhong Leng*: It literally means cold in the chest; however, it actually refers to deficiency cold in the stomach.

Interpretations

The pulse is faint and rapid at the *Cunkou* position. A faint pulse indicates deficiency of *Wei*-defensive qi. Deficiency of *Wei*-defensive qi causes deficiency of *Ying*-nutrients qi. Deficiency of *Ying*-nutrients qi causes deficiency of qi and blood. Deficiency of qi and blood causes deficiency cold in the stomach (nausea and vomiting).

*****

[05] 趺阳脉浮而涩[1]，浮则为虚，涩则伤脾，脾伤则不磨，朝食暮吐，暮食朝吐，宿食不化，名曰胃反[2]。脉紧而涩[3]，其病难治。

Annotations

[1] *Fu Yang Mai Fu Er Se*: The pulse is superficial and hesitant at Chongyang (ST 42). A superficial pulse indicates stomach qi deficiency and a hesitant pulse indicates damage to spleen yin and impaired function in transportation and transformation.

[2] *Wei Fan*: A condition characterized by poor digestion, eating in the morning but vomiting in the evening, or eating in the evening but vomiting in the morning. It is similar to pyloric obstruction in modern medicine.

[3] *Mai Jin Er Se*: The pulse is tight and hesitant. A tight pulse means severe cold and a hesitant pulse indicates damage to body fluids. The condition is hard to treat if patients experience severe vomiting and constipation.

Interpretations

The pulse is superficial and hesitant at Chongyang (ST 42). A superficial pulse indicates stomach qi deficiency. A hesitant pulse indicates damage to body fluids. Impaired functions of the spleen and stomach in transportation and transformation may cause eating in the morning but vomiting in the evening or eating in the morning but vomiting in the morning with undigested food. A tight, hesitant pulse (frequent vomiting, loss of appetite and constipation) indicates the disease is hard to treat.

*****

[06] 病人欲吐者，不可下之。

Interpretations

Patients with nausea and vomiting cannot be treated with draining downward method.

*****

[07] 哕〔1〕而腹满，视其前后〔2〕，知何部不利，利之即愈。

Annotations

[1] *Hui*: Hiccups
[2] *Qian Hou*: Bladder and bowel movements.

Interpretations

For patients with hiccups and abdominal fullness, it's important to inquire about their bladder and bowel movements and use methods to promote urination or bowel movements. Hiccups will stop afterwards.

*****

[08] 呕而胸满〔1〕者，茱萸汤〔2〕主之。
茱萸汤方：
吴茱萸一升人参三两生姜六两大枣十二枚　右四味，以水五升，煮取三升。温服七合，日三服。

Annotations

[1] *Xiong Man*: Stomach fullness and distension.
[2] *Zhu Yu Tang* (Evodia Decoction): A formula to warm the stomach, reinforce the body, dissipate cold and down-regulate qi.

Interpretations

Vomiting with stomach fullness and distension should be treated with *Zhu Yu Tang* (Evodia Decoction).

Zhu Yu Tang

[Ingredients]

吴茱萸	*wú zhū yú*	1 *shēng*	Fructus Evodiae (2 *shēng* in other text)
人参	*rén shēn*	3 *liǎng*	Radix et Rhizoma Ginseng
生姜	*shēng jiāng*	6 *liǎng*	Rhizoma Zingiberis Recens
大枣	*dà zǎo*	12 pieces	Fructus Jujubae (10 pieces in other text)

Decoct the four ingredients in 5 *shēng* of water to get 3 *shēng* (2 *shēng* in *Shang Han Lun*). Take 0.7 *shēng* for each dose when it is warm, 3 doses a day.

*****

[09] 干呕〔1〕，吐涎沫，头痛〔2〕者，茱萸汤主之。方见上。

Annotations

[1] *Gan Ou*: Retching.
[2] *Tou Tong:* Vertex headache.

Interpretations

Retching, vomiting of foamy saliva and vertex headache can be treated with *Zhu Yu Tang* (Evodia Decoction) (the formula is discussed in line 8).

*****

[10] 呕而肠鸣，心下痞[1]者，半夏泻心汤[2]主之。

半夏泻心汤方：

半夏半升，洗黄芩干姜人参各三两黄连一两大枣十二枚甘草三两，炙右七味，以水一斗，煮取六升，去滓，再煮取三升。温服一升，日三服。

Annotations

[1] *Xin Xia Pi*: Stomach discomfort.

[2] *Ban Xia Xie Xin Tang* (Pinellia Heart-Draining Decoction): A formula to harmonize the stomach. Of the ingredients, *Ban Xia* (Rhizoma Pinelliae) is used as the monarch ingredient; *Gan Jiang* (Rhizoma Zingiberis) unblocks qi; *Huang Qin* (Radix Scutellariae) and *Huang Lian* (Rhizoma Coptidis) reduce fire; and *Ren Shen* (Radix et Rhizoma Ginseng) and *Gan Cao* (Radix et Rhizoma Glycyrrhizae) tonify qi.

Interpretations

Vomiting with bowel sounds and stomach discomfort can be treated with *Ban Xia Xie Xin Tang* (Pinellia Heart-Draining Decoction).

Ban Xia Xie Xin Tang

[Ingredients]

半夏	*bàn xià*	0.5 *shēng*	Rhizoma Pinelliae (0.5 *jīn* in other text)
黄芩	*huáng qín*	3 *liǎng*	Radix Scutellariae
干姜	*gān jiāng*	3 *liǎng*	Rhizoma Zingiberis
人参	*rén shēn*	3 *liǎng*	Radix et Rhizoma Ginseng
黄连	*huáng lián*	1 *liǎng*	Rhizoma Coptidis
大枣	*dà zǎo*	12 pieces	Fructus Jujubae
甘草	*gān cǎo*	3 *liǎng*	Radix et Rhizoma Glycyrrhizae Preparata

Decoct the seven ingredients in 1 *dòu* of water to get 6 *shēng*. Remove the dregs and re-decoct to get 3 *shēng*. Take 1 *shēng* for each dose when it is warm, 3 doses a day.

*****

[11] 干呕而利[1]者，黄芩加半夏生姜汤[2]主之。

黄芩加半夏生姜汤方：

黄芩三两甘草二两炙芍药二两半夏半升生姜三两大枣二十枚右六味，以水一斗，煮取三升，去滓。温服一升，日再夜一服。

Annotations

[1] *Gan Ou Er Li*: Retching with diarrhea due to pathogenic heat affecting the stomach and intestines.

[2] *Huang Qin Jia Ban Xia Sheng Jiang Tang* (Scutellaria Decoction plus Pinellia and Fresh Ginger): A modified formula of *Huang Qin Tang* (Scutellaria Decoction). It acts to clear heat, stop diarrhea, harmonize the stomach and down-regulate qi.

Interpretations

Retching with diarrhea can be treated with *Huang Qin Jia Ban Xia Sheng Jiang Tang* (Scutellaria Decoction plus Pinellia and Fresh Ginger).

Huang Qin Jia Ban Xia Sheng Jiang Tang

[Ingredients]

黄芩	*huáng qín*	3 *liǎng*	Radix Scutellariae
甘草	*gān cǎo*	2 *liǎng*	Radix et Rhizoma Glycyrrhizae Preparata
芍药	*sháo yào*	2 *liǎng*	Radix Paeoniae (3 *liǎng* in other text)

半夏	*bàn xià*	0.5 *shēng*	Rhizoma Pinelliae
生姜	*shēng jiāng*	3 *liǎng*	Rhizoma Zingiberis Recens (4 *liǎng* in other text)
大枣	*dà zǎo*	20 pieces	Fructus Jujubae (12 pieces in other text)

Decoct the six ingredients in 1 *dòu* of water to get 3 *shēng*. Take 1 *shēng* for each dose when it is warm, 2 doses during the day and 1 dose at night.

*****

[12] 诸呕吐，谷不得下[1]者，小半夏汤[2]主之。方见痰饮中。

Annotations

[1] *Gu Bu De Xia*: Unable to eat because of severe vomiting.

[2] *Xiao Ban Xia Tang* (Minor Pinellia Decoction): A formula to resolve water fluids and down-regulate qi. It is a major formula to stop vomiting.

Interpretations

All types of vomiting with an inability to eat food can be treated with *Xiao Ban Xia Tang* (Minor Pinellia Decoction) (for the ingredients and usage of the formula, see chapter 12, line 28).

*****

[13] 呕吐而病在膈上[1]，后思水者[2]，解，急与之。思水者，猪苓散[3]主之。

猪苓散方：

猪苓茯苓白术各等分右三味，杵为散，饮服方寸匕，日三服。

Annotations

[1] *Ge Shang*: It literally means above the diaphragm; it actually refers to the stomach.

[2] *Hou Si Shui Zhe*: This is the aforementioned "thirst after vomiting".

[3] *Zhu Ling San* (Polyporus Powder): A formula to fortify the spleen and promote urination. Of the ingredients, *Zhu Ling* (Polyporus) promotes urination and drains dampness; and *Bai Zhu* (Rhizoma Atractylodis Macrocephalae) and *Fu Ling* (Poria) fortify the spleen and promote urination.

Interpretations

Stomach problems with vomiting and desire to drink water after vomiting predicts a high chance that vomiting will stop. It's advisable to drink a small amount of water immediately. Excessive thirst with a desire to drink water can be managed by *Zhu Ling San* (Polyporus Powder).

Zhu Ling San

[Ingredients]

猪苓	*zhū líng*	Polyporus
茯苓	*fú líng*	Poria
白术	*bái zhú*	Rhizoma Atractylodis Macrocephalae

Grind the three ingredients into a powder. Take 1 square-inch spoon for each dose with water, 3 doses a day.

*****

[14] 呕而脉弱，小便复利〔1〕，身有微热，见厥者〔2〕，难治，四逆汤〔3〕主之。

四逆汤方：

附子一枚，生用干姜一两半甘草二两，炙 右三味，以水三升，煮取一升二合，去滓。分温再服，强人可大附子一枚、干姜三两。

Annotations

[1] *Ou Er Mai Ruo, Xiao Bian Fu Li*: Retching with a weak pulse (indicating deficiency cold) and normal urination.

[2] *Shen You Wei Re, Jian Jue Zhe*: Low-grade fever with cold limbs.

[3] *Si Ni Tang* (Frigid Extremities Decoction): A formula to restore yang and prevent collapse.

Interpretations

Retching with a weak pulse, normal urination, and a low-grade fever but cold limbs are life-threatening and should be treated with *Si Ni Tang* (Frigid Extremities Decoction).

Si Ni Tang

[Ingredients]

附子	*fù zǐ*	1 piece	Radix Aconiti Lateralis Praeparata
甘草	*gān cǎo*	2 *liǎng*	Radix et Rhizoma Glycyrrhizae Preparata
干姜	*gān jiāng*	1.5 *liǎng*	Rhizoma Zingiberis

Decoct the three ingredients in 3 *shēng* of water to get 1.2 *shēng*. Remove the dregs and take in two divided doses. A large piece of *Fu Zi* and 3 *liǎng* of *Gan Jiang* can be used for patients with a strong body.

*****

[15] 呕而发热〔1〕者，小柴胡汤〔2〕主之。

小柴胡汤方：

柴胡半斤黄芩三两人参三两甘草三两半夏半斤生姜三两大枣十二枚右七味，以水一斗二升，煮取六升，去滓，再煎取三升。温服一升，日三服。

Annotations

[1] *Ou Er Fa Re*: Vomiting due to pathogenic heat. Patients may experience alternating fever and chills, pain in the subcostal region and poor appetite.

[2] *Xiao Chai Hu Tang* (Minor Bupleurum Decoction): A formula to clear heat, supplement healthy qi and down-regulate qi.

Interpretations

Vomiting with fever should be treated with *Xiao Chai Hu Tang* (Minor Bupleurum Decoction).

Xiao Chai Hu Tang

[Ingredients]

柴胡	*chái hú*	0.5 *jīn*	Radix Bupleuri (8 *liǎng* in *Shang Han Lun*)
黄芩	*huáng qín*	3 *liǎng*	Radix Scutellariae
人参	*rén shēn*	3 *liǎng*	Radix et Rhizoma Ginseng
甘草	*gān cǎo*	3 *liǎng*	Radix et Rhizoma Glycyrrhizae (2 *liǎng* in other text)
半夏	*bàn xià*	0.5 *jīn*	Rhizoma Pinelliae (0.5 *shēng* in other text)
生姜	*shēng jiāng*	3 *liǎng*	Rhizoma Zingiberis Recens
大枣	*dà zǎo*	12 pieces	Fructus Jujubae

Decoct the seven ingredients in 1.2 *dòu* of water to get 6 *shēng*. Remove the dregs and re-decoct to get 3 *shēng*. Take 1 *shēng* for each dose when it is warm, 3 doses a day.

*****

[16] 胃反呕吐〔1〕者，大半夏汤〔2〕主之。《千金》云：治胃反不受食，食入即吐。《外台》云：治呕，心下痞鞕者。

大半夏汤方：

半夏二升，洗完用人参三两白蜜一升右三味，以水一斗二升，和蜜扬之二百四十遍，煮药取升半。温服一升，余分再服。

Annotations

[1] *Wei Fan Ou Tu*: It includes symptoms such as eating in the morning but vomiting in the evening, eating in the evening but vomiting in the morning, and poor digestion.

[2] *Da Ban Xia Tang* (Major Pinellia Decoction): A formula to harmonize the stomach, down-regulate qi, reinforce the body and moisten dryness.

Interpretations

Stomach discomfort with vomiting (eating in the morning but vomiting in the evening or eating in the evening but vomiting in the morning) can be treated with *Da Ban Xia Tang* (Major Pinellia Decoction). The *Qian Jin Yao Fang* (Important Formulas Worth a Thousand Gold Pieces) states, "This formula is indicated for an inability to eat food and vomiting immediately after eating". The *Wai Tai Mi Yao* (Arcane Essentials from the Imperial Library) states, "This formula is indicated for vomiting with epigastric hardness and masses".

Da Ban Xia Tang

[Ingredients]

半夏	*bàn xià*	2 *shēng*	Rhizoma Pinelliae (washed)
人参	*rén shēn*	3 *liǎng*	Radix et Rhizoma Ginseng
白蜜	*bái mì*	1 *shēng*	White honey

Blend the honey into 1.2 *dòu* of water, stir 240 times and decoct with the other two ingredients to get 2.5 *shēng*. Take 1 *shēng* when it is warm for the first dose. Divide the rest decoction into two doses and take when it is warm.

*****

[17] 食已即吐〔1〕者，大黄甘草汤〔2〕主之。《外台》方：又治吐水。

大黄甘草汤方：

大黄四两甘草一两右二味，以水三升，煮取一升。分温再服。

Annotations

[1] *Shi Yi Ji Tu*: Vomiting immediately after eating food due to excess heat in the stomach.

[2] *Da Huang Gan Cao Tang* (Rhubarb and Licorice Decoction): A formula to clear heat and reduce fire.

Interpretations

Vomiting immediately after eating food should be treated with *Da Huang Gan Cao Tang* (Rhubarb and Licorice Decoction). The *Wai Tai Mi Yao* (Arcane Essentials from the Imperial Library) states, “This formula is also indicated for vomiting immediately after drinking water”.

Da Huang Gan Cao Tang

[Ingredients]

大黄	*dà huáng*	4 *liǎng*	Radix et Rhizoma Rhei
甘草	*gān cǎo*	1 *liǎng*	Radix et Rhizoma Glycyrrhizae

Decoct the two ingredients in 3 *shēng* of water to get 1 *shēng*. Divide into two doses and drink when it is warm.

*****

[18] 胃反，吐而渴欲饮水〔1〕者，茯苓泽泻汤〔2〕主之。

茯苓泽泻汤方《外台》云：治消渴〔3〕脉绝，胃反吐食之，有小麦一升 茯苓半斤泽泻四两 甘草二两桂枝二两白术三两生姜四两

右六味，以水一斗，煮取三升，内泽泻，再煮取二升半。温服八合，日三服。

Annotations

[1] *Tu Er Ke Yu Yin Shui*: Persistent vomiting—drinking after vomiting and vomiting again after drinking. This is caused by retained fluid in the stomach.

[2] *Fu Ling Ze Xie Tang* (Poria and Alisma Decoction): A formula to resolve water fluids, promote urination, harmonize the stomach, and down-regulate qi.

[3] *Xiao Ke*: Here it refers to thirst with a desire to drink water but vomit immediately after drinking.

Interpretations

Stomach discomfort with persistent vomiting after drinking (then drinking again but vomiting immediately after drinking) should be treated with *Fu Ling Ze Xie Tang* (Poria and Alisma Decoction). The *Wai Tai Mi Yao* (Arcane Essentials from the Imperial Library) states, "This formula is indicated for thirst with a desire to drink water but vomit immediately after drinking, an extremely faint pulse (can hardly be felt). It also includes 1 *shēng* (2 *shēng* in other texts) of wheat".

Fu Ling Ze Xie Tang

[Ingredients]

茯苓	*fú líng*	0.5 *jīn*	Poria
泽泻	*zé xiè*	4 *liǎng*	Rhizoma Alismatis
甘草	*gān cǎo*	2 *liǎng*	Radix et Rhizoma Glycyrrhizae
桂枝	*guì zhī*	2 *liǎng*	Ramulus Cinnamomi
白术	*bái zhú*	3 *liǎng*	Rhizoma Atractylodis Macrocephalae
生姜	*shēng jiāng*	3 *liǎng*	Rhizoma Zingiberis Recens

Decoct *Fu Ling* (Poria), *Gan Cao* (Radix et Rhizoma Glycyrrhizae), *Gui Zhi* (Ramulus Cinnamomi), *Bai Zhu* (Rhizoma Atractylodis Macrocephalae) and *Sheng Jiang* (Rhizoma Zingiberis Recens) in 1 *dòu* of water to get 3 *shēng*. Then add *Ze Xie* (Rhizoma Alismatis) and decoct to get 2.5 *shēng*. Take 0.8 *shēng*for each dose when it is warm, 3 doses a day.

*****

[19] 吐后，渴欲得水而贪饮〔1〕者，文蛤汤〔2〕主之。兼主微风，脉紧，头痛〔3〕。

文蛤汤方：

文蛤五两麻黄甘草生姜各三两石膏五两杏仁五十枚大枣十二枚

右七味，以水六升，煮取二升。温服一升。汗出愈。

Annotations

[1] *Tu Hou, Ke Yu De Shui Er Tan Yin*: Excessive drinking after vomiting. This is caused by internal heat.

[2] *Wen Ge Tang* (Meretrix Clam Shell Decoction): A formula to induce sweating, clear heat and stop thirst. Of the ingredients, *Wen Ge* (Meretricis Concha) clears the lung, regenerates fluids and stops thirst, *Yue Bi Tang* (Maidservant From Yue Decoction) is combined to induce sweating and release the exterior.

[3] *Jian Zhu Wei Feng, Mai Jin, Tou Tong*: Exterior wind syndrome with a tight pulse and headache.

Interpretations

Excessive thirst and drinking after vomiting can be treated with *Wen Ge Tang* (Meretrix Clam Shell Decoction). This formula is also indicated for exterior wind syndrome with a tight pulse and headache.

Wen Ge Tang

[Ingredients]

文蛤	*wén gé*	5 *liǎng*	Meretricis Concha
麻黄	*má huáng*	3 *liǎng*	Herba Ephedrae
甘草	*gān cǎo*	3 *liǎng*	Radix et Rhizoma Glycyrrhizae
生姜	*shēng jiāng*	3 *liǎng*	Rhizoma Zingiberis Recens
石膏	*shí gāo*	5 *liǎng*	Gypsum Fibrosum
杏仁	*xìng rén*	50 pieces	Semen Armeniacae Amarum
大枣	*dà zǎo*	20 pieces	Fructus Jujubae

Decoct the seven ingredients in 6 *shēng* of water to get 2 *shēng*. Take 1 *shēng* for each dose when it is warm. Patients may recover after sweating.

*****

[20] 干呕，吐逆，吐涎沫，半夏干姜散[1]主之。

半夏干姜散方：

半夏干姜各等分右二味，杵为散，取方寸匕，浆水一升半，煎取七合。顿服之。

Annotations

[1] *Ban Xia Gan Jiang San* (Pinellia and Dried Ginger Powder): A formula to warm the spleen and stomach and down-regulate qi.

Interpretations

Retching, vomiting or vomiting of foamy saliva can be treated with *Ban Xia Gan Jiang San* (Pinellia and Dried Ginger Powder).

Ban Xia Gan Jiang San

[Ingredients]

半夏	*bàn xià*	Rhizoma Pinelliae
干姜	*gān jiāng*	Rhizoma Zingiberis

Grind the two ingredients into a powder. Decoct one square-inch spoon of the powder in 1.5 *shēng* of millet water to get 0.7 *shēng*. Drink up at a draught.

*****

[21] 病人胸中似喘不喘，似呕不呕，似哕不哕，彻心中愦愦[1]然无奈者，生姜半夏汤[2]主之。

生姜半夏汤方：

半夏半斤生姜汁一升右二味，以水三升，煮半夏，取二升，内生姜汁，煮取一升半。小冷，分四服，日三夜一服。止，停后服。

Annotations

[1] *Xin Zhong Kui Kui*: Indescribable heart discomfort.

[2] *Sheng Jiang Ban Xia Tang* (Fresh Ginger and Pinellia Decoction): A formula to unblock yang, eliminate masses, resolve water fluid and down-regulate qi. It's advisable to take a small dose in multiple times when it is cold. The *Yi Zong Jin Jian* (Golden Mirror of the Medical Tradition) states, "This formula is similar to the previous *Ban Xia Gan Jiang San* (Pinellia and Dried Ginger Powder); however, the other one uses dried ginger to warm qi of the spleen and stomach and this one uses fresh ginger to resolve water fluid. In addition, the other one is taken at a draught to aggressively down-regulate qi and stop vomiting, whereas this one is taken in small doses at multiple times to gradually resolve cold retention".

Interpretations

Indescribable heart discomfort symptoms that resemble panting, nausea/vomiting or hiccups can be treated with *Sheng Jiang Ban Xia Tang* (Fresh Ginger and Pinellia Decoction).

Sheng Jiang Ban Xia Tang

[Ingredients]

半夏	*bàn xià*	0.5 *jīn*	Rhizoma Pinelliae
姜汁	*jiāng zhī*	1 *shēng*	Fresh ginger juice

Decoct *Ban Xia* (Rhizoma Pinelliae) first in 3 *shēng* of water to get 2 *shēng*, add fresh ginger juice to decoct and get 1.5 *shēng*. Drink in four times when it is cold—3 times during the day and one time at night. Stop taking the formula once vomiting stops.

*****

[22] 干呕，哕，若手足厥[1]者，橘皮汤[2]主之。

橘皮汤方：

橘皮四两生姜半斤右二味，以水七升，煮取三升。温服一升，下咽即愈。

Annotations

[1] *Shou Zu Jue*: Cold limbs due to obstruction of yang qi.

[2] *Ju Pi Tang* (Tangerine Peel Decoction): A formula to unblock yang, dissipate cold, down-regulate qi and harmonize the stomach.

Interpretations

Retching or hiccups with cold limbs should be treated with *Ju Pi Tang* (Tangerine Peel Decoction).

Ju Pi Tang

[Ingredients]

橘皮	*jú pí*	4 *liǎng*	Pericarpium Citri Reticulatae
生姜	*shēng jiāng*	0.5 *jīn*	Rhizoma Zingiberis Recens

Decoct the two ingredients in 7 *shēng* of water to get 3 *shēng*. Take 1 *shēng* when it is warm. The patients may recover once they swallow down the decoction.

*****

[23] 哕逆者，橘皮竹茹汤[1]主之。

橘皮竹茹汤方：

橘皮二升竹茹二升大枣三十个生姜半斤甘草五两人参一两右六味，以水一斗，煮取三升。温服一升，日三服。

Annotations

[1] *Ju Pi Zhu Ru Tang* (Tangerine Peel and Bamboo Shavings Decoction): A formula to supplement healthy qi, clear heat, down-regulate qi and harmonize the stomach.

Interpretations

Retching or hiccups with cold limbs should be treated with *Ju Pi Tang* (Tangerine Peel Decoction).

Ju Pi Tang

[Ingredients]

橘皮	*jú pí*	2 *shēng*	Pericarpium Citri Reticulatae
竹茹	*zhú rú*	2 *shēng*	Caulis Bambusae in Taenia (2 *jīn* in other text)
大枣	*dà zǎo*	30 pieces	Fructus Jujubae
生姜	*shēng jiāng*	0.5 *jīn*	Rhizoma Zingiberis Recens
甘草	*gān cǎo*	5 *liǎng*	Radix et Rhizoma Glycyrrhizae
人参	*rén shēn*	1 *liǎng*	Radix et Rhizoma Ginseng

Decoct the six ingredients in 1 *dòu* of water to get 3 *shēng*. Take 1 *shēng* for each dose, 3 doses a day.

*****

[24] 夫六腑气绝于外者，手足寒，上气，脚缩；五脏气绝于内者，利不禁，下甚者，手足不仁。

Interpretations

Yang qi deficiency of the zang-fu organs manifests as cold limbs, rapid breathing and curled toes externally and persistent, severe diarrhea with limb numbness internally.

*****

[25] 下利脉沉弦者，下重[1]；脉大者，为未止；脉微弱数者，为欲自止，虽发热不死。

Annotations

[1] *Xia Zhong*: Tenesmus in patients with diarrhea.

Interpretations

Diarrhea with a deep, wiry pulse indicates tenesmus; diarrhea with a large, surging pulse indicates unresolved diarrhea; and diarrhea with a weak, rapid pulse predicts a fast recovery—patients may have fever but the condition is not severe.

*****

[26] 下利手足厥冷，无脉者，灸之不温，若脉不还，反微喘者，死；少阴负趺阳[1]者，为顺也。

Annotations

[1] *Shao Yin Fu Fu Yang*: A smaller pulse at Taixi (KI 3) than Chongyang (ST 42) indicates a favorable prognosis with undamaged stomach yang.

Interpretations

For diarrhea with cold limbs and a pulse that can hardly be felt, cold limbs and impalpable pulse after moxibustion coupled with mild panting indicate a life-threatening condition. A faint, thready pulse at Taixi (KI 3) but steady and smaller than Chongyang (ST 42) indicates a high chance that patients may get better.

*****

[27] 下利有微热而渴，脉弱者，今自愈。

Interpretations

Diarrhea (due to deficiency cold) with a low-grade fever, thirst and a weak pulse predicts a favorable prognosis.

*****

[28] 下利脉数，有微热，汗出，今自愈；设脉紧为未解。

Interpretations

Diarrhea (due to deficiency cold) with a rapid pulse, low-grade fever and sweating predicts a favorable prognosis; diarrhea with a tight pulse indicates it still takes time for the patients to get better.

*****

[29] 下利脉数而渴者，今自愈。设不差，必清脓血〔1〕，以有热故也。

Annotations

[1] *Qing Nong Xue*: Pus and blood in stools.

Interpretations

Diarrhea (due to deficiency cold) with a rapid pulse and thirst predicts a favorable prognosis; persistent diarrhea may cause stools containing pus or blood, this is caused by retained heat in the body.

*****

[30] 下利脉反弦，发热，身汗者，自愈。

Interpretations

Diarrhea (due to deficiency cold) with a wiry pulse, fever and sweating predicts a favorable prognosis.

*****

[31] 下利气〔1〕者，当利其小便。

Annotations

[1] *Xia Li Qi*: Diarrhea with flatus.

Interpretations

Diarrhea with flatus should be treated by inducing urination.

*****

[32] 下利，寸脉反浮数〔1〕，尺中自涩者〔2〕，必清脓血。

Annotations

[1] *Cun Mai Fa Fu Shuo*: A superficial, rapid pulse at the *Cun* position. Here it refers to heat-related diarrhea.

[2] *Chi Zhong Zi Se Zhe*: A hesitant pulse at the *Chi* position, indicating blood stagnation due to heat.

Interpretations

Diarrhea with a superficial, rapid pulse at the *Cun* position and a hesitant pulse at the *Chi* position indicates pus or blood in the stools.

*****

[33] 下利清谷〔1〕，不可攻其表，汗出必胀满。

Annotations

[1] *Xia Li Qing Gu*: Diarrhea with stools that contain undigested food, indicating the diarrhea is caused by deficiency cold.

Interpretations

Diarrhea with stools that contain undigested food (even if there is an exterior syndrome) cannot be treated by inducing sweating; otherwise, patients may experience abdominal fullness and distension.

*****

[34] 下利脉沉而迟，其人面少赤，身有微热，下利清谷者，必郁冒〔1〕，汗出而解，病人必微热〔2〕，所以然者，其面戴阳〔3〕，下虚故也。

Annotations

[1] *Yu Mao*: Dizziness and blurred vision.

[2] *Wei Re*: It might be a wrong spelling of *Wei Jue*, meaning cold limbs.

[3] *Dai Yang*: Floating yang that often presents with a pale complexion with rosy cheeks.

Interpretations

Patients with diarrhea may present with a deep, slow pulse, a slightly red face, a low-grade fever, passing of stools that contain undigested food, dizziness and blurred vision. The symptoms may alleviate upon sweating but patients may have cold limbs. This is called floating yang in the face but deficiency cold in the spleen and stomach.

*****

[35] 下利后脉绝，手足厥冷，晬时〔1〕脉还，手足温者生；脉不还者死。

Annotations

[1] *Zui Shi*: Here it refers to one day (24 fours).

Interpretations

For diarrhea (due to deficiency cold) with cold limbs and a faint, thready pulse that can hardly be felt, restoration of the pulse with warm limbs within a day indicates a favorable prognosis; otherwise, it can be life threatening.

*****

[36] 下利腹胀满，身体疼痛者，先温其里，乃攻其表。温里宜四逆汤，攻表宜桂枝汤〔1〕。

四逆汤方方见上。

桂枝汤方：

桂枝三两，去皮芍药三两甘草二两，炙 生姜三两大枣十二枚 右五味，咀，以水七升，微火煮取三升，去滓。适寒温服一升，服已须臾，啜稀粥一升，以助药力。温覆令一时许，遍身漐漐微似有汗者，益佳。不可令如水淋漓。若一服汗出病差，停后服。

Annotations

[1] *Gui Zhi Tang* (Cinnamon Twig Decoction): A formula to release the exterior, dissipate cold and harmonize the *Ying*-nutrients and *Wei*-defense.

Interpretations

For diarrhea (due to deficiency cold) with abdominal fullness and distension (interior syndrome) and body ache (exterior syndrome), the treatment strategy should be to warm the interior first with *Si Ni Tang* (Frigid Extremities Decoction) and then release the exterior with *Gui Zhi Tang* (Cinnamon Twig Decoction).

For ingredients and usage of *Si Ni Tang* (Frigid Extremities Decoction), see line 14 in this chapter.

Gui Zhi Tang

[Ingredients]

桂枝	*guì zhī*	3 *liǎng*	Ramulus Cinnamomi (skin removed)
芍药	*sháo yào*	3 *liǎng*	Radix Paeoniae
甘草	*gān cǎo*	2 *liǎng*	Radix et Rhizoma Glycyrrhizae Preparata (3 *liǎng* in other text)
生姜	*shēng jiāng*	3 *liǎng*	Rhizoma Zingiberis Recens
大枣	*dà zǎo*	12 pieces	Fructus Jujubae

Slice the five ingredients and decoct in 7 *shēng* of water with mild fire to get 3 *shēng*. Remove the dregs and take 1 *shēng* when it is warm. After a while drink 1 *shēng* of congee to enhance the efficacy. Stay warm for approximately 2 hours to induce mild, persistent sweating instead of profuse sweating. Do not take the rest of the decoction if patients sweat and fully recover after one dose.

*****

[37] 下利三部〔1〕脉皆平，按之心下坚〔2〕者，急下之，宜大承气汤。

Annotations

[1] *San Bu*: Three positions to feel the pulse: *Cun*, *Guan* and *Chi*.
[2] *Xin Xia Jian*: Epigastric hardness and fullness.

Interpretations

Diarrhea with a forceful pulse at all three (*Cun*, *Guan* and *Chi*) positions and epigastric fullness and hardness should immediately be treated with *Da Cheng Qi Tang* (Major Purgative Decoction) to drain downward.

*****

[38] 下利脉迟而滑者，实也，利未欲止，急下之，宜大承气汤。

Interpretations

Diarrhea with a slow, slippery pulse indicates stagnation in the intestine and should be immediately treated with *Da Cheng Qi Tang* (Major Purgative Decoction) to drain downward.

*****

[39] 下利脉反滑者，当有所去[1]，下乃愈，宜大承气汤。

Annotations

[1] *Dang You Suo Qu*: Internal retention of undigested food.

Interpretations

Diarrhea with a slippery pulse indicates internal retention of undigested food. This can be treated with *Da Cheng Qi Tang* (Major Purgative Decoction) to drain downward.

*****

[40] 下利已差，至其年月日，时复发[1]者，以病不尽故也。当下之，宜大承气汤。

大承气汤方见痉病中

Annotations

[1] *Zhi Qi Nian Yue Ri, Shi Fu Fa*: Intermittent recurrences of heat-related diarrhea due to incomplete recovery. It is known as bacterial dysentery in modern medicine.

Interpretations

Intermittent recurrences of heat-related diarrhea due to incomplete recovery should be treated with *Da Cheng Qi Tang* (Major Purgative Decoction) to drain downward.

The ingredients and usage of this formula is discussed in chapter 2 (line 13).

*****

[41] 下利谵语[1]者，有燥屎也，小承气汤主之。

小承气汤方：

大黄四两厚朴二两，炙枳实大者三枚，炙 右三味，以水四升，煮取一升二合，去滓。分温二服得利则止。

Annotations

[1] *Xia Li Zhan Yu*: Inarticulate speeches during sleep.

Interpretations

Diarrhea with inarticulate speeches during sleep indicates retained dry feces (due to excess heat in the stomach and intestines) (probably in combination with fecal impaction with watery diarrhea, abdominal fullness, foul smelling stools and a slippery, rapid pulse) should be treated with *Xiao Cheng Qi Tang* (Minor Purgative Decoction) (to promote bowel movements and eliminate dry feces).

Xiao Cheng Qi Tang

[Ingredients]

大黄	*dà huáng*	4 *liǎng*	Radix et Rhizoma Rhei
厚朴	*hòu pò*	2 *liǎng*	Cortex Magnoliae Officinalis
枳实	*zhǐ shí*	3 pieces	Fructus Aurantii Immaturus (fried)

Decoct the three ingredients in 4 *shēng* of water to get 1.2 *shēng*. Remove the dregs, divided into two doses and take when it is warm.

*****

[42] 下利，便脓血者[1]，桃花汤[2]主之。

桃花汤方：

赤石脂一斤（一半锉，一半筛末）干姜一两粳米一升 右三味，以水七升，煮米令熟，去滓。温七合，内赤石脂末方寸匕，日三服；若一服愈，余勿服。

Annotations

[1] *Xia Li, Bian Nong Xue Zhe*: Chronic diarrhea (due to deficiency cold) may cause stools that contain mucus or dark, purple blood.

[2] *Tao Hua Tang* (Peach Blossom Decoction): A formula to warm the spleen and stomach and astringe the intestine. It's called peach blossom decoction because its major ingredient *Chi Shi Zhi* (Halloysitum Rubrum) (pink in color) resembles peach blossom.

Interpretations

Chronic diarrhea (due to deficiency cold) with stools that contain mucus, pus or dark, purple blood should be treated with *Tao Hua Tang* (Peach Blossom Decoction).

Tao Hua Tang

[Ingredients]

赤石脂	*chì shí zhī*	1 *jīn*	Halloysitum Rubrum (half rasped, half sifted)
干姜	*gān jiāng*	1 *liǎng*	Rhizoma Zingiberis
粳米	*jīng mǐ*	1 *shēng*	Oryza Sativa L.

Decoct the three ingredients (except for halloysite powder) in 7 *shēng* of water until the non-glutinous rice is fully cooked. Remove the dregs and mix 1 square-inch spoon of halloysite powder with 0.7 *shēng* of warm decoction for each dose, 3 doses a day. If patients fully recover after the first dose, do not take the rest of the decoction.

*****

[43] 热利重下者，白头翁汤〔1〕主之。

白头翁汤方：

白头翁二两黄连黄柏秦皮各三两右四味，以水七升，煮取二升，去滓。温服一升。不愈，更服。

Annotations

[1] *Bai Tou Weng Tang* (Pulsatilla Decoction): A formula to clear heat and dry dampness. It is still used today for bacterial dysentery.

Interpretations

Heat-related diarrhea with tenesmus (stools containing mucus, pus or blood, abdominal pain and fever) can be treated with *Bai Tou Weng Tang* (Pulsatilla Decoction).

Bai Tou Weng Tang

[Ingredients]

白头翁	*bái tóu wēng*	2 *liǎng*	Radix Pulsatillae
黄连	*huáng lián*	3 *liǎng*	Rhizoma Coptidis
黄柏	*huáng bǎi*	3 *liǎng*	Cortex Phellodendri Chinensis
秦皮	*qín pí*	3 *liǎng*	Cortex Fraxini

Decoct the four ingredients in 7 *shēng* of water to get 2 *shēng*. Remove the dregs and take 1 *shēng* for each dose when it is warm. If patients do not fully recover, take another dose (1 *shēng*).

*****

[44] 下利后更烦，按之心下濡者，为虚烦〔1〕也。栀子豉汤〔2〕主之。

栀子豉汤方：

栀子十四枚 香豉四合，绵裹右二味，以水四升，先煮栀子，得二升半，内豉，煮取一升半，去滓。分二服，温进一服，得吐则止。

Annotations

[1] *Xu Fan*: Intangible pathogenic heat.

[2] *Zhi Zi Chi Tang* (Gardenia and Fermented Soybean Decoction): A formula to clear unresolved heat.

Interpretations

Low-grade fever after diarrhea with epigastric softness is caused by retained intangible heat and can be treated with *Zhi Zi Chi Tang* (Gardenia and Fermented Soybean Decoction).

Zhi Zi Chi Tang

[Ingredients]

栀子	*zhī zǐ*	14 pieces	Fructus Gardeniae
香豉	*xiāng chǐ*	0.4 *shēng*	Semen Sojae Praeparatum (wrapped in cotton gauze)

Decoct *Zhi Zi* (Fructus Gardeniae) first in 4 *shēng* of water to get 2.5 *shēng*, and then add *Xiang Chi* (Semen Sojae Praeparatum) to get 1.5 *shēng*. Divide into two doses and drink when it is warm. In case vomiting occurs after the first dose, do not take the second dose.

*****

[45] 下利清谷，里寒外热，汗出而厥〔1〕者，通脉四逆汤〔2〕主之。

通脉四逆汤方：

附子大者一枚，生用干姜三两，强人可四两 甘草二两，炙右三味，以水三升，煮取一升二合，去滓。分温再服。

Annotations

[1] *Li Han Wai Re, Han Chu Er Jue*: Diarrhea indicates interior cold and sweating indicates exterior sweating. Here it refers to true cold with false heat due to floating of deficiency yang.

[2] *Tong Mai Si Ni Tang* (Channel-Unblocking for Frigid Extremities Decoction): A formula to restore yang and prevents collapse.

Interpretations

Stools that contain undigested food, sweating and cold limbs indicate a life-threatening true cold with false heat and should be immediately treated with *Tong Mai Si Ni Tang* (Channel-Unblocking for Frigid Extremities Decoction).

Tong Mai Si Ni Tang

[Ingredients]

附子	*fù zǐ*	1 piece	Radix Aconiti Lateralis (large)
干姜	*gān jiāng*	3 *liǎng*	Rhizoma Zingiberis (4 *liǎng* for those with a strong body)
甘草	*gān cǎo*	2 *liǎng*	Radix et Rhizoma Glycyrrhizae Preparata

Decoct the three ingredients in 3 *shēng* of water to get 1.2 *shēng*. Remove the dregs, divide into two doses and drink when it is warm.

*****

[46] 下利肺痛[1]，紫参汤[2]主之。

紫参汤方：

紫参半斤甘草三两右二味，以水五升，先煮紫参，取二升，内甘草，煮取一升半。分温三服疑非仲景方。

Annotations

[1] *Xia Li Fei Yong*: Chronic diarrhea followed by pain in the lung (probably in combination with cough with blood-stained sputum).

[2] *Zi Shen Tang* (Salviae Decoction): A formula to break and resolve masses. *Zi Shen* is also named as *Shi Jian Chuan* (Herba Salviae Chinensis). (See chapter 7, line 9 for reference).

Interpretations

Loose stools followed by pain in the lung (probably in combination with cough with blood-stained sputum) should be treated with *Zi Shen Tang* (Salviae Decoction).

Huang Qin Tang

[Ingredients]

紫参	*zǐ shēn*	0.5 *jīn*	Herba Salviae Chinensis
甘草	*gān cǎo*	3 *liǎng*	Radix et Rhizoma Glycyrrhizae

Decoct *Zi Shen* (Herba Salviae Chinensis) in 5 *shēng* of water to get 2 *shēng*. Add *Gan Cao* (Radix et Rhizoma Glycyrrhizae) to decoct to 1.5 *shēng*. Divide into three doses and take when it is warm (some suspect it's not an original formula of Zhang Zhongjing).

*****

[47] 气利〔1〕，诃梨勒散〔2〕主之。
诃梨勒散方：
诃梨勒十枚，煨右一味，为散。粥饮和，顿服疑非仲景方。

Annotations

[1] *Qi Li*: Passing out of stools during flatus; however, there is no mucus or foul smelling. This is caused by chronic diarrhea.

[2] *He Li Le San* (Chebulae Powder): A formula to warm the meridians and astringe the intestine.

Interpretations

In patients with chronic diarrhea, passing out stools during flatus should be treated with *He Li Le San* (Chebulae Powder).

Method: Grind 10 pieces of *He Zi* (Fructus Chebulae) into a fine powder, mix with congee, and drink up at a draught (some suspect that it's not an original formula of Zhang Zhongjing).

*****

Annex formula # 1 Qian Jin Yi Fang *Xiao Cheng Qi Tang*

《千金翼》小承气汤，治大便不通，哕数谵语。方见上。

Interpretations

The *Xiao Cheng Qi Tang* (Minor Purgative Decoction) in the *Qian Jin Yi Fang* (Supplement to 'Important Formulas Worth a Thousand Gold Pieces') is indicated for constipation, frequent hiccups, and delirium (the ingredients and usage of the formula, see line 41).

*****

Annex formula # 2 Wai Tai *Huang Qin Tang* (Scutellaria Decoction)

《外台》黄芩汤[1]，治干呕下利。

黄芩人参干姜各三两桂枝一两大枣十二枚半夏半升右六味，以水七升，煮取三升。温分三服。

Annotations

[1] *Huang Qin Tang* (Scutellaria Decoction): A formula to clear the intestine, stop diarrhea, and strengthen the spleen and stomach.

Interpretations

The *Huang Qin Tang* (Scutellaria Decoction) in *Wai Tai Mi Yao* (Arcane Essentials from the Imperial Library) is indicated for retching and diarrhea.

Huang Qin Tang

[Ingredients]

黄芩	*huáng qín*	3 *liǎng*	Radix Scutellariae (2 *liǎng* in other text)
人参	*rén shēn*	3 *liǎng*	Radix et Rhizoma Ginseng (2 *liǎng* in other text)
干姜	*gān jiāng*	3 *liǎng*	Rhizoma Zingiberis (2 *liǎng* in other text)
桂枝	*guì zhī*	1 *liǎng*	Ramulus Cinnamomi
大枣	*dà zǎo*	12 pieces	Fructus Jujubae
半夏	*bàn xià*	0.5 *shēng*	Rhizoma Pinelliae

Decoct the six ingredients in 7 *shēng* of water to get 3 *shēng*. Divide into three doses and take when it is warm.

疮痈肠痈浸淫病脉证并治第十八
Chapter 18 Skin Abscesses, Intestinal Abscesses, and Wet Spreading Sores—Pulses, Patterns and Treatment

Overview

This chapter is exclusively dedicated to four external conditions—skin abscesses, intestinal abscesses, incised wounds and wet-spreading sores.

*****

[01] 诸浮数脉，应当发热，而反洒淅恶寒，若有痛处，当发其痈〔1〕。

Annotations

[1] *Yong*: A purulent condition (due to toxic heat) characterized by local redness, swelling, warmth and pain. It can internally affect the zang-fu organs and externally affect the skin.

Interpretations

Normally, patients with a superficial, rapid pulse have fever; however, they may also experience aversion to cold as if there is cold water spraying on the body. Localized pain (in combination with redness, swelling and warmth) indicates the formation of abscess.

*****

[02] 师曰：诸痈肿，欲知有脓无脓，以手掩肿上，热者为有脓，不热者为无脓。

Interpretations

The Master said, "For all types of abscesses, there is one way to tell whether they are purulent or not—gently touch the swollen area: a warm sensation indicates there is pus; otherwise there is no pus".

*****

[03] 肠痈[1]之为病，其身甲错[2]，腹皮急[3]，按之濡，如肿状[4]，腹无积聚，身无热，脉数，此为腹内有痈脓，薏苡附子败酱散[5]主之。

薏苡附子败酱散方：

薏苡仁十分附子二分败酱五分右三味，杵为末，取方寸匕，以水二升，煎减半。顿服小便[6]当下。

Annotations

[1] *Chang Yong*: Intestinal abscess. It is characterized by lower abdominal pain, pain upon pressure, tensing of the abdominal wall, fever and chills. It is similar to acute appendicitis or appendicular abscess in modern medicine.

[2] *Qi Shen Jia Cuo*: Rough, scaly skin of the body.

[3] *Fu Pi Ji*: Tensing of the lower abdominal skin. It is similar to abdominal guarding in modern medicine.

[4] *An Zhi Ru, Ru Zhong Zhuang*: Feeling of soft masses with heavy pressure, indicating the formation of abscess.

[5] *Yi Yi Fu Zi Bai Jiang San* (Coix, Aconite and Patrinia Powder): A formula to remove toxins, drain pus, break stasis and resolve masses.

[6] *Xiao Bian*: Urine. However, it should be a wrong spelling of bowel movements.

Interpretations

Patients with intestinal abscess may present with (dry) rough, scaly skin and tensing of lower abdominal skin with gentle pressure but soft masses with heavy pressure. However, there is no abdominal masses. Although they do not have fever, the pulse is rapid. This indicates the formation of abscess inside the abdomen and should be treated with *Yi Yi Fu Zi Bai Jiang San* (Coix, Aconite and Patrinia Powder).

Yi Yi Fu Zi Bai Jiang San

[Ingredients]

薏苡仁	*yì yǐ rén*	10 *fēn*	Semen Coicis
附子	*fù zǐ*	2 *fēn*	Radix Aconiti Lateralis Praeparata
败酱	*bài jiàng*	5 *fēn*	Herba Patriniae

Grind the three ingredients into a fine powder. Decoct 1 square-inch spoon in 2 *shēng* of water to get 1 *shēng*. Drink up at a draught (the pus should be discharged through bowel movements).

*****

[04] 肠痈者，少腹肿痞，按之即痛如淋〔1〕，小便自调，时时发热，自汗出，复恶寒。其脉迟紧者，脓未成，可下之〔2〕，当有血。脉洪数者，脓已成，不可下也〔3〕。大黄牡丹汤〔4〕主之。

大黄牡丹汤方：

大黄四两牡丹一两桃仁五十个瓜子半升芒硝三合 右五味，以水六升，煮取一升，去滓，内芒硝，再煎沸。顿服之。有脓当下；如无脓，当下血。

Annotations

[1] *Chang Yong Zhe...Ji Tong Ru Lin*: Local symptoms in early stage intestinal abscess: Lower abdominal swelling or bulging with palpable masses, pain upon heavy pressure, and lower abdominal pain that radiates to the umbilicus as in strangury.

[2] *Nong Wei Cheng, Ke Xia Zhi*: *Da Huang Mu Dan Tang* (Rhubarb and Moutan Decoction) can be used to drain downward before the formation of abscess.

[3] *Mai Hong Shuo Zhe...Bu Ke Xia Ye*: Draining downward method is prohibited after the formation of abscess; otherwise, perforation may occur. The previously discussed *Yi Yi Fu Zi Bai Jiang San* (Coix, Aconite and Patrinia Powder) can be used instead to drain pus and remove toxins.

[4] *Da Huang Mu Dan Tang* (Rhubarb and Moutan Decoction): A formula to clear heat, break stasis, resolve masses and eliminate abscess. It is a common formula for acute appendicitis.

Interpretations

Patients with intestinal abscess may first present with lower abdominal swelling or bulging with palpable masses and pain upon pressure as in strangury (tensing and pain of lower abdominal skin that radiate to the umbilicus); however, they have normal urination (no dribbling urination). In addition, they have fever, sweating, aversion to cold, and a slow, tight pulse. This indicates there is no formation of abscess yet and can be treated with *Da Huang Mu Dan Tang* (Rhubarb and Moutan Decoction) to drain downward. Normally there should be blood in stools after taking the formula. A surging, rapid pulse indicates the formation of abscess. In such case, the formula cannot be used.

Da Huang Mu Dan Tang

[Ingredients]

大黄	*dà huáng*	4 *liǎng*	Radix et Rhizoma Rhei
牡丹	*mŭ dān*	1 *liǎng*	Cortex Moutan
桃仁	*táo rén*	50 pieces	Semen Persicae
瓜子	*guā zĭ*	0.5 *shēng*	Semen Benincasae
芒硝	*máng xiāo*	0.3 *shēng*	Natrii Sulfas

Decoct the first four ingredients in 6 *shēng* of water to get 1 *shēng*. Remove the dregs and add *Man Xiao* (Natrii Sulfas) to bring it to a boil. Drink up at a draught. There should be pus or blood in stools after taking the formula.

*****

[05] 问曰：寸口脉浮微而涩，然当亡血若汗出[1]。设不汗者云何？答曰：若身有疮，被刀斧所伤，亡血故也。

Annotations

[1] *Mai Fu Wei Er Se, Ran Dan Wang Xue Ruo Han Chu*: A faint, superficial pulse indicates qi deficiency. Normally this pulse should be seen in people after heavy bleeding or profuse sweating.

Interpretations

Question: Normally a superficial, weak and hesitant pulse is seen in people after heavy bleeding or profuse sweating. If there is no blood loss or sweating, what is the cause?

Answer: This is caused by blood loss due to incised wounds.

*****

[06] 病金疮〔1〕，王不留行散〔2〕主之。

王不留行散方：

王不留行十分，八月八日采 蒴藋细叶十分，七月七日采桑东南根白皮，十分，三月三日采甘草十八分川椒三分，除目及闭口者汗黄芩二分干姜二分芍药二分厚朴二分 右九味，桑根皮以上三味烧灰存性，勿令灰过，各别杵筛，合治之为散。服方寸匕。小疮即粉之，大疮但服之。产后亦可服。如风寒，桑东根勿取之。前三物皆阴干百日。

Annotations

[1] *Bing Jin Chuan*: Incised wounds or cuts by metallic weapons or instruments.

[2] *Wang Bu Liu Xing San* (Vaccaria Powder): A formula to move blood, resolve stasis, heal wounds and stop bleeding.

Interpretations

Incised wounds can be treated with *Wang Bu Liu Xing San* (Vaccaria Powder).

Wang Bu Liu Xing San

[Ingredients]

王不留行	*wáng bù liú xíng*	10 *fēn*	Radix et Rhizoma Rhei (harvested on Aug. 8)
蒴藋细叶	*shuò dí xì yè*	10 *fēn*	Radix Schefflerae Arboricolae (harvested on July 7)
桑白皮	*sāng bái pí*	10 *fēn*	Cortex Mori
甘草	*gān cǎo*	18 *fēn*	Radix et Rhizoma Glycyrrhizae (10 *fēn* in other text)
川椒	*chuān jiāo*	3 *fēn*	Pericarpium Zanthoxyli

Wang Bu Liu Xing San

[Ingredients]

黄芩	*huáng qín*	2 *fēn*	Radix Scutellariae
干姜	*gān jiāng*	2 *fēn*	Rhizoma Zingiberis
芍药	*sháo yào*	2 *fēn*	Radix Paeoniae
厚朴	*hòu pò*	2 *fēn*	Cortex Magnoliae Officinalis

Char the first three ingredients into ashes without destroying their medicinal nature. Grind and sift the rest of the ingredients into a fine powder separately and then mix together. Take a square-inch spoon for each dose. Apply the medicinal powder to small wounds. Take it orally for large wounds. New mothers after childbirth can also take this formula. Remove *Sang Bai Pi* (Cortex Mori) if patients contracted wind cold.

[Cautionary note] The first three ingredients need to be dried in the shade for a hundred days (avoid fire or direct sun exposure).

*****

[07] 排脓散〔1〕方：

枳实十六枚芍药六分桔梗二分 右三味，杵为散，取鸡子黄一枚，以药散与鸡黄相等，揉和令相得。饮和服之，日一服。

Annotations

[1] *Pai Nong San* (Pus-Drainage Powder): A formula to move qi, drain pus, harmonize blood and supplement healthy qi. The major ingredient is *Jie Geng* (Radix Platycodonis).

Pai Nong San

[Ingredients]

枳实	*zhǐ shí*	16 pieces	Fructus Aurantii Immaturus
芍药	*sháo yào*	6 *fēn*	Radix Paeoniae
桔梗	*jié gěng*	2 *fēn*	Radix Platycodonis

Grind the three ingredients into a fine powder. Then blend one egg yolk with an equal amount of the powder. Take with water, once a day.

*****

[08] 排脓汤〔1〕方：

甘草二两桔梗三两一两大枣十枚右四味，以水三升，煮取一升。温服五合，日再服。

Annotations

[1] *Pai Nong Tang* (Pus-Drainage Decoction): A formula to remove toxins and drain pus.

Pai Nong Tang

[Ingredients]

甘草	*gān cǎo*	2 *liǎng*	Radix et Rhizoma Glycyrrhizae
桔梗	*jié gěng*	3 *liǎng*	Radix Platycodonis
生姜	*shēng jiāng*	1 *liǎng*	Rhizoma Zingiberis Recens
大枣	*dà zǎo*	12 pieces	Fructus Jujubae

Decoct the four ingredients in 3 *shēng* of water and get 1 *shēng*. Take 0.5 *shēng* for each dose, two doses a day.

*****

[09] 浸淫疮，从口流向四肢者，可治；从四肢流来入口者，不可治。

Interpretations

Wet spreading sores that start from the mouth and extend to the limbs are not severe and easy to treat; sores that start from the limbs and extend to the mouth are severe and hard to treat.

*****

[10] 浸淫疮，黄连粉〔1〕主之。方未见。

Annotations

[1] *Huang Lian Fen* (Coptis Powder): There is no detailed information about the formula. It probably contains a single ingredient *Huang Lian* (Rhizoma Coptidis). It acts to clear heat, dry dampness, reduce fire and remove toxins.

Interpretations

Wet Spreading Sores can be treated with *Huang Lian Fen* (Coptis Powder). No formula is provided in the text.

跌蹶手指臂肿转筋阴狐疝蚘虫病脉证治第十九

Chapter 19 Dorsal Muscle Spasticity of the Foot, Swelling in Fingers/Arms, Cramping, Groin Hernia and Roundworms—Pulses, Patterns and Treatment

Overview

This chapter discusses five conditions—dorsal muscle spasticity of the foot, swelling in the fingers and arms, cramping, groin and hernia and roundworms. They are discussed together because they are all associated with sinews.

*****

[01] 师曰：病趺蹶〔1〕，其人但能前，不能却，刺腨〔2〕入二寸，此太阳经伤也。

Annotations

[1] *Fu Jue*: Dorsal muscle spasticity of the foot due to damage to the bladder meridian. With this condition, patients can only move forward.

[2] *Ci Shuan*: Needling Chengshan (BL 57).

Interpretations

The Master said, "With dorsal muscle spasticity of the foot, patients can only move forward. This is caused by damage to the bladder meridian and can be treated by needling 2 cun into Chengshan (BL 57).

*****

[02] 病人常以手指臂肿动[1]，此人身体[2]者，藜芦甘草汤[3]主之。

藜芦甘草汤方未见。

Annotations

[1] *Shou Zhi Bi Zhong Dong*: Swelling and involuntary twitching in the fingers and arms due to wind phlegm affecting the muscles or sinews.

[2] *Shen Ti*: Here it refers to mild twitching in the fingers or arms.

[3] *Li Lu Gan Cao Tang* (Veratrum and Licorice Decoction): A formula to induce sweating, resolve phlegm and extinguish wind. Since *Li Lu* (Veratrum Nigrum) is toxic, only a smaller dose can be used. Later this formula has been made into powder.

Interpretations

Swelling in the fingers and arms as well as mild involuntary twitching can be treated with *Li Lu Gan Cao Tang* (Veratrum and Licorice Decoction). The formula was not provided in the text.

*****

[03] 转筋[1]之为病，其人臂脚直，脉上下行，微弦[2]。转筋入腹者，鸡屎白散[3]主之。

鸡屎白散方：

鸡屎白 右一味，为散，取方寸匕，以水六合和。温服。

Annotations

[1] *Zhuan Jin*: Cramping of the arms and legs due to heat damaging yin.

[2] *Mai Shang Xia Xing, Wei Xian*: A slightly wiry pulse at all three positions (*Cun, Guan and Chi*).

[3] *Ji Shi Bai San* (White Chicken Poop Powder): A formula to promote digestion and resolve dampness.

Interpretations

Cramping may cause rigidity and spasm of the arms and legs, along with a slight wiry pulse in all three positions (*Cun, Guan* and *Chi*). In severe cases, cramping may radiate to the lower abdomen. This can be treated with *Ji Shi Bai San* (White Chicken Poop Powder).

Method: Grind the white chicken poop into a powder. Mix a square-inch spoon with 0.6 *shēng* of water. Bring it to boil and take when it is warm.

*****

[04] 阴狐疝气〔1〕者，偏有小大，时时上下，蜘蛛散〔2〕主之。

蜘蛛散方：

蜘蛛[3]十四枚，熬焦桂枝半两二味，为散。取八分一匕，饮和服，日再服。蜜丸亦可。

Annotations

[1] *Yin Hu Shan Qi*: Groin hernia that bulges on one side of the scrotum and moves up and down. It is caused by cold qi stagnation in the genital area along the pathway of the liver meridian.

[2] *Zhi Zhu San* (Spider Powder): A formula to break stasis, resolve masses, unblock yang, and dissipate cold.

[3] *Zhi Zhu*: Spider. It acts to remove wind, resolve swelling and remove toxins.

Interpretations

Groin hernia bulges on one side of the scrotum and moves up and down. The bulge becomes more prominent when standing up or walking and disappears on lying down. This can be treated with *Zhi Zhu San* (Spider Powder).

Zhi Zhu San

[Ingredients]

蜘蛛	*zhī zhu*	14 pieces	Spider (boil until parched)
桂枝	*guì zhī*	0.5 *liǎng*	Ramulus Cinnamomi

Grind the two ingredients into a fine powder. Take the mixture of 1/8 square-inch spoon with water for each dose, 2 doses a day. Alternatively, the powder can be mixed with honey to make into pills.

*****

[05] 问曰：病腹痛有虫，其脉何以别之？师曰：腹中痛，其脉当沉若弦。反洪大，故有蛔虫。

Interpretations

Question: How do you diagnose abdominal pain caused by roundworms from the pulse?

Answer: Normally, abdominal pain causes a deep (interior cold) or wiry (qi stagnation) pulse; a large, surging pulse often indicates moving of roundworms.

*****

[06] 蛔虫〔1〕之为病，令人吐涎，心痛发作有时，毒药不止〔2〕，甘草粉蜜汤〔3〕主之。

甘草粉蜜汤方：

甘草二两 粉一两重 蜜四两 右三味，以水三升，先煮甘草，取二升，去滓，内粉、蜜，搅令和，煎如薄粥。温服一升，差即止。

Annotations

[1] *Hui Chong*: Roundworms. Here it refers to roundworms-induced problems that are characterized by paroxysmal intense abdominal pain and vomiting.

[2] *Du Yao Bu Zhi*: Persistent stomach discomfort after taking harsh, roundworm-expelling medicinals.

[3] *Gan Cao Fen Mi Tang* (Licorice, Rice Flour and Honey Decoction): A formula to harmonize the stomach and alleviate the side effects of roundworm-expelling medicinals.

Interpretations

Roundworms cause vomiting of foamy saliva, paroxysmal, intense abdominal pain; however, harsh roundworm-expelling medicinals may cause persistent stomach discomfort. This can be treated with *Gan Cao Fen Mi Tang* (Licorice, Rice Flour and Honey Decoction).

Gan Cao Fen Mi Tang

[Ingredients]

甘草	*gān cǎo*	2 *liǎng*	Radix et Rhizoma Glycyrrhizae
粉	*fěn*	1 *liǎng*	Rice flour
蜜	*mì*	4 *liǎng*	Honey

Decoct *Gan Cao* (Radix et Rhizoma Glycyrrhizae) first in 3 *shēng* of water to get 2 *shēng*. Remove the dregs and mix with the rice flour and honey thoroughly. Re-decoct until it looks like thin congee. Take 1 *shēng* for each dose when it is warm and stop upon a full recovery.

*****

[07] 蛔厥[1]者，当吐蛔。令病者静，而复时烦[2]，此为藏寒，蛔上入膈，故烦，须臾复止。得食而呕，又烦者，蛔闻食臭出，其人常自吐蛔。

Annotations

[1] *Hui Jue*: A condition caused by roundworms. It is characterized by paroxysmal, intense abdominal pain, restlessness and vomiting of roundworms. It is similar to biliary ascariasis in modern medicine.

[2] *Fan*: Restlessness, uneasiness.

Interpretations

For patients with intestinal roundworms, roundworms normally appear in the vomitus. They experience alternating calmness with restlessness, because the roundworms ascend to the diaphragm and subcostal region to escape away from the cold in the intestine. After eating food, they feel uneasy and vomit again because the roundworms start to move at the smell of food. As a result, roundworms appear in the vomitus.

*****

[08] 蛔厥者，乌梅丸[1]主之。乌梅丸方：

乌梅三百个细辛六两干姜十两黄连一斤当归四两附子六两，炮川椒四两，去汗桂枝六两人参黄柏各六两　右十味，异捣筛，合治之，以苦酒渍乌梅一宿，去核，蒸之五升米[2]下，饭熟捣成泥，和药令相得，内臼中，与蜜杵二千下，丸如梧子大。先食，饮服十丸，三服，稍加至二十丸。禁生冷、滑臭等食。

Annotations

[1] *Wu Mei Wan* (Mume Pill): A formula to calm the roundworms and relieve pain. It is now commonly used for biliary ascariasis.

Interpretations

Intestinal roundworms can be treated with *Wu Mei Wan* (Mume Pill).

Wu Mei Wan

[Ingredients]

乌梅	*wū méi*	300 Pieces	Fructus Mume
细辛	*xì xīn*	6 *liǎng*	Radix et Rhizoma Asari
干姜	*gān jiāng*	10 *liǎng*	Rhizoma Zingiberis
黄连	*huáng lián*	1 *jīn*	Rhizoma Coptidis (16 *liǎng* in *Shang Han Lun*)
当归	*dāng guī*	4 *liǎng*	Radix Angelicae Sinensis
附子	*fù zǐ*	6 *liǎng*	Radix Aconiti Lateralis Praeparata
花椒	*huā jiāo*	4 *liǎng*	Pericarpium Zanthoxyli Praeparata (seed-removed)
桂枝	*guì zhī*	6 *liǎng*	Ramulus Cinnamomi (skin-removed)
人参	*rén shēn*	6 *liǎng*	Radix et Rhizoma Ginseng
黄柏	*huáng bǎi*	6 *liǎng*	Cortex Phellodendri Chinensis

Grind the ten ingredients separately and then mix together. Soak the *Wu Mei* (Fructus Mume) in vinegar overnight, remove the kernels and steam under five *shēng* of rice. When the rice is fully cooked, pound it into a paste, mix with the rest of the ingredients, and place into a mortar. Add some honey and pound 2,000 times to make into pills the size of firmiana seeds. Take 10 pills for each dose before meals, 3 doses a day. Gradually increase the dose to 20 pills. Stay away from raw, stimulating food (such as mutton, fish, shrimps, etc.).

妇人妊娠病脉证并治第二十
Chapter 20 Pregnancy-Related Problems—Pulses, Patterns and Treatment

Overview

Gynecological diseases are commonly involved with menstruation, leucorrhea, pregnancy and childbirth. This chapter specifically discusses pregnancy-related disorders—uterine bleeding, abdominal pain, vomiting, difficult urination and water qi (swelling).

*****

[01] 师曰：妇人得平脉，阴脉小弱〔1〕，其人渴〔2〕，不能食，无寒热，名妊娠，桂枝汤主之方见利中。于法六十日当有此证，设有医治逆者，却一月加吐下者，则绝之。

Annotations

[1] *Fu Ren De Ping Mai, Yin Mai Xiao Ruo*: The *Ping Mai* means a normal pulse. The *Yin Mai* refers to pulse felt at the *Chi* position.

[2] *Ke*: It originally means thirst; however, it might be a wrong spelling of *Ou*, which means vomiting.

Interpretations

The Master said, "During early stage pregnancy, women have a normal pulse, just slightly weak at the *Chi* position; however, they experience vomiting (thirst in the text) that affects the appetite with an absence of fever or chills. This is called nausea and vomiting of pregnancy (aka morning sickness). Typically these symptoms occur after 60 days of pregnancy and can be managed with *Gui Zhi Tang* (Cinnamon Twig Decoction) (to harmonize the spleen and stomach) (the formula is described in chapter 17). If this condition was mistakenly treated as a disease, inducing vomiting or draining downward is prohibited within another month.

*****

[02] 妇人宿有症病，经断未及三月〔1〕，而得漏下不止〔2〕，胎动在脐上者，为症痼害。妊娠六月动者，前三月经水利时，胎下血者，后断三月衃〔3〕也。所以血不止者，其症不去故也，当下其症。桂枝茯苓丸〔4〕主之。

桂枝茯苓丸方：

桂枝茯苓牡丹去心桃仁去皮、尖，熬芍药各等分右五味，末之，炼蜜和丸，如兔屎大。每日食前服一丸。不知，加至三丸。

Annotations

[1] *Su You Zheng Bing, Jing Duan Wei Ji San Yue*: The word *Zheng* means abdominal masses (similar to uterine fibroids).

[2] *Bu Zhi*: Persistent bleeding.

[3] *Pai*: Dark red blood clots.

[4] *Gui Zhi Fu Ling Wan* (Cinnamon Twig and Poria Pill): A formula to resolve stasis and eliminate masses. Of the ingredients, *Gui Zhi* (Ramulus Cinnamomi) warms blood and unblocks blood vessels; *Tao Ren* (Semen Persicae), *Dan Pi* (Cortex Moutan) and *Chi Shao* (Radix Paeoniae Rubra) circulate blood and resolve stasis; and *Fu Ling* (Poria) supplements healthy qi and fortifies the spleen. It's advisable to start with a small dose and gradually increase to resolve masses without damaging the fetus.

Interpretations

Because of the pre-existing abdominal masses (aka uterine fibroids), women may present with persistent bleeding during the first three months after pregnancy, along with fetal movement around the umbilicus. This is caused by abdominal masses impairing the fetal development. Patients have normal fetal movements in the sixth month of pregnancy but bleeding during the first three months. Due to coagulation of stagnant blood, bleeding stopped between the third and sixth months. The persistent bleeding is caused by retained abdominal masses and should be treated with *Gui Zhi Fu Ling Wan* (Cinnamon Twig and Poria Pill).

Gui Zhi Fu Ling Wan

[Ingredients]

桂枝	*guì zhī*	Ramulus Cinnamomi
茯苓	*fú líng*	Poria
牡丹皮	*mŭ dān pí*	Cortex Moutan (core removed)
桃仁	*táo rén*	Semen Persicae (boiled with skin and tips removed)
芍药	*sháo yào*	Radix Paeoniae Rubra

Grind the five ingredients into a fine powder and mix with processed honey to make into pills the size of rabbit droppings. Take one pill a day before meals. If no efficacy is noticed, gradually increase to 3 pills.

*****

[03] 妇人怀娠六七月，脉弦发热，其胎愈胀〔1〕，腹痛恶寒者，少腹如扇，所以然者，子脏开故也〔2〕。当以附子汤〔3〕温其脏。方未见。

Annotations

[1] *Qi Tai Yu Zhang*: Aggravated abdominal distension.
[2] *Zi Zang Kai*: It is similar to incompetent or weakened cervix.

[3] *Fu Zi Tang* (Aconite Decoction): No formula is provided here. According to the *Shang Han Lun* (Treatise on Cold Damage), its ingredients include *Fu Zi* (Radix Aconiti Lateralis Praeparata), *Fu Ling* (Poria), *Ren Shen* (Radix et Rhizoma Ginseng), *Bai Zhu* (Rhizoma Atractylodis Macrocephalae) and *Shao Yao* (Radix Paeoniae). Of the ingredients, *Fu Zi* warms meridians and dissipates cold; *Fu Ling* and *Bai Zhu* tonify qi and secure the fetus; and *Shao Yao* alleviates spasm and stops pain.

Interpretations

In women with 6 or 7 months of pregnancy, a wiry pulse, fever, abdominal pain and distension, aversion to cold, and a sensation of wind blowing on the surface of the lower abdomen as if being fanned are caused by weakened cervix. These symptoms should be treated with *Fu Zi Tang* (Aconite Decoction) to warm the uterus. No formula is provided here.

*****

[04] 师曰：妇人有漏下者，有半产〔1〕后因续下血都不绝者，有妊娠下血者。假令妊娠腹中痛，为胞阻〔2〕，胶艾汤〔3〕主之。

芎归胶艾汤方一方加干姜一两，胡治治妇人胞动，无干姜：

芎劳阿胶甘草各二两艾叶当归各三两芍药四两干地黄六两右七味，以水五升，清酒三升，合煮，取三升，去滓，内胶，令消尽。温服一升，日三服。不差，更作。

Annotations

[1] *Ban Chan*: Miscarriage after three months of pregnancy.

[2] *Bao Zu*: It literally means obstructed fetal development—a condition characterized by uterine bleeding and cramping. It is similar to threatened miscarriage.

[3] *Jiao Ai Tang* (Donkey-Hide Gelatin and Mugwort Decoction): A formula to regulate and reinforce the *Chong* and *Ren*, nourish blood

and secure the fetus. Of the ingredients, *E Jiao* (Colla Corii Asini) and *Ai Ye* (Folium Artemisiae Argyi) nourish blood and stop bleeding; *Dang Gui* (Radix Angelicae Sinensis), *Di Huang* (Radix Rehmanniae), *Chuan Xiong* (Rhizoma Chuanxiong) and *Shao Yao* (Radix Paeoniae Rubra) are later known as the four ingredients of a well-known blood-nourishing formula—*Si Wu Tang* (Four Ingredients Decoction).

Interpretations

The Master said, "Women may experience prolonged menstrual bleeding, persistent bleeding after miscarriage or bleeding during pregnancy. Additional abdominal pain indicates obstructed fetal development and should be treated with *Jiao Ai Tang* (Donkey-Hide Gelatin and Mugwort Decoction) (the formula in other text also contains 1 *liǎng* of dried ginger; however, it is removed for threatened miscarriage).

Jiao Ai Tang

[Ingredients]

川芎	*chuān xiōng*	2 *liǎng*	Rhizoma Chuanxiong
阿胶	*ē jiāo*	2 *liǎng*	Colla Corii Asini
甘草	*gān cǎo*	2 *liǎng*	Radix et Rhizoma Glycyrrhizae
艾叶	*ài yè*	3 *liǎng*	Folium Artemisiae Argyi
当归	*dāng guī*	3 *liǎng*	Radix Angelicae Sinensis
芍药	*sháo yào*	4 *liǎng*	Radix Paeoniae Rubra
干地黄	*gān dì huáng*	6 *liǎng*	Radix Rehmanniae

Decoct the ingredients except *E Jiao* (Colla Corii Asini) in 5 *shēng* of water and 3 *shēng* (5 *shēng* in other text) of rice wine to get 3 *shēng*. Remove dregs and add *E Jiao* to allow it to thoroughly dissolve. Take 1 *shēng* for each dose when it is warm, 3 doses a day. It's advisable to take the same formula until a full recovery.

*****

[05] 妇人怀娠，腹中绞痛[1]，当归芍药散〔2〕主之。

当归芍药散方：

当归三两芍药一斤　茯苓四两白术四两泽泻半斤芎藭半斤，一作三两 右六味，杵为散。取方寸匕，酒和。日三服。

Annotations

[1] *Jiao Tong*: Acute abdominal pain.

[2] *Dang Gui Shao Yao San* (Chinese Angelica and Peony Powder): A formula to soothe the liver, fortify the spleen and harmonize qi and blood. Of the ingredients, *Dang Gui* (Radix Angelicae Sinensis) and *Shao Yao* (Radix Paeoniae) move blood and stop pain. This formula is later modified into the well-known *Xiao Yao San* (Free Wanderer Powder).

Interpretations

Acute abdominal pain during pregnancy can be treated with *Dang Gui Shao Yao San* (Chinese Angelica and Peony Powder).

Dang Gui Shao Yao San

[Ingredients]

当归	*dāng guī*	3 *liǎng*	Radix Angelicae Sinensis
芍药	*sháo yào*	1 *jīn*	Radix Paeoniae
茯苓	*fú líng*	4 *liǎng*	Poria
白术	*bái zhú*	4 *liǎng*	Rhizoma Atractylodis Macrocephalae
泽泻	*zé xiè*	0.5 *jīn*	Rhizoma Alismatis
川芎	*chuān xiōng*	0.5 *jīn*	Rhizoma Chuanxiong (3 *liǎng* in other text)

Grind the six ingredients into a powder. Take one square-inch spoon mixed with wine for each dose, 3 doses a day.

*****

[06] 妊娠呕吐不止〔1〕，干姜人参半夏丸〔2〕主之。

干姜人参半夏丸方：

干姜人参各一两半夏二两右三味，末之，以生姜汁糊为丸，如梧子大。饮服十丸，日三服。

Annotations

[1] *Ren Shen Ou Tu Bu Zhi*: Severe, persistent morning sickness in early pregnancy. It is similar to hyperemesis gravidarum in modern medicine.

[2] *Gan Jiang Ren Shen Ban Xia Wan* (Dried Ginger, Ginseng and Pinellia Pill): A formula to warm the spleen and stomach and down-regulate qi. Of the ingredients, *Gan Jiang* (Rhizoma Zingiberis) warms the spleen and stomach, dissipates cold and activates stomach yang, *Ban Xia* (Rhizoma Pinelliae) resolves fluid retention, stop vomiting and down-regulate stomach qi, and *Ren Shen* (Radix et Rhizoma Ginseng) supplements qi and fortifies the spleen and stomach.

Interpretations

Persistent, severe nausea and vomiting in early pregnancy should be treated with *Gan Jiang Ren Shen Ban Xia Wan* (Dried Ginger, Ginseng and Pinellia Pill).

Gan Jiang Ren Shen Ban Xia Wan

[Ingredients]

干姜	*gān jiāng*	1 *liǎng*	Rhizoma Zingiberis
人参	*rén shēn*	1 *liǎng*	Radix et Rhizoma Ginseng
半夏	*bàn xià*	2 *liǎng*	Rhizoma Pinelliae

Grind the three ingredients into a fine powder and mix with fresh ginger juice to make into pills the size of firmiana seeds. Take 10 pills for each dose with water, 3 doses a day.

*****

[07] 妊娠，小便难〔1〕，饮食如故〔2〕，归母苦参丸〔3〕主之。

当归贝母苦参丸方男子加滑石半两：

当归贝母苦参各四两右三味，末之，炼蜜丸，如小豆大，饮服三丸，加至十丸。

Annotations

[1] *Xiao Bian Nan*: Dribbling, hesitant and painful urination, along with urinary urgency and frequency. This often occurs in late pregnancy due to damp heat affecting the urinary bladder. It is later known as stranguria during pregnancy.

[2] *Yin Shi Ru Gu*: Normal eating and drinking. This indicates normal functioning of the spleen and stomach and the symptom is caused by damp heat in the urinary bladder.

[3] *Gui Mu Ku Shen Wan* (Chinese Angelica, Fritillaria and Flavescent Sophora Pill): A formula to clear heat, moisten dryness and alleviate stranguria. It can also be used for dribbling, painful urination in men.

Interpretations

Difficult urination (a dribbling, hesitant, painful urination with urinary urgency and frequency) with normal eating and drinking in pregnancy can be treated with *Gan Jiang Ren Shen Ban Xia Wan* (Dried Ginger, Ginseng and Pinellia Pill) (add 0.5 *liǎng* of talcum for men).

Gui Mu Ku Shen Wan

[Ingredients]

当归	*dāng guī*	4 *liǎng*	Radix Angelicae Sinensis
贝母	*bèi mǔ*	4 *liǎng*	Bulbus Fritillaria
苦参	*kǔ shēn*	4 *liǎng*	Radix Sophorae Flavescentis

Grind the three ingredients into a fine powder and mix with honey to make into pills the size of small beans. Take 3 pills for each dose with water, and gradually increase to 10 pills for each dose.

*****

[08] 妊娠有水气〔1〕，身重，小便不利，洒淅恶寒，起即头眩，葵子茯苓散〔2〕主之。

葵子茯苓散方：

葵子一斤茯苓三两右二味，杵为散。饮服方寸匕，日三服。小便利则愈。

Annotations

[1] *Shui Qi*: Edema in late pregnancy. It is often accompanied by body heaviness and dysuria.

[2] *Kui Zi Fu Ling San* (Mallow Seed and Poria Powder): A formula to promote urination and unblock yang.

Interpretations

Water qi disorder in late pregnancy with body heaviness, difficult urination, aversion to cold and dizziness and blurred vision when standing up from sitting or lying down should be treated with *Kui Zi Fu Ling San* (Mallow Seed and Poria Powder).

Kui Zi Fu Ling San

[Ingredients]

葵子	*kuí zǐ*	1 *jīn*	Fructus Malvae
茯苓	*fú líng*	3 *liǎng*	Poria

Grind the three ingredients into a fine powder. Take one square-inch spoon for each dose with water, 3 doses a day. The symptoms alleviate with normal bladder movements.

*****

[09] 妇人妊娠，宜常服当归散[1]主之。

当归散方：

当归黄芩芍药芎䓖各一斤白术半斤右五味，杵为散。酒饮服方寸匕，日再服。妊娠常服即易产，胎无苦疾。产后百病悉主之。

Annotations

[1] *Dang Gui San* (Chinese Angelica Powder): A formula to nourish blood, clear heat and secure the fetus. Of the ingredients, *Huang Qin* (Radix Scutellariae) and *Bai Zhu* (Rhizoma Atractylodis Macrocephalae) are two major ingredients to secure the fetus.

Interpretations

Women in pregnancy should regularly take *Dang Gui San* (Chinese Angelica Powder).

Dang Gui San

[Ingredients]

当归	*dāng guī*	1 *jīn*	Radix Angelicae Sinensis
黄芩	*huáng qín*	1 *jīn*	Radix Scutellariae

Dang Gui San

[Ingredients]

芍药	*sháo yào*	1 *jīn*	Radix Paeoniae
川芎	*chuān xiōng*	1 *jīn*	Rhizoma Chuanxiong
白术	*bái zhú*	0.5 *jīn*	Rhizoma Atractylodis Macrocephalae

Grind the five ingredients into a fine powder. Take one square-inch spoon for each dose with rice wine for each dose, 2 doses a day. Taking this formula regularly during pregnancy benefits a smooth delivery and a healthy baby. It also helps with health problems after childbirth.

*****

[10] 妊娠养胎，白术散〔1〕主之。

白术散方见《外台》：

白术芎䓖蜀椒三分，汗 牡蛎右四味，杵为散。酒服一钱匕，日三服，夜一服。但苦痛，加芍药；心下毒痛，倍加芎䓖；心烦吐痛，不能食饮，加细辛一两、半夏大者二十枚。服之后，更以醋浆水服之；若呕，以醋浆水服之；复不解者，小麦汁服之；已后渴者，大麦粥服之。病虽愈，服之勿置。

Annotations

[1] *Bai Zhu San* (Atractylodes Macrocephala Powder): A formula to warm and fortify the spleen, and nourish and secure the fetus. It is recorded in the *Wai Tai Mi Yao* (Arcane Essentials from the Imperial Library).

Interpretations

Bai Zhu San (Atractylodes Macrocephala Powder) is recommended for women in pregnancy (especially those with abdominal pain and vomiting) to nourish and secure the fetus.

Bai Zhu San

[Ingredients]

白术	*bái zhú*	4 *fēn*	Rhizoma Atractylodis Macrocephalae
川芎	*chuān xiōng*	4 *fēn*	Rhizoma Chuanxiong
花椒	*huā jiāo*	3 *fēn*	Pericarpium Zanthoxyli (oil removed)
牡蛎	*mŭ lì*	2 *fēn*	Concha Ostreae

Grind the four ingredients into a powder. Take one square-inch spoon for each dose with rice wine for each dose, 3 doses during the day and 1 dose at night.

Modifications

✓ For abdominal pain alone, add *Shao Yao* (Concha Ostreae).

✓ For intense pain below the heart, double the dose of *Chuan Xiong* (Rhizoma Chuanxiong).

✓ For stomach discomfort/pain and vomiting, add 1 *liǎng* of *Xi Xin* (Radix et Rhizoma Asari) and 20 large pieces of *Ban Xia* (Rhizoma Pinelliae); and drink fermented millet porridge after taking the decoction.

✓ For vomiting, take the powder with fermented millet porridge.

✓ For persistent vomiting, take wheatgrass juice.

✓ For thirst after vomiting, take barley gruel. It's recommended to continue taking the barley gruel even after all symptoms disappear.

*****

[11] 妇人伤胎，怀身腹满，不得小便〔1〕，从腰以下重，如有水气状。怀身七月，太阴当养不养，此心气实〔2〕。当刺泻劳宫〔3〕及关元，小便微利则愈。见《玉函》。

Annotations

[1] *Fu Ren Shang Tai…Bu De Xiao Bian*: Lower abdominal distension and fullness with urine retention during pregnancy.

[2] *Huai Shen Qi Yue...Ci Xin Qi Shi*: In the 7th month of pregnancy, the fetus is supposed to be nourished through the lung meridian. If hyperactive heart qi overacts lung qi and affects the lung's function in regulating waterways, women in pregnancy may experience abdominal fullness and lower body heaviness due to urine retention.

[3] Laogong (PC 8): An acupuncture point located in the centre of the palm, between the 2nd and 3rd metacarpal bones.

Interpretations

Damage to the fetal qi in late pregnancy may cause lower abdominal distension and fullness, urine retention and lower body heaviness like water qi disorder. This is caused by hyperactive heart qi affecting the lung's function in regulating waterways and impairing the fetal nourishment through the lung meridian in the 7th month of pregnancy. It should be treated by applying reducing needling technique to Laogong (PC 8) and Guanyuan (CV 4). The symptoms alleviate with normal bladder movements [see *Jin Kui Yu Han Jing* (the Jade Case Classic of the Golden Cabinet) for reference].

妇人产后病脉证治第二十一
Chapter 21 Postpartum Diseases—Pulses, Patterns and Treatment

Overview

This chapter discusses postpartum diseases. These include three major conditions—tetany, childbed fever and constipation, along with abdominal pain, wind attacking the Taiyang meridian, diarrhea and hiccups.

*****

[01] 问曰：新产妇人有三病：一者病痓〔1〕，二者病郁冒〔2〕，三者大便难。何谓也？师曰：新产血虚，多汗出，喜中风，故令病痓。亡血复汗，寒多，故令郁冒。亡津液，胃燥，故大便难。

Annotations

[1] *Jing*: Tetany after childbirth. It is caused by blood deficiency, sweating, malnourishment of muscles or meridians and exposure to wind. It is similar to postpartum tetanus.

[2] *Yu Mao*: A condition after childbirth characterized by fever, absence of sweating and loss of consciousness due to blood deficiency, loss of fluids and exposure to cold. It is similar to postpartum childbed fever.

Interpretations

Question: New mothers after childbirth are susceptible to three conditions—tetany, childbed fever and difficulty passing of stools. Why is that?

Answer: Due to blood deficiency and profuse sweating, new mothers after childbirth are susceptible to tetany when exposed to wind. Due to loss of blood and sweating, they are susceptible to childbed fever when exposed to cold. Due to loss of bodily fluids and intestinal dryness, they are susceptible to difficulty passing of stools.

*****

[02] 产妇郁冒，其脉微弱，不能食，大便反坚，但头汗出。所以然者，血虚而厥，厥而必冒[1]。冒家欲解，必大汗出。以血虚下厥，孤阳上出，故头汗出。所以产妇喜汗出者，亡阴血虚，阳气独盛，故当汗出，阴阳乃复[2]。大便坚，呕不能食，小柴胡汤主之。方见呕吐中。

Annotations

[1] *Chan Fu Yu Mao...Jue Er Bi Mao*: The pulse is weak due to deficiency of qi and blood after childbirth. Other symptoms include vomiting, hard stools, sweating on the head, fever, chills, and loss of consciousness.

[2] *Mao Jia Yu Jie...Yin Yang Nai Fu*: Patients cannot recover until sweating all over the body, for sweating is the only way to restore yin-yang balance.

Interpretations

Postpartum childbed fever causes a feeble, weak pulse, (fever, chills, vomiting), poor appetite, hard stools, sweating on the head and loss of consciousness. These symptoms are caused by floating of yang due to deficiency of yin blood. Patients need to sweat all over the body to restore yin-yang balance. They can take *Xiao Chai Hu Tang* (Minor Bupleurum Decoction). For ingredients and usage of this formula, see Chapter 17.

*****

[03] 病解能食，七八日更发热者，此为胃实[1]。大承气汤主之。方见痉中。

Annotations

[1] *Wei Shi*: Excess stomach heat. Patients may experience fever, abdominal fullness/pain and constipation.

Interpretations

The postpartum childbed fever went away and the appetite became better; however, the fever came back after 7 or 8 days. This indicates the retention of excess stomach heat (abdominal fullness/pain and constipation), which should be treated with *Da Cheng Qi Tang* (Major Purgative Decoction). For ingredients and usage of this formula, see Chapter 13.

*****

[04] 产后腹中叫㽲痛[1]，当归生姜羊肉汤主之。并治腹中寒疝，虚劳不足。当归生姜羊肉汤方见寒疝中。

Annotations

[1] *Jiao Tong*: Dull pain caused by internal cold due to blood deficiency.

Interpretations

Dull abdominal pain after childbirth can be treated with *Dang Gui Sheng Jiang Yang Rou Tang* (Chinese Angelica, Fresh Ginger and Goat Meat Decoction). This formula is also indicated for acute peri-umbilical pain and general deficiency. For ingredients and usage of this formula, see Chapter 10.

*****

[05] 产后腹痛，烦满不得卧[1]，枳实芍药散[2]主之。枳实芍药散方：枳实烧令黑，勿太过芍药等分右二味，杵为散。服方寸匕，日三服。并主痈脓，以麦粥下之。

Annotations

[1] *Chan Hou Fu Tong, Fan Man Bu De Wo*: Abdominal pain, distension and fullness that affect sleep. This is caused by stagnation of qi and blood and lochia retention.

[2] *Zhi Shi Shao Yao San* (Immature Bitter Orange and Peony Powder): A formula to move qi and harmonize blood. *Zhi Shi* (Fructus Aurantii Immaturus) moves qi and alleviates pain. When burnt, it moves qi in the blood. *Shao Yao* (Radix Paeoniae) harmonizes blood and alleviates pain.

Interpretations

Abdominal pain, distension and fullness that disturb sleep after childbirth should be treated with *Shi Zhi Shao Yao San* (Immature Bitter Orange and Peony Powder).

Zhi Shi Shao Yao San

[Ingredients]

枳实	*zhǐ shí*	Fructus Aurantii Immaturus (burn until black, but not excessively)
芍药	*sháo yào*	Radix Paeoniae

Grind the two ingredients into a powder. Take a square-inch spoon for each dose, 3 doses a day. This formula is also indicated for sores, ulcers or abscesses—drink with barley congee.

*****

[06] 师曰：产妇腹痛，法当以枳实芍药散。假令不愈者，此为腹中有干血著脐下[1]，宜下瘀血汤[2]主之。亦主经水不利。

下瘀血汤方：大黄二两桃仁二十枚蛰虫二十枚，熬，去足右三味，末之，炼蜜和为四丸。以酒一升，煎一丸，取八合。顿服之。新血下如豚肝[3]。

Annotations

[1] *Chan Fu Fu Tong...Ci Wei Fu Zhong You Gan Xue Zhuo Qi Xia*: Abdominal pain after childbirth is often caused by stagnation of qi and blood; it's therefore treated with *Shi Zhi Shao Yao San* (Immature Bitter Orange and Peony Powder) to move qi and harmonize blood. If it doesn't work, the pain is probably caused by retention of stagnant blood. Symptoms may include retained lochia and lower abdominal hardness and fullness that aggravate upon pressure.

[2] *Xia Yu Xue Tang* (Stasis-Resolving Decoction): A formula to break blood and resolve stasis. Honey is used to moderate its harsh property.

[3] *Xie Xue Xia Ru Tun Gan*: Discharge of blood in dark red color (lochia) that resemble pork liver.

Interpretations

The Master said, "Abdominal pain after childbirth is often treated with *Zhi Shi Shao Yao San* (Immature Bitter Orange and Peony Powder) to move qi and harmonize blood. If it doesn't work, the pain is probably caused by retention of stagnant blood and should be treated with *Xia Yu Xue Tang* (Stasis-Resolving Decoction). This formula is also indicated for irregular menstruation due to blood stasis.

Xia Yu Xue Tang

[Ingredients]

大黄	*dà huáng*	2 *liǎng*	Radix et Rhizoma Rhei
桃仁	*táo rén*	20 pieces	Semen Persicae
蛰虫	*zhé chóng*	20 pieces	Eupolyphaga seu Steleophaga

Grind the three ingredients into a fine powder. Mix with processed honey to make into four pills. Decoct one pill in 1 *shēng* of liquor to get 0.8 *shēng*. Drink up at one draught. After taking the decoction, the patient may discharge blood in dark red color that resembles pork liver.

*****

[07] 产后七八日，无太阳证，少腹坚痛[1]，此恶露不尽；不大便，烦躁发热，切脉微实。再倍发热，日晡时烦躁者，不食，食则谵语，至夜即愈[2]，宜大承气汤主之。热在里，结在膀胱也[3]。方见痉病中。

Annotations

[1] *Shao Fu Jian Tong*: Lower abdominal hardness and pain.

[2] *Zai Bei Fa Re...Zhi Ye Zi Yu*: Aggravated fever between 3 and 5 pm, restlessness and delirium; reduced fever and discontinuation of delirium at night.

[3] *Re Zai Li, Jie Zai Pang Guang Ye*: Interior (lower abdomen) heat. *Pang Guang* literally means the urinary bladder; however, here it refers to the uterus. This condition is similar to endometritis in modern medicine.

Interpretations

An absence of Taiyang exterior syndrome with lower abdominal hardness and pain 7 or 8 days after childbirth indicate lochia retention. Other symptoms include constipation, heat, restlessness and a mildly replete pulse. Patients may experience aggravated fever, restlessness, an inability to eat food and delirium in the afternoon, followed by reduced fever and discontinuation of delirium at night. This should be treated with *Da Cheng Qi Tang* (Major Purgative Decoction). For ingredients and usage of this formula, see Chapter 2. This is caused by heat retained in the lower abdomen.

*****

[08] 产后风续之数十日不解[1]，头微痛，恶寒，时时有热，心下闷，干呕，汗出，虽久，阳旦证[2]续在耳，可与阳旦汤。即桂枝汤。方见下利中。

Annotations

[1] *Chan Hou Feng Xu Zhi Shu Shi Ri Bu Jie*: Unresolved wind attack of Taiyang meridian dozens of days after childbirth.

[2] *Yang Dan Zheng*: Taiyang exterior syndrome characterized by fever, chills, sweating and headache, etc.

Interpretations

Unresolved wind attack of Taiyang meridian dozens of days after childbirth may cause mild headache, chills, fever, chest tightness, retching, and sweating. Despite the long duration, as long as there is Taiyang exterior syndrome, *Yang Dan Tang*, i.e., *Gui Zhi Tang* (Cinnamon Twig Decoction) can still be used. For ingredients and usage of this formula, see Chapter 17.

*****

[09] 产后中风，发热，面正赤，喘而头痛[1]，竹叶汤[2]主之。

竹叶汤方：竹叶一把 葛根三两防风一两桔梗桂枝人参甘草各一两附子一枚，炮大枣十五枚 生姜五两 右十味，以水一斗，煮取二升半。分温三服。温覆使汗出。颈项强，用大附子一枚，破之如豆大，煎药，扬去沫。呕者，加半夏半升洗。

Annotations

[1] *Chan Hou Zhong Feng...Chuan Er Tou Tong*: Exposure to wind after childbirth with fever and headache (exterior) as well as a red face and rapid breathing (a warning sign of tetany).

[2] *Zhu Ye Tang* (Lophatherum Decoction): A formula to clear heat, remove wind, supplement qi, and expel pathogenic factors.

Interpretations

Exposure to wind after childbirth with fever, a red face, rapid breathing and headache should be treated with *Zhu Ye Tang* (Lophatherum Decoction).

Zhu Ye Tang

[Ingredients]

竹叶	*zhú yè*	1 handful	Folium Phyllostachydis Henonis
葛根	*gé gēn*	3 *liǎng*	Radix Puerariae Lobatae
防风	*fáng fēng*	1 *liǎng*	Radix Saposhnikoviae
桔梗	*jié gěng*	1 *liǎng*	Radix Platycodonis
桂枝	*guì zhī*	1 *liǎng*	Ramulus Cinnamomi
人参	*rén shēn*	1 *liǎng*	Radix et Rhizoma Ginseng
甘草	*gān cǎo*	1 *liǎng*	Radix et Rhizoma Glycyrrhizae
附子	*fù zǐ*	1 piece	Radix Aconiti Lateralis Praeparata
大枣	*dà zǎo*	15 pieces	Fructus Jujubae
生姜	*shēng jiāng*	5 *liǎng*	Rhizoma Zingiberis Recens

Decoct the ten ingredients in 1 *dòu* of water to get 2.5 *shēng* and take in three divided doses. Stay warm to induce sweating. For neck stiffness, add 1 large piece of *Fu Zi* (Radix Aconiti Lateralis Praeparata), cracked to bean-sized pieces, decoct and skim off the foam. For vomiting, add 0.5 *shēng* of washed *Ban Xia* (Rhizoma Pinelliae).

*****

[10] 妇人乳中虚，烦乱呕逆，安中益气，竹皮大丸[1]主之。

竹皮大丸方：生竹茹二分石膏二分桂枝一分甘草七分白薇一分

右五味，末之，枣肉和丸，弹子大。以饮服一丸，日三夜二服。有热者，倍白薇。烦喘者，加柏实一分。

Annotations

[1] *Zhu Pi Da Wan* (Major Bamboo Shavings Pill): A formula to clear deficiency heat and tonify spleen qi. A big dose of *Gan Cao* (Radix et Rhizoma Glycyrrhizae) is used in combination with jujube paste to benefit qi of the spleen and stomach.

Interpretations

Restlessness and hiccups (due to interior deficiency) during the postpartum period should be treated with *Zhu Pi Da Wan* (Major Bamboo Shavings Pill) to benefit qi of the spleen and stomach.

Zhu Pi Da Wan

[Ingredients]

竹茹	*zhú rú*	2 *fēn*	Caulis Bambusae in Taenia
石膏	*shí gāo*	2 *fēn*	Gypsum Fibrosum
桂枝	*guì zhī*	1 *fēn*	Ramulus Cinnamomi
甘草	*gān cǎo*	7 *fēn*	Radix et Rhizoma Glycyrrhizae
白薇	*bái wēi*	1 *fēn*	Radix et Rhizoma Cynanchi Atrati

Decoct the five ingredients into a fine powder and mix with jujube paste to make into pills the size of slingshot ball. Take 1 pill with water for each dose, 3 doses a day and 2 doses at night. For a low-grade fever, double the dose of *Bai Wei* (Radix et Rhizoma

Cynanchi Atrati). For shortness of breath, add 1 *fēn* of *Bai Zi Ren* (Semen Platycladi).

*****

[11] 产后下利〔1〕虚极〔2〕，白头翁加甘草阿胶汤〔3〕主之。

白头翁加甘草阿胶汤方：

白头翁二两黄连蘗皮秦皮各三两甘草二两阿胶二两右六味，以水七升，煮取二升半，内胶令消尽。分温三服。

Annotations

[1] *Xia Li*: Here it refers to heat-related diarrhea. Patients may have tenesmus and presence of pus or blood in stools.

[2] *Xu Ji*: Fatigue, exhausted.

[3] *Bai Tou Weng Jia Gan Cao E Jiao Tang* (Pulsatillae Decoction plus Licorice and Donkey-Hide Gelatin): A formula to clear heat, dry dampness, tonify qi and nourish blood.

Interpretations

Heat-related diarrhea (tenesmus and presence of pus or blood in stools) and exhaustion during postpartum period should be treated with *Bai Tou Weng Jia Gan Cao E Jiao Tang* (Pulsatillae Decoction plus Licorice and Donkey-Hide Gelatin).

Bai Tou Weng Jia Gan Cao E Jiao Tang

[Ingredients]

白头翁	*bái tóu wēng*	2 *liǎng*	Radix Pulsatillae
黄连	*huáng lián*	3 *liǎng*	Rhizoma Coptidis
黄柏	*huáng bǎi*	3 *liǎng*	Cortex Phellodendri Chinensis
秦皮	*qín pí*	3 *liǎng*	Cortex Fraxini
甘草	*gān cǎo*	2 *liǎng*	Radix et Rhizoma Glycyrrhizae
阿胶	*ē jiāo*	2 *liǎng*	Colla Corii Asini

Decoct the first five ingredients in 7 *shēng* of water and get 2.5 *shēng*. Add E Jiao (Colla Corii Asini) and re-decoct until it completely dissolves. Take in three divided doses.

*****

Annex formula # 1 *San Wu Huang Qin Tang* (Three Ingredients Scutellariae Decoction)

《千金》三物黄芩汤〔1〕：治妇人在草蓐〔2〕，自发露得风〔3〕，四肢苦烦热〔4〕。头痛者，与小柴胡汤〔5〕；头不痛但烦者，此汤主之。右三味，以水八升，煮取二升。温服一升。多吐下虫。

Annotations

[1] *San Wu Huang Qin Tang* (Three Ingredients Scutellariae Decoction): A formula to clear heat, dry dampness and cool blood. *Huang Qin* (Radix Scutellariae) and *Ku Shen* (Radix Sophorae Flavescentis) clear heat and dry dampness. *Gan Di Huang* (Radix Rehmanniae) cools blood.

[2] *Cao Ru*: In labor.

[3] *Zi Fa Lou De Feng*: Exposure to wind-heat during labor.

[4] *Si Zhi Ku Fan Re*: General feverish sensation.

[5] *Tou Tong Zhe, Yu Xiao Chai Hu Tang*: Fever and headache due to exposure to wind should be treated with *Xiao Chai Hu Tang* (Minor Bupleurum Decoction) to harmonize and release Shaoyang meridian, supplement qi and remove pathogenic factors.

Interpretations

San Wu Huang Qin Tang (Three Ingredients Scutellariae Decoction) in the *Qian Jin Yao Fang* (Important Formulas Worth a Thousand Gold Pieces) can be used to treat body fever due to exposure to wind during labor. For fever with headache, use *Xiao Chai Hu Tang* (Minor Bupleurum Decoction). For fever alone, use *San Wu Huang Qin Tang* (Three Ingredients Scutellariae Decoction).

San Wu Huang Qin Tang

[Ingredients]

黄芩	*huáng qín*	1 *liǎng*	Radix Scutellariae
苦参	*kǔ shēn*	2 *liǎng*	Radix Sophorae Flavescentis
干地黄	*gān dì huáng*	4 *liǎng*	Radix Rehmanniae

Decoct the three ingredients in 8 *shēng* of water to get 2 *shēng*. Take 1 *shēng* when it is warm. After taking the formula, some patients may throw up worms or discharge worms through stools.

*****

Annex formula # 2 *Nei Bu Dang Gui Jian Zhong Tang* (Middle Jiao-Fortifying Decoction Plus Chinese Angelica)

《千金》内补当归建中汤〔1〕：治妇人产后虚羸不足，腹中刺痛不止，吸吸少气〔2〕，或苦少腹中急，摩痛引腰背〔3〕，不能食饮。产后一月日，得服四五剂为善，令人强壮宜。

当归四两桂枝三两芍药六两生姜三两甘草二两大枣十二枚右六味，以水一斗，煮取三升。分温三服，一日令尽。若大虚，加饴糖六两，汤成，内之，于火上暖令饴消。若去血过多，崩伤内衄不止，加地黄六两、阿胶二两，合八味，汤成，内阿胶。若无当归，以芎䓖代之；若无生姜，以干姜代之。

Annotations

[1] *Nei Bu Dang Gui Jian Zhong Tang* (Chinese Angelica Middle Jiao-Fortifying Decoction): This formula is made up of *Xiao Jian Zhong Tang* (Minor Middle Jiao-Fortifying Decoction) plus *Dang Gui* (Radix Angelicae Sinensis). It acts to nourish blood, warm the middle jiao and alleviate pain.

[2] *Fu Zhong Ci Tong Bu Zhi, Hu Xi Shao Qi*: Persistent stabbing abdominal pain with rapid breathing or shortness of breath.

[3] *Ku Shao Fu Zhong Ji, Mo Tong Yin Yao Bei*: Lower abdominal contracture and pain that radiate towards the low back.

Interpretations

Nei Bu Dang Gui Jian Zhong Tang (Middle Jiao-Fortifying Decoction Plus Chinese Angelica) in the *Qian Jin Yao Fang* (Important Formulas Worth a Thousand Gold Pieces) can be used to treat postpartum weakness, deficiency of qi and blood, persistent stabbing abdominal pain, shortness of breath or lower abdominal contracture and pain that radiate towards the low back, and a poor appetite. It is recommended to take 4 or 5 formulas within one month after childbirth, which help to strengthen the body.

Dang Gui Jian Zhong Tang

[Ingredients]

当归	*dāng guī*	4 *liǎng*	Radix Angelicae Sinensis
桂枝	*guì zhī*	3 *liǎng*	Ramulus Cinnamomi
芍药	*sháo yào*	6 *liǎng*	Radix Paeoniae
生姜	*shēng jiāng*	3 *liǎng*	Rhizoma Zingiberis Recens
甘草	*gān cǎo*	2 *liǎng*	Radix et Rhizoma Glycyrrhizae
大枣	*dà zǎo*	12 pieces	Fructus Jujubae

Decoct the six ingredients in 1 *dòu* of water to get 3 *shēng*. Take in 3 divided doses a day when it is warm. Modifications: For general weakness, add 6 *liǎng* of malt sugar and heat until it completely dissolves; for heavy bleeding or persistent internal bleeding after childbirth, add 6 *liǎng* of *Di Huang* (Radix Rehmanniae) and 2 *liǎng* of *E Jiao* (Colla Corii Asini) (add to the decoction later). If there is no *Dang Gui* (Radix Angelicae Sinensis), use *Chuan Xiong* (Rhizoma Chuanxiong) instead. If there is no fresh ginger, use dried ginger.

妇人杂病脉证并治第二十二
Chapter 22 Women's Miscellaneous Diseases—Pulses, Patterns and Treatment

Overview

This chapter discusses women's miscellaneous diseases. These include problems involving menstruation, leucorrhea, blood heat, emotions and external genitalia.

*****

[01] 妇人中风〔1〕，七八日续来寒热，发作有时，经水适断，此为热入血室〔2〕。其血必结，故使如疟状，发作有时。小柴胡汤主之。方见呕吐中。

Annotations

[1] *Fu Ren Zhong Feng*: Exposure to wind cold.

[2] *Re Ru Xue Shi*: It literally means heat entering the uterus. An acute condition during menstruation or after childbirth characterized by fever, chills, alternating fever and chills, lower abdominal pain, vaginal bleeding and mental confusion associated with high fever. It is similar to acute endometritis.

Interpretations

Upon exposure to wind (fever and chills), women may experience alternating fever and chills at regular intervals for 7 or

8 days and interrupted menstrual period. This is caused by retained blood heat in the uterus, which explains the malaria-like alternating fever and chills with regular intervals. As a result, it should be treated with *Xiao Chai Hu Tang* (Minor Bupleurum Decoction). For ingredients and usage of this formula, see chapter 17.

*****

[02] 妇人伤寒发热〔1〕，经水适来，昼日明了，暮则语，如见鬼状者，此为热入血室。治之无犯胃气及上二焦〔2〕，必自愈。

Annotations

[1] *Shang Han Fa Re*: Fever due to exposure to wind cold.

[2] *Wu Fan Wei Ji Shang Er Jiao*: Do not treat the upper and middle jiao, but to treat the lower jiao.

Interpretations

Upon exposure to wind cold, women may experience fever (chills), menstrual period, a clear mind during the day but talking nonsense in the evening. This is caused by blood entering the uterus. It should be treated from the lower jiao instead of the upper and middle jiao.

*****

[03] 妇人中风，发热恶寒，经水适来，得七八日，热除， 脉迟，身凉和，胸胁满如结胸〔1〕状，语者，此为热入血室也。当刺期门〔2〕，随其实而取之。

Annotations

[1] *Jie Xiong*: Heat-related pain in the subcostal region.

[2] *Qimen* (LR 14): An acupuncture point located below the nipple, in the 6th intercostal space. It is the front-Mu point of the liver.

Interpretations

Upon exposure to wind cold, women may experience fever, chills, menstrual period, reduced fever after 7 or 8 days, a slow pulse, and mildly warm skin; however, they have subcostal distension, fullness and pain, and talk nonsense. This is also caused by heat entering the uterus. It should be treated by needling Qimen (LR 14) in combination with *Xiao Chai Hu Tang* (Minor Bupleurum Decoction) according to deficiency or excess.

*****

[04] 阳明病，下血〔1〕，语者，此为热入血室。但头汗出，当刺期门，随其实而泻之，濈然〔2〕汗出者愈。

Annotations

[1] *Xia Xue*: Menstrual blood.
[2] *Ji Ran*: Fast sweating.

Interpretations

Excess heat in Yangming meridian may cause menstrual bleeding and delirium. This is known as heat entering the uterus. Sweating on the head should be treated by needling Qimen (LR 14) with reducing manipulation. This can cause fast sweating all over the body and speed up the recovery.

*****

[05] 妇人咽中如有炙脔〔1〕，半夏厚朴汤[2]主之。

半夏厚朴汤方《千金》作胸满，心下坚，咽中怗怗如有炙肉，吐之不出，吞之不下：

半夏一升厚朴三两茯苓四两生姜五两干苏叶二两右五味，以水七升，煮取四升。分温四服，日三夜一服。

Annotations

[1] *Yan Zhong Ru You Zhi Luan*: A foreign body sensation stuck in the throat, like a piece of roasted meat that cannot be swallowed or expectorated. It is known as globus hystericus.

[2] *Ban Xia Hou Po Tang* (Pinellia and Officinal Magnolia Bark Decoction): A formula to relieve stagnation, resolve phlegm and down-regulate qi.

Interpretations

A sensation like a piece of roasted meat in the throat in women should be treated with *Ban Xia Hou Po Tang* (Pinellia and Officinal Magnolia Bark Decoction). According to *Qian Jin Yao Fang* (Important Formulas Worth a Thousand Gold Pieces), this formula is indicated for chest fullness, hardness below the heart, and a sensation of a piece of roasted meat in throat that cannot be swallowed or expectorated.

Ban Xia Hou Po Tang

[Ingredients]

半夏	*bàn xià*	1 *shēng*	Rhizoma Pinelliae
厚朴	*hòu pò*	3 *liǎng*	Cortex Magnoliae Officinalis
茯苓	*fú líng*	4 *liǎng*	Poria
生薑	*shēng jiāng*	5 *liǎng*	Rhizoma Zingiberis Recens
苏叶	*sū yè*	2 *liǎng*	Folium Perillae (dried)

Decoct the five ingredients in 7 *shēng* of water to get 4 *shēng*. Take in four divided doses—3 doses during the day and 1 dose at night.

*****

[06] 妇人脏躁〔1〕，喜悲伤欲哭，象如神灵所作，数欠伸，甘麦大枣汤〔2〕主之。甘草小麦大枣汤方：

甘草三两小麦一升大枣十枚右三味，以水六升，煮取三升。温分三服，亦补脾气。

Annotations

[1] *Zang Zao*: Ungovernable emotional excess (hysteria) characterized by unexplained laughing and crying and mood swings. It is caused by deficiency of the heart and spleen.

[2] *Gan Mai Da Zao Tang* (Licorice, Wheat and Jujube Decoction): A formula to alleviate spasm and calm the heart mind.

Interpretations

Hysteria in women with unexplained laughing and crying as if possessed by spirits, and frequent yawning and stretching should be treated with *Gan Mai Da Zao Tang* (Licorice, Wheat and Jujube Decoction).

Gan Mai Da Zao Tang

[Ingredients]

甘草	*gān cǎo*	3 *liǎng*	Radix et Rhizoma Glycyrrhizae
小麦	*xiǎo mài*	1 *shēng*	Fructus Tritici
大枣	*dà zǎo*	10 pieces	Fructus Jujubae

Decoct the three ingredients in 6 *shēng* of water to get 3 *shēng*. Take in three divided doses when it is warm. This formula also tonifies spleen qi.

*****

[07] 妇人吐涎沫〔1〕，医反下之，心下即痞〔2〕，当先治其吐涎沫，小青龙汤主之；涎沫止，乃治痞，泻心汤主之。

小青龙汤方见肺痈中。泻心汤方见惊悸中。

Annotations

[1] *Tu Xian Mo*: Cough with thin, foamy sputum due to cold fluid in the lung. It should be treated with *Xiao Qing Long Tang* (Minor Green Dragon Decoction) to warm and resolve the retained cold fluids.

[2] *Xin Xia Ji Pi*: Gastric or abdominal stuffiness.

Interpretations

The wrong use of draining downward therapy for coughing with thin sputum in women may cause gastric or abdominal stuffiness. This should first be treated with *Xiao Qing Long Tang* (Minor Green Dragon Decoction) (see chapter 7) to resolve phlegm and then with *Xie Xin Tang* (Heart-Draining Decoction) (see chapter 16) to relieve gastric or abdominal stuffiness.

*****

[08] 妇人之病，因虚、积冷、结气，为诸经水断绝〔1〕，至有历年，血寒积结，胞门〔2〕寒伤，经络凝坚。在上呕吐涎唾，久成肺痈，形体损分。在中盘结，绕脐寒疝，或两胁疼痛，与脏相连；或结热中，痛在关元〔3〕，脉数无疮，肌若鱼鳞。时着男子，非止女身〔4〕。在下未多，经候不匀，令阴掣痛，少腹恶寒；或引腰脊，下根气街〔5〕，气冲急痛，膝胫疼烦；奄忽眩冒〔6〕，状如厥癫〔7〕；或有忧惨，悲伤多嗔，此皆带下〔8〕，非有鬼神。久则羸瘦，脉虚多寒。三十六病〔9〕，千变万端，审脉阴阳，虚实紧

弦〔10〕。行其针药，治危得安，其虽同病，脉各异源，子当辨记，勿谓不然。

Annotations

[1] *Yin Xu, Ji Leng, Jie Qi, Wei Zhu Jing Shui Duan Jue*: Three major causes of women's diseases: Deficiency of qi and blood, cold retention and qi stagnation. All three factors can impair menstruation and, in severe cases, result in amenorrhea.

[2] *Bao Men*: The uterus.

[3] *Guanyuan* (CV 4): An acupuncture point located 3 cun below the umbilicus. Here it refers to the lower abdomen.

[4] *Zai Shang Ou Tu Xian Tuo…Fei Zhi Nǚ Shen*: In addition to problems of the lower jiao, the above three causes (deficiency, cold retention and qi stagnation) may also cause problems of the upper and middle jiao—lung decline characterized by vomiting of foamy saliva; pre-umbilical pain; lower abdominal pain, a rapid pulse and dry, scaly skin. These symptoms may also affect men.

[5] *Qijie/Qichong* (ST 30): An acupuncture point located at the lateral superior side of the pubic tubercle, 2 cun lateral to the median line of the abdomen in the upper inguinal region, medial to the common iliac artery. Here it refers to the lateral lower abdomen.

[6] *Yan Hu Xuan Mao*: Sudden dizziness and blurred vision.

[7] *Jue Dian*: Sudden collapse, loss of consciousness, and epileptic seizures.

[8] *Dai Xia*: A general term for gynecological diseases, including problems of menstruation and leucorrhea.

[9] *San Shi Liu Bing*: Thirty-six women's conditions discussed in chapter 1.

[10] *Shen Mai Yin Yang, Xu Shi Jin Xian*: Identification of cold, heat, deficiency and excess. A tight pulse indicates cold retention and a wiry pulse indicates qi stagnation.

Interpretations

There are three main causes for women's diseases—deficiency of qi and blood, retained cold qi, and qi stagnation. All three factors may impair menstruation, and in severe cases, result in an absence of menstrual period. Over time, cold retention may cause blood stagnation, impair the uterus, obstruct the meridians and lead to irregular menstruation.

The aforementioned three factors (deficiency of qi and blood, retained cold qi, and qi stagnation) may cause lung decline characterized by coughing with thin, foamy sputum and weight loss (upper jiao), peri-umbilical pain or pain in the subcostal region, and intestinal abscess with bilateral lower abdominal pain, a superficial, rapid pulse, and dry, scaly skin (middle jiao). These symptoms may also be present among men. As for problems of the lower jiao, women may experience irregular menstruation, genital pain and a cold sensation in the lower abdomen. Some may have lower abdominal contracture and pain that radiate towards the low back, and pain in the knees and legs. Some may experience sudden dizziness and blurred vision that resemble collapse or epilepsy. Some may present with melancholy, frustration, sadness and frequent anger. These are all women's diseases and not caused by spirit possession.

Over time, these conditions may cause weight loss and deficiency cold of the meridians. Although there are a variety of women's diseases (36 conditions), they can be treated with acupuncture or herbal formula upon a clear identification of the yin-yang property of the pulse, cold, heat, deficiency and excess, and root cause (cold retention or qi stagnation). It is important to differentiate the root cause of these conditions prior to treatment.

*****

[09] 问曰：妇人年五十所，病下利数十日不止〔1〕，暮即发热，少腹里急、腹满，手掌烦热，唇口干燥，何也？师曰：此病属带下，何以故？曾经半产，瘀血在少腹不去，何以知之？其证唇口干燥，故知之。当以温经汤〔2〕主之。

温经汤方：

吴茱萸三两当归芎䓖芍药各二两人参桂枝阿胶牡丹去心生姜甘草各二两半夏半升麦门冬一升，去心右十二味，以水一斗，煮取三升。分温三服。亦主妇人少腹寒，久不受胎，兼取崩中去血或月水来过多，及至期不来。

Annotations

[1] *Fu Ren Nian Wu Shi Suo, Bing Xia Li Shu Shi Ri Bu Zhi*: Women in their 50s experience vaginal bleeding for dozens of days.

[2] *Wen Jing Tang* (Meridian-Warming Decoction): A formula to warm meridians and resolve stasis. *Wu Zhu Yu* (Fructus Evodiae) is used as the chief ingredient. Animal studies have proven that it can induce uterine contraction.

Interpretations

Question: Women in their 50s experience vaginal bleeding for dozens of days, fever in the late afternoon, lower abdominal contracture, distension and fullness, feverish sensations in the palms, soles and chest, and a dry mouth and lips. What is this?

Answer: This is a gynecological disease. It is caused by retention of stagnant blood in the uterus after miscarriage. We can diagnose this from the dry mouth and lips. This condition should be treated with *Wen Jing Tang* (Meridian-Warming Decoction).

Wen Jing Tang

[Ingredients]

吴茱萸	*wú zhū yú*	3 *liǎng*	Fructus Evodiae
当归	*dāng guī*	2 *liǎng*	Radix Angelicae Sinensis
川芎	*chuān xiōng*	2 *liǎng*	Rhizoma Chuanxiong

芍药	*sháo yào*	2 *liǎng*	Radix Paeoniae
人参	*rén shēn*	2 *liǎng*	Radix et Rhizoma Ginseng
桂枝	*guì zhī*	2 *liǎng*	Ramulus Cinnamomi
阿胶	*ē jiāo*	2 *liǎng*	Colla Corii Asini
牡丹皮	*mǔ dān pí*	2 *liǎng*	Cortex Moutan (core removed)
生姜	*shēng jiāng*	2 *liǎng*	Rhizoma Zingiberis Recens
甘草	*gān cǎo*	2 *liǎng*	Radix et Rhizoma Glycyrrhizae
半夏	*bàn xià*	0.5 *shēng*	Rhizoma Pinelliae
麦冬	*mài dōng*	1 *shēng*	Radix Ophiopogonis

Decoct the twelve ingredients in 1 *dòu* of water and get 3 *shēng*. Take in three divided doses. This formula is also indicated for difficulty getting pregnant due to deficiency cold of the uterus, metrorrhagia, metrostaxis, heavy menstruation or delayed period.

*****

[10] 带下经水不利，少腹满痛，经一月再见者〔1〕，土瓜根散〔2〕主之。

土瓜根散方：阴癞肿〔3〕亦主之。

土瓜根芍药桂枝䗪虫各三分右四味，杵为散。酒服方寸匕，日三服。

Annotations

[1] *Jing Yi Yue Zai Jian Zhe*: Two periods in a month.

[2] *Tu Gua Gen San* (Thladiantha Powder): A formula to circulate blood and resolve stasis.

[3] *Yin Dian Zhong*: Scrotal swelling.

Interpretations

Inhibited menstrual flow, lower abdominal fullness, distension and pain, and two periods in a month should be treated with *Tu Gua Gen San* (Thladiantha Powder).

Tu Gua Gen San

[Ingredients]

土瓜根	*tǔ guā gēn*	3 *fēn*	Radix Trichosanthis Cucumeroidis
芍药	*sháo yào*	3 *fēn*	Radix Paeoniae
桂枝	*guì zhī*	3 *fēn*	Ramulus Cinnamomi
蛰虫	*zhé chóng*	3 *fēn*	Eupolyphaga seu Steleophaga

Grind the four ingredients into a powder. Take 1 square-inch spoon with liquor for each dose, 3 doses a day.

*****

[11] 寸口脉弦而大，弦则为减，大则为芤。减则为寒，芤则为虚，寒虚相搏，此名曰革，妇人则半产漏下，旋复花汤〔1〕主之。

旋复花汤方：

旋复花三两葱十四茎新绛少许右三味，以水三升，煮取一升。顿服之。

Annotations

[1] *Xuan Fu Hua Tang* (Inula Decoction): A formula to move qi, circulate blood, fortify the spleen and stomach and stop bleeding. This formula is indicated for liver stagnation in chapter 11.

Interpretations

The pulse is wiry and large at the *Cunkou* area. The 'wiry' here is weak due to cold. The 'large' here is hollow due to deficiency. This wiry, large pulse is called tympanic pulse and can be seen in women after miscarriage or with metrorrhagia and metrostaxis. This should be treated with *Xuan Fu Hua Tang* (Inula Decoction).

Xuan Fu Hua Tang

[Ingredients]

旋复花	*xuán fù huā*	3 *liǎng*	Flos Inulae
葱白	*cōng bái*	14 pieces	Bulbus Allii Fistulosi
茜草	*qiàn cǎo*	A small amount	Radix et Rhizoma Rubiae

Decoct the three ingredients in 3 *shēng* of water to get 1 *shēng*. Drink up at one draught.

*****

[12] 妇人陷经〔1〕，漏下黑不解，胶姜汤〔2〕主之。臣亿等校诸本，无胶姜汤方，想是前妊娠中胶艾汤。

Annotations

[1] *Xian Jing*: Persistent vaginal bleeding with dark-colored blood.

[2] *Jiao Jiang Tang* (Donkey-hide Gelatin and Mugwort Decoction): A formula to regulate Chong and Ren, warm the spleen and stomach, and nourish blood.

Interpretations

Chronic, dribbling vaginal bleeding of dark-colored blood should be treated with *Jiao Jiang Tang* (Donkey-hide Gelatin and

Mugwort Decoction). Chen Yi et al checked all the versions and did not find any formula named *Jiao Ai Tang*. They assumed this refers to the formula for pregnancy in chapter 21.

*****

[13] 妇人少腹满如敦〔1〕状，小便微难而不渴，生后者〔2〕，此为水与血并结在血室也。大黄甘遂汤〔3〕主之。

大黄甘遂汤方：

大黄四两甘遂二两阿胶二两右三味，以水三升，煮取一升。顿服之。其血当下。

Annotations

[1] *Dun*: An ancient food utensil, similar to a bowl.

[2] *Sheng Hou Zhe*: Postpartum women.

[3] *Da Huang Gan Sui Tang* (Rhubarb and Kansui Decoction): A formula to break blood, expel water, nourish blood and strengthen the body.

Interpretations

Lower abdominal distension, fullness and bulging like a bowl, mild dysuria and absence of thirst in postpartum women are caused by retained water and blood in the uterus. This should be treated with *Da Huang Gan Sui Tang* (Rhubarb and Kansui Decoction).

Da Huang Gan Sui Tang

[Ingredients]

大黄	*dà huáng*	4 *liǎng*	Radix et Rhizoma Rhei
甘遂	*gān suì*	2 *liǎng*	Radix Kansui
阿胶	*ē jiāo*	2 *liǎng*	Colla Corii Asini

Decoct the three ingredients in 3 *shēng* of water to get 1 *shēng*. Drink up at one draught. Patients may restore normal menstruation afterwards.

*****

[14] 妇人经水不利下〔1〕，抵党汤〔2〕主之。亦治男子膀胱满急，有瘀血者。

抵党汤方：

水蛭三十个，熬虻虫三十，熬，去翅、足桃仁廿个，去皮、尖大黄三两，酒浸右四味，为末，以水五升，煮取三升，去滓。温服一升。

Annotations

[1] *Fu Ren Jing Shui Bu Li Xia*: Amenorrhea with lower abdominal hardness, fullness and pain with tenderness.

[2] *Di Dang Tang* (Resistance Decoction): A formula to break blood and resolve stasis. *Shui Zhi* (Hirudo) and *Meng Chong* (Tabanus) resolve stasis. *Da Huang* (Radix et Rhizoma Rhei) and *Tao Ren* (Semen Persicae) circulate blood.

Interpretations

Amenorrhea (lower abdominal hardness and fullness) should be treated with *Di Dang Tang* (Resistance Decoction). This formula is also indicated for men with urinary bladder distension, fullness, contracture and pain due to retention of stagnant blood.

Di Dang Tang

[Ingredients]

水蛭	*shuǐ zhì*	30 pieces	Hirudo (boiled)
虻虫	*méng chóng*	30 pieces	Tabanus (boiled, wings/legs removed)

Di Dang Tang

[Ingredients]

桃仁	*táo rén*	20 pieces	Semen Persicae (skin and tips removed)
大黄	*dà huáng*	3 *liǎng*	Radix et Rhizoma Rhei (soaked in liquor)

Grind the four ingredients into a powder. Decoct in 5 *shēng* of water to get 3 *shēng*. Remove the dregs and take 1 *shēng* when it is warm.

*****

[15] 妇人经水闭不利，藏[1]坚癖不止，中有干血，下白物[2]，矾石丸[3]主之。

矾石丸方：

矾石三分，烧 杏仁一分右二味，末之，炼蜜和丸，枣核大。内脏中[4]，剧者再内之。

Annotations

[1] *Zang*: It refers to the uterus.

[2] *Bai Wu:* Leucorrhea. Itchiness of the vulva may also be present.

[3] *Fan Shi Wan* (Alum Pill): A formula to clear heat and dry dampness. Alum acts to dry dampness and relieve itching.

[4] *Nei Zang Zhong*: External genitalia.

Interpretations

Amenorrhea, hard masses with dry blood in the uterus, and whitish vaginal discharges can be treated externally with *Fan Shi Wan* (Alum Pill). Method: Grind 3 *fēn* of *Fan Shi* (Alumen) and 1 *fēn* of *Xing Ren* (Semen Armeniacae Amarum) into a powder.

Mix with processed honey and make into pills the size of jujube pit. Insert into the vagina. In severe cases, insert a second one.

*****

[16] 妇人六十二种风〔1〕，及腹中血气刺痛〔2〕，红蓝花酒〔3〕主之。

红蓝花〔2〕酒方：疑非仲景方。红蓝花一两右一味，以酒一大升，煎减半。顿服一半，未止再服。

Annotations

[1] *Liu Shi Er Zhong Feng*: Sixty-two types of wind, indicating wind can cause a variety of conditions.

[2] *Ji Fu Zhong Xue Qi Ci Tong:* Stabbing abdominal pain and inhibited menstrual flow upon exposure to wind during period or after childbirth.

[3] *Hong Lan Hua Jiu* (Carthamus liquor): A formula to circulate blood and remove wind. This is an example of "moving blood before stopping wind".

[4] *Hong Lan Hua*: Carthami Flos. It acts to move blood, unblock meridians, resolve stasis and alleviate pain.

Interpretations

Wind-induced abdominal pain and stabbing abdominal pain due to stagnation of qi and blood in women can be treated with *Hong Lan Hua Jiu* (Carthamus liquor).

Formula of *Hong Lan Hua Jiu* (Carthamus liquor) (It is doubtful that this is Zhongjing's formula): Decoct *Hong Lan Hua* (Carthami Flos) in a large *shēng* of liquor to get half of the liquor. Take half for one dose. If the pain remains, take the other half.

*****

[17] 妇人腹中诸疾痛，当归芍药散主之。
当归芍药散方：见前妊娠中。

Interpretations

Abdominal pain due to disharmony between qi and blood can be treated with *Dang Gui Shao Yao San* (Chinese Angelica and Peony Powder). For ingredients and usage of the formula, see chapter 20.

*****

[18] 妇人腹中痛[1]，小建中汤主之。
小建中汤方：见前虚劳中。

Annotations

[1] *Fu Ren Fu Zhong Tong*: Dull abdominal pain that alleviates upon warmth and pressure. Other symptoms include a lusterless complexion, and general fatigue. As a result, *Xiao Jian Zhong Tang* (Minor Middle Jiao-Fortifying Decoction) is used to tonify qi and blood.

Interpretations

Dull abdominal pain can be treated with *Xiao Jian Zhong Tang* (Minor Middle Jiao-Fortifying Decoction). For ingredients and usage of the formula, see chapter 6.

*****

[19] 问曰：妇人病饮食如故，烦热不得卧，而反倚息〔1〕者，何也？师曰：此名转胞〔2〕，不得溺也。以胞系了戾，故致此病，但利小便则愈，宜肾气丸〔3〕主之。

肾气丸方:

干地黄八两薯蓣四两山茱萸四两泽泻三两茯苓三两牡丹皮三两桂枝附子炮，各一两右八味，末之，炼蜜和丸，梧子大。酒下十五丸，加至二十五丸，日再服。

Annotations

[1] *Yin Shi Ru Gu ... Er Fan Yi Xi*: Normal appetite indicates the problem is not located in the middle jiao but in the lower jiao (urinary bladder). Patients experienced severe lower abdominal distension and fullness with an inability to lie flat.

[2] *Zhuan Bao*: Twisted urinary bladder characterized by inhibited urination and lower abdominal distension and fullness due to kidney qi deficiency and impaired qi transformation of the urinary bladder. It is similar to urine retention.

[3] *Shen Qi Wan* (Kidney Qi Pill): See *Cui Shi Ba Wei Wan* (Cui's Eight Ingredients Pill) in chapter 5, *Ba Wei Shen Qi Wan* (Eight Ingredients Kidney Qi Pill) in chapter 6, and *Shen Qi Wan* (Kidney Qi Pill) in chapter 12. These formulas share the same name but have different functions. Here it acts to warm the kidney, transform qi and induce urination.

Interpretations

Questions: Women have a normal appetite; however they have a feverish sensation, restlessness and an inability to lie flat. What is this?

Answer: This is called twisted bladder with urine retention. This results from twisting of the bladder connections. It should be treated with *Shen Qi Wan* (Kidney Qi Pill).

Shen Qi Wan

[Ingredients]

干地黄	*gān dì huáng*	8 *liǎng*	Radix Rehmanniae
山药	*shān yào*	4 *liǎng*	Rhizoma Dioscoreae

Shen Qi Wan

[Ingredients]

山茱萸	*shān zhū yú*	2 *liǎng*	Fructus Corni
泽泻	*zé xiè*	3 *liǎng*	Rhizoma Alismatis
茯苓	*fú líng*	3 *liǎng*	Poria
牡丹皮	*mǔ dān pí*	3 *liǎng*	Cortex Moutan
桂枝	*guì zhī*	1 *liǎng*	Ramulus Cinnamomi
附子	*fù zǐ*	1 *liǎng*	Radix Aconiti Lateralis Praeparata

Grind the eight ingredients into a fine powder and mix with the processed honey to make into pills the size of firmiana seeds. Take 15 pills with liquor for each dose, and gradually increase to 25 pills, 2 doses a day.

*****

[20] 蛇床子散〔1〕方，温阴中坐药〔2〕。

蛇床子仁右一味，末之，以白粉〔3〕少许，和令相得，如枣大。绵裹内之，自然温。

Annotations

[1] *She Chuang Zi San* (Cnidium Fruit Powder): An externally used formula to warm the vagina and dry cold dampness.

[2] *Zuo Yao*: Externally used suppository.

[3] *Bai Fen*: Rice powder.

Interpretations

The *She Chuang Zi San* (Cnidium Fruit Powder) is an externally used suppository to warm the vagina. Method: Grind *She Chuang*

Zi (Fructus Cnidii) into a fine powder and mix with rice powder to make into suppositories the size of a jujube. Wrap with cotton and insert into the vagina.

*****

[21] 少阴脉滑而数者，阴中即生疮，阴中蚀疮烂者〔1〕，狼牙汤〔2〕洗之。

狼牙〔3〕汤方：

狼牙三两右一味，以水四升，煮取半升，以绵缠箸如茧。浸汤沥阴中，日四遍。

Annotations

[1] *Shao Yin Mai Hua Er Shuo Zhe…Yin Zhong Shi Chuang Lan Zhe*: *Shao Yin Mai* refers to the pulse of the kidney felt at Taixi (KI 3). A slippery and rapid pulse at Taixi (KI 3) indicates damp heat in the lower jiao. Damp heat accumulating in the external genitalia may cause sores or ulcers.

[2] *Lang Ya Tang* (Hairy Vein Agrimonia Decoction): An externally used lotion to clear heat and dry dampness.

[3] *Lang Ya*: *Xian He Cao* (Herba Agrimoniae). It acts to clear heat, dry dampness and kill parasites.

Interpretations

A slippery, rapid pulse at Taixi (KI 3) with sores and ulcers in the external genitalia can be washed by *Lang Ya Tang* (Hairy Vein Agrimonia Decoction). Method: Decoct 3 *liǎng* of *Xian He Cao* (Herba Agrimoniae) in 4 *shēng* of water to get 0.5 *shēng*. Wrap a piece of cotton around a chopstick like a cocoon, soak it in the decoction and trickle into the inside of the vagina, four times a day.

*****

[22] 胃气下泄〔1〕，阴吹〔2〕而正喧，此谷气之实也。膏发煎〔3〕导之。膏发煎方见黄疸中。

Annotations

[1] *Wei Qi Xia Xie*: Downward draining of intestinal qi.

[2] *Yin Chui*: Vaginal flatulence.

[3] *Gao Fa Jian* (Lard and Human Hair Decoction): A formula to moisten the intestines and unblock the Fu-organs.

Interpretations

Downward draining of intestinal qi with incessant vaginal flatulence is caused by intestinal obstruction and constipation. It should be treated with *Gao Fa Jian* (Lard and Human Hair Decoction) to moisten the intestines and promote bowel movements. The formula is discussed in chapter 15.

*****

[23] 小儿疳虫蚀齿〔1〕方：疑非仲景方。

雄黄葶苈右二味，末之，取腊日猪脂熔，以槐枝绵裹头四五枝，点药烙之。

Annotations

[1] *Gan Chong Shi Chi*: Ulcerated gums and tooth decay due to stomach heat.

Interpretations

A formula for infantile tooth decay and ulcerated gums (It is doubtful that this is Zhongjing's formula): Grind *Xiong Huang* (Realgar) and *Ting Li* (Semen Lepidii) into a powder, melt in pork lard in the twelfth month of the lunar year. Wrap 4 or 5 pagoda tree twigs with the tips wrapped in cotton. Dip the medicinal powder in it and ignite to fumigate the affected teeth.

杂疗方第二十三
Chapter 23 Miscellaneous Formulas—Pulses, Patterns and Treatment

Overview

This chapter discusses emergency treatments for miscellaneous diseases, both internal and external. Most of these formulas have no commentaries. Miscellaneous diseases in this chapter are all life threatening. These include sudden collapse, suicide by hanging, sunstroke, drowning and traumatic injuries.

*****

[01] 退五脏虚热〔1〕，四时加减柴胡饮子〔2〕方。

冬三月加柴胡八分白术八分 大腹槟榔四枚，并皮、子用 陈皮五分生姜五分桔梗七分 春三月加枳实减白术共六味。夏三月加生姜三分枳实五分甘草三分，共八味。秋三月加陈皮三分，共六味。

右各㕮咀，分为三贴。一贴以水三升，煮取二升。分温三服，如人行四五里进一服。如四体壅，添甘草少许。每贴分作三小贴，每小贴以水一升，煮取七合，温服。再合滓为一服，重煮都成四服疑非仲景方。

Annotations

[1] *Tui Wu Zang Xu Re*: Resolve fever due to deficiency of the five-zang organs.

[2] *Si Shi Jia Jian Chai Hu Yin Zi* (Seasonally Modified Bupleurum Decoction): A formula to soothe the liver and fortify the spleen. It is the

original version of modified *Xiao Yao San* (Free Wanderer Powder) or *Si Ni San* (Frigid Extremities Powder).

Interpretations

Deficiency heat of the five-zang organs can be treated with *Si Shi Jia Jian Chai Hu Yin Zi* (Seasonally Modified Bupleurum Decoction).

In three winter months:

Si Shi Jia Jian Chai Hu Yin Zi

[Ingredients]

柴胡	*chái hú*	8 *fēn*	Radix Bupleuri
白术	*bái zhú*	8 *fēn*	Rhizoma Atractylodis Macrocephalae
槟榔	*bīng láng*	4 pieces	Semen Arecae (including skin and seed)
陈皮	*chén pí*	5 *fēn*	Pericarpium Citri Reticulatae
生姜	*shēng jiāng*	5 *fēn*	Rhizoma Zingiberis Recens
桔梗	*ié gěng*	7 *fēn*	Radix Platycodonis

In the three spring months, add *Zhi Shi* (Fructus Aurantii Immaturus) and remove *Bai Zhu* (Rhizoma Atractylodis Macrocephalae) (6 ingredients in total).

In the three summer months, add an additional 3 *fēn* (i.e., 8 *fēn* in total) of *Sheng Jiang* (Rhizoma Zingiberis Recens), 5 *fēn* of *Zhi Shi* (Fructus Aurantii Immaturus) and 3 *fēn* of *Gan Cao* (Radix et Rhizoma Glycyrrhizae) (8 ingredients in total).

In the three autumn months, add an additional 3 *fēn* (i.e., 8 *fēn* in total) of *Chen Pi* (Pericarpium Citri Reticulatae) (6 ingredients in total).

Chop the above ingredients into pieces and divide into three packets. Decoct each packet in 3 *shēng* of water to get 2 *shēng*. Take in three divided doses when it is warm. The time interval between two doses is equal to the time it takes one to walk 2000 to 2500 meters.

For limb edema, add a small amount of *Gan Cao* (Radix et Rhizoma Glycyrrhizae). Divide each packet into three portions and decoct each portion in 1 *shēng* of water to get 0.7 *shēng*. Drink the decoction when it is warm. Then combine the dregs to make another packet and re-decoct to make a fourth dose. It is doubtful whether this is Zhongjing's formula.

*****

[02] 长服诃梨勒丸〔1〕方疑非仲景方。

诃梨勒煨陈皮各三两右三味，末之，炼蜜丸如梧子大。酒饮服二十丸，加至三十丸。

Annotations

[1] *He Li Le Wan* (Chebulae Pill): A formula to fortify the spleen, move qi, unblock six-Fu organs, and harmonize the qi and blood. Of the ingredients, *He Zi* (Fructus Chebulae) warms the stomach and astringes the intestines, *Chen Pi* (Pericarpium Citri Reticulatae) and *Hou Po* (Cortex Magnoliae Officinalis) move qi and relieve stagnation.

Interpretations

Take the *He Li Le Wan* (Chebulae Pill) for an extended period. It is doubtful whether this is Zhongjing's formula.

He Li Le Wan

[Ingredients]

诃子	*hē zǐ*	3 *liǎng*	Fructus Chebulae
陈皮	*chén pí*	3 *liǎng*	Pericarpium Citri Reticulatae
厚朴	*hòu pò*	3 *liǎng*	Cortex Magnoliae Officinalis

Grind the three ingredients into a powder and mix with processed honey to make into pills the size of firmiana seeds. Take 20 pills for each dose with liquor and increase to 30 pills.

*****

[03] 三物备急丸〔1〕方：见《千金》司空裴秀为散用亦可。先和成汁，乃倾口中，令从齿间得入，至良验。

大黄一两干姜一两巴豆一两，去皮、心，熬，外研如脂

右药各须精新。先捣大黄，干姜为末，研巴豆内中，合治一千杵。用为散，蜜和丸亦佳，蜜器中贮之，莫令歇。主心腹诸卒暴百病。若中恶客忤，心腹胀满，卒痛如锥刺〔2〕，气急口噤，停尸卒死者，以缓水若酒服大豆许三四丸。或不下，捧头起，灌令下咽，须臾当差。如未差，更与三丸，当腹中鸣，即吐下便差。若口噤，亦须折齿灌之。

Annotations

[1] *San Wu Bei Ji Wan* (Three Ingredient Emergency Pill): A formula to promote bowel movements and remove toxins. Of the ingredients, *Da Huang* (Radix et Rhizoma Rhei) and *Ba Dou* (Fructus Crotonis) cleanse the intestine and stomach.

[2] *Zu Tong Ru Zhui Ci*: Acute pain like being stabbed by an awl.

Interpretations

San Wu Bei Ji Fang (Three Ingredient Emergency Pill). According to the *Qian Jin Yao Fang* (Important Formulas Worth a Thousand Gold Pieces), PEI Xiu (an official titled Si Kong in the Wei-Jin dynast) made into powder and mixed with water to pour into the mouth through the teeth. This helped to achieve a good effect.

San Wu Bei Ji Wan

[Ingredients]

大黄	*dà huáng*	*1 liǎng*	Radix et Rhizoma Rhei
干姜	*gān jiāng*	*1 liǎng*	Rhizoma Zingiberis
巴豆	*bā dòu*	*1 liǎng*	Fructus Crotonis (remove the skin and core, boil and make into fat paste)

All ingredients need to be fresh and of high quality. First grind *Da Huang* (Radix et Rhizoma Rhei) and *Gan Jiang* (Rhizoma Zingiberis) into a powder. Then smash *Ba Dou* (Fructus Crotonis), mix with the powder and pound 1,000 times. Either use as a powder or make into honey pills. Place in an airtight container to preserve the medicinal smell.

It is indicated for sudden, severe heart and abdominal conditions, such as cardiac or abdominal distension and fullness upon exposure to toxic qi with acute pain like being stabbed by an awl, rapid breathing and trismus and sudden rigor. The method is to take 3-4 pills the size of a soybean with warm water or liquor. If patients are unable to swallow the pills, dissolve the pills in water, lift up the head and pour the liquid into the mouth. They should get better after a while. If not, give three more pills. The condition will significantly alleviate with bowel sounds and subsequent vomiting or diarrhea. With a clenched jaw, if necessay, one can knock out the teeth to pour the liquid containing dissolved pills.

*****

[04] 治伤寒令愈不复，紫石寒食散[1]方见《千金翼》：

紫石英白石英赤石脂钟乳碓，炼 栝蒌根防风桔梗文蛤鬼臼各十分太一余粮十分，烧干姜附子炮，去皮桂枝去皮，各四分　右十三味，杵为散。酒服方寸匕。

Annotations

[1] *Zi Shi Han Shi San* (Fluorite Heat-Inducing Powder): A formula to warm kidney yang and remove toxins. It is a modified formula of *Feng Yin Tang* (Wind-Extinguishing Decoction) (chapter 5).

Interpretations

Si Shi Han Shi Fang (Fluorite Heat-Inducing Powder) can be used to prevent relapse of a recovered cold damage. The formula is recorded in the *Qian Jin Yi Fang* (Supplement to 'Important Formulas Worth a Thousand Gold Pieces').

Zi Shi Han Shi San

[Ingredients]

紫石英	*zǐ shí yīng*	10 *fēn*	Fluoritum
白石英	*bái shí yīng*	10 *fēn*	Quartz Album
赤石脂	*chì shí zhī*	10 *fēn*	Halloysitum Rubrum
钟乳石	*zhōng rǔ shí*	10 *fēn*	Stalactitum
栝蒌根	*guā lóu gēn*	10 *fēn*	Radix Trichosanthis
防风	*fáng fēng*	10 *fēn*	Radix Saposhnikoviae
桔梗	*ié gěng*	10 *fēn*	Radix Platycodonis
文蛤	*wén gé*	10 *fēn*	Concha Meretricis seu Cyclinae
鬼臼	*gǔ jiù*	10 *fēn*	Rhizoma Dysosnae Versipellis
禹余粮	*yǔ yú liáng*	10 *fēn*	Limonitum (burnt)
干姜	*gān jiāng*	4 *fēn*	Rhizoma Zingiberis
附子	*fù zǐ*	4 *fēn*	Radix Aconiti Lateralis Praeparata
桂枝	*guì zhī*	4 *fēn*	Ramulus Cinnamomi

Grind the thirteen ingredients into a powder and take a square-inch spoon with liquor.

*****

[05] 救卒死方：

薤捣汁灌鼻中。又方：雄鸡冠割取血，管吹内鼻中。猪脂如鸡子大，苦酒一升，煮沸灌喉中。鸡肝及血涂面上，以灰围四旁，立起。大豆二七粒，以鸡子白并酒和，尽以吞之。

Interpretations

Formulas to rescue sudden collapse:

Crush long stamen onion bulb and pour the juice into the nose. Alternatively, cut off a rooster's comb and take the blood. Use a tube to blow it into the nose.

Boil the lard the size of an egg in 1 *shēng* of vinegar and then pour into the throat.

Apply the chicken liver (or chicken comb blood) and chicken blood on the face and surround it with ash. Patients can regain consciousness immediately.

Mix 14 (2×7) soybeans with egg white or liquor and swallow all of it.

*****

[06] 救卒死而壮热者方：

矾石半斤，以水一斗半，煮消，以渍脚，令没踝。

Interpretations

A formula for sudden collapse with a strong fever: Decoct 0.5 *jīn* of alum in 1.5 *dòu* of water until it completely dissolved. Soak the feet into the decoction up to the ankles.

*****

[07] 救卒死而目闭者方：
骑牛临面，捣薤汁灌耳中，吹皂荚末鼻中，立效。

Interpretations

A formula for sudden collapse with closed eyes: Ride on the patients' body like riding on an ox, pour the smashed long stamen onion bulb into the ears and blow the powder of Chinese honey locust fruit into the nostrils. This can get an immediate effect.

*****

[08] 救卒死而张口反折者方：
灸手足两爪后十四壮了，饮以五毒诸膏散[1]有巴豆者。

Annotations

[1] *Wu Du Zhu Gao San* (Five Toxins Powder): Five poisonous medicinals include *Wu Tou* (Chinese monkshood), *Fu Zi* (Radix Aconiti Lateralis), *Shu Jiao* (Pericarpium Zanthoxyli), *Ba Dou* (Fructus Crotonis) and *Da Huang* (Radix et Rhizoma Rhei). Powders that contain poisonous medicinals are *Wu Tou Jian* (Chinese monkshood Decoction), *Fu Zi Jian* (Aconiti Decoction) and *San Wu Bei Ji Fang* (Three Ingredient Emergency Pill), etc.

Interpretations

A formula for sudden collapse with an open mouth (eyes in other texts) and opisthotonos: First apply 14 cones of moxibustion to finger/toe nails and then drink the *Wu Du Zhu Gao San* (Five Toxins Powder) that contains *Ba Dou* (Fructus Crotonis).

*****

[09] 救卒死而四肢不收，失便者方：

马屎一升，水三斗，煮取二斗，以洗之；又取牛洞稀粪也一升，温酒灌口中，灸心下一寸、脐上三寸、脐下四寸各一百壮，差。

Interpretations

A formula for sudden shock with slack limbs and bladder and bowel incontinence:

Boil 1 *shēng* of horse feces in 3 *dòu* of water to get 2 *dòu*. Use this to wash the patients' body or feet. Then mix 1 *shēng* of cow sloppy stool with warm liquor to pour into the patient's mouth. At the same time, apply 100 cones of moxibustion to Juque (CV 14), Jianli (CV 11) and Zhongji (CV 3). After this, the patient can regain consciousness.

*****

[10] 小儿卒死而吐利，不知是何病方：

狗屎一丸，绞取汁，以灌之。无湿者，水煮干者取汁。

Interpretations

A formula for sudden, unexplained vomiting, diarrhea and faint in children:

Wring out a piece of dog feces to pour into the child's mouth. If there is no wet stool, decoct a dry one in water.

*****

[11] 尸蹶[1]脉动而无气，气闭不通，故静而死也，治方脉证见上卷：

菖蒲屑，内鼻两孔吹之，令人以桂屑着舌下。

又方：剔取左角发方寸烧末，酒和灌令入喉，立起。

Annotations

[1] *Shi Jue*: A condition characterized by sudden collapse, loss of consciousness, cold limbs and faint breathing.

Interpretations

A formula to treat sudden collapse with pulsations but no breathing, blocked airway and lie motionless (for the pulses and signs, see chapter 1):

Blow the flakes of acorus into the nostrils and place the cinnamon flakes under the tongue.

Another option: Scrape off a square-inch hair from the left corner of the head, burn into a powder and then mix with liquor. Pour it into the patient's throat. The patient can regain consciousness immediately.

*****

[12] 救卒死，客忤死，还魂汤主之方《千金方》云：主卒忤鬼击飞尸，诸奄忽气绝，无复觉，或已无脉，口噤拗不开，去齿下汤。汤下口不下者，分病人发左右，捉肩引之，药下复增取一升，须臾立苏：

麻黄三两，去节。一方四两杏仁去皮、尖，七十个甘草一两炙《千金》用桂心二两

右三味，以水八升，煮取三升，去滓。分令咽之，通治诸感忤。

又方：

韭根一把乌梅二七个吴茱萸半升，炒右三味，以水一斗煮之，以病人栉内中，三沸，栉浮者 生，沉者死。煮取三升，去滓。分饮之。

Interpretations

Sudden collapse or exposure to toxic qi can be treated with *Huan Hun Tang* (Ethereal Soul-Returning Decoction). The *Qian Jin Yao Fang* (Important Formulas Worth a Thousand Gold Pieces) states, "This formula is indicated for sudden faint, demon possession, flying corpse, sudden stop of breathing, loss of unconsciousness, and absence of pulses." In case of a clenched jaw, knock out the teeth and pour the decoction into the mouth. If the decoction fails to be swallowed, separate the patient's hair and grasp it on both sides, and pull the patient's shoulder to guide the decoction down. After the decoction is swallowed, add 1 additional *shēng* more. The patient can soon regain consciousness.

麻黄	*má huáng*	3 *liǎng*	Herba Ephedrae (4 *liǎng* in another formula)
杏仁	*xìng rén*	70 pieces	Semen Armeniacae Amarum (skin and tip removed)
甘草	*gān cǎo*	1 *liǎng*	Radix et Rhizoma Glycyrrhizae (fried)

There is 2 *liǎng* of *Gui Xin* (shaved cinnamon bark) in the *Qian Jin Yao Fang*.

Decoct the three ingredients in 8 *shēng* of water to get 3 *shēng*. Remove the dregs and have the patient swallow it in divided portions. This formula can be used for all kinds of problems upon exposure to pathogenic qi.

Alternative formula

韭根	*jiǔ gēn*	A handful	Radix Allii Tuberosi
乌梅	*wū méi*	14 pieces	Fructus Mume
吴茱萸	*wú zhū yú*	0.5 *shēng*	Fructus Evodiae (fried)

Decoct the three ingredients in 1 *dòu* of water. Add the patient's wood comb and bring to boil three times. If the comb floats, the patient lives; if the comb sinks, the patient dies. Decoct to get 3 *shēng*, remove the dregs and drink in divided portions.

*****

[13] 救自缢死，旦至暮，虽已冷，必可治；暮至旦，小难也，恐此当言阴气盛故也。然夏时夜短于昼，又热，犹应可治。又云：心下若微温者，一日以上，犹可治之方。

徐徐抱解，不得截绳，上下安被卧之。一人以脚踏其两肩，手少挽其发，常弦弦勿纵之，一人以手按据胸上，数动之。一人摩捋臂胫屈伸之，若已僵，但渐渐强屈之，并按其腹。如此一炊顷，气从口出，呼吸眼开，而犹引按莫置，亦勿苦劳之。须臾，可少桂汤及粥清含与之，令濡喉，渐渐能咽，及稍止。若向令两人，以管吹其两耳，冞好。此法最善，无不活者。

Interpretations

To rescue someone from hanging, if it has happened from dawn till dusk, even if the body is already cold, the patient still have a chance; if it has happened from dusk until dawn, the patient has a slim chance, probably because of excess yin qi. However, it is easier to rescue in summer because it is hot and the night is shorter than the daytime. It's also said that, even after more than one day, patients with a mildly warm chest still have a chance.

The rescue method is to gently place the person down to the ground; do not cut off the rope too soon. Have one person step on the patient's shoulders with feet and grasp the patient's hair with both hands, hold it tightly and do not release. Have another person to press the chest continuously and rhythmically. Have another person to flex the patient's arms and legs with gradually increased force in case of rigor. At the same time, knead and press the patient's abdomen as long as it takes to cook a meal. When the patient restores breathing and opens the eyes, do not stop and keep on pressing; however, it's important not to make the patient tired. After a while, prepare a small amount of cinnamon twig decoction or congee, have the patient to hold it in the throat and swallow slowly. Gradually stop pressing the patient's chest. A better effect can be achieved if two people blow into the patient's ears with a pen tube. This is the best rescue method for suicide by hanging.

*****

[14] 凡中暍死，不可使得冷，得冷便死，疗之方。

屈草带，绕暍人脐，使三两人溺其中，令温。亦可用热泥和屈草。亦可扣瓦碗底，按及车缸，以着暍人，取令溺，须得流去。此谓道路穷，卒无汤，当令溺其中，欲使多人溺，取令温，若汤，便可与之。不可泥及车缸，恐此物冷。暍既在夏月，得热泥土、暖车缸，亦可用也。

Interpretations

Do not use cold water for heat stroke, for cold water makes the condition worse. A method for heat stroke: Make a rope out of grass and encircle it around the patient's umbilicus. Have two or three people urinate in the center to warm the umbilical region. Alternatively, mix hot mud with the grass rope. You can also cover the patient's umbilicus with the bottom of a ceramic bowl or axle of a cart, have people urinate and try to keep the urine in it. This is a roadway method where there is no hot water: to have more people to urinate (functioning as hot water) to warm the grass rope. Do not let the patient to expose to the cold axle. As heatstroke happens in summer, hot mud and warm axle are both available.

*****

[15] 救溺死方：

取灶中灰两石余，以埋人，从头至足，水出七孔，即活。

右疗自缢、溺、暍之法，并出自张仲景为之，其意殊绝，殆非常情所及，本草所能关，实救人之大术矣。伤寒家数有暍病，非此遇热之暍见《外台》、《肘后》目。

Interpretations

A formula to treat drowning: Take two *dàn* or more of ashes from inside a cooking stove and bury the patient's body from head to toes. The patient lives when water flows out of the mouth or noses.

The above treatment methods for hanging, drowning and sunstroke are developed by Zhang Zhongjing. These methods are beyond common knowledge or explanations and truly extraordinary, life-saving skills. Some physicians on cold damage believed heatstroke is not limited to exposure to heat. See *Wai Tai Mi Yao* (Arcane Essentials from the Imperial Library) and *Zhou Hou Bei Ji Fang* (Emergency Formulas to Keep Up One's Sleeve).

*****

[16] 治马坠及一切筋骨损方：见《肘后方》。

大黄一两，切，浸汤成下 绯帛如手大，烧灰乱发如鸡子大，烧灰用久用炊单布一尺，烧灰 败蒲一握三寸桃仁四十九个，去皮、尖，熬甘草如中指节，炙，锉 右七味，以童子小便量多少，煎汤成，内酒一大盏，次下大黄，去滓。分温三服。先锉败蒲席半领，煎汤浴，衣被覆复，斯须通利数行，痛楚立差。利及浴水赤，勿怪，即瘀血也。

Interpretations

A formula to treat fall from a horse or all traumatic injuries involving the sinews and bones and see the formula in *Zhou Hou Bei Ji Fang* (Emergency Formulas to Keep Up One's Sleeve):

大黄	*dà huáng*	1 *liǎng*	Radix et Rhizoma Rhei
绯帛	*fēi bó*	1 piece (hand-sized)	Red silk (burnt)
乱发	*luàn fā*	1 egg-sized piece	Human hair
炊单布	*chui dān bù*	1 *chǐ*	Used cotton in a steamer
败蒲	*bài pú*	1 handful	Livistona Chinensis
桃仁	*táo rén*	49 pieces	Semen Persicae (skin and tip removed, boiled)
甘草	*gān cǎo*	A piece the size of the middle finger joint	Radix et Rhizoma Glycyrrhizae

First decoct the six ingredients (excluding *Da Huang*) in a child's urine. Then add a large cup of liquor and *Da Huang* (Radix et Rhizoma Rhei) to decoct. Remove the dregs and take in three divided doses. In addition, decoct a part of Livistona Chinensis mat half the size of a cloth, bathe in the decoction, and then cover up with a quilt afterwards. After a while, the patient may have bowel movements and the pain relieved. Do not be surprised if the stool and the bath water turn red, this is caused by discharge of stagnant blood.

禽兽鱼虫禁忌并治第二十四
Chapter 24 Poultry, Fowl, Fish and Insects—Contraindications and Treatment

Overview

This chapter discusses the contraindications of poultry, fowl, fish and insects and prevention and treatment of food poisoning.

*****

[01] 凡饮食滋味，以养于生。食之有妨，反能为害。自非服药炼液[1]，焉能不饮食乎？切见时人，不闲调摄，疾疢竞起[2]，若不因食而生。苟全其生，须知切忌者矣。所食之味，有与病相宜，有与身为害。若得宜，则益体；害则成疾，以此致危，例皆难疗。凡煮药饮汁，以解毒者，虽云救急，不可热饮，诸毒病得热更甚，宜冷饮之。

Annotations

[1] *Fu Yao Lian Ye*: This refers to ingesting medicinals or Daoist fasting.
[2] *Ji Chen Jing Qi*: Illnesses occur one after another.

Interpretations

All types of food provide nutritional support for our body. However, poor selection of food may be harmful to the body. Other than ingestion of medicinals or Daoist fasting, how could anyone live without eating and drinking? Many people have little knowledge on health cultivation and food selection. As a result, illnesses occur one after another. It's essential to understand the selection and contraindications of food to stay safe and healthy. Some food are beneficial to disease treatment, whereas some are harmful. Good selection of food benefits the body. Poor selection of food may cause illnesses or aggravate pre-existing illnesses, making them more difficult to treat. Do not take toxin-removing decoctions when they are hot, even in emergency, for poisoning conditions are aggravated by hot drinks. It is therefore important to take toxin-removing decoctions when they are cold.

*****

[02] 肝病禁辛，心病禁咸，脾病禁酸，肺病禁苦，肾病禁甘[1]。春不食肝，夏不食心，秋不食肺，冬不食肾，四季不食脾。辨曰：春不食肝者，为肝气王，脾气败，若食肝，则又补肝，脾气败尤甚，不可救。又肝王之时，不可以死气[2]入肝，恐伤魂也。若非王时即虚，以肝补之佳，余藏准此。

Annotations

[1] *Gan Bing Jin Xin...Shen Bing Jin Gan*: Contraindications of food according to the interactions among the five elements, five zang-organs and five flavors. According to the five-element theory, wood promotes fire, fire promotes earth, earth promotes metal, metal promotes water and water promotes wood; wood restricts earth, earth restricts water, water restricts fire, fire restricts metal and metal restricts wood. As (lung) metal restricts (liver) wood and pungent food enters the lung, pungent food is contraindicated for liver problems.

[2] *Si Qi*: Food or medicinals that consume liver qi.

Interpretations

Pungent food is contraindicated for liver problems, salty food is contraindicated for heart problems, sour food is contraindicated for spleen problems, bitter food is contraindicated for lung problems and sweet food is contraindicated for kidney problems. Do not eat liver in spring. Do not eat heart in summer. Do not eat lung in autumn. Do not eat kidney in winter. Do not eat spleen in all seasons. Explanations: In spring, liver qi flourishes and spleen qi declines. Eating liver may further damage spleen qi to a point where it cannot be recovered. In addition, do not eat food or medicinals that consume liver qi when liver qi is in excess, for it may damage the ethereal soul. It's recommended to reinforce the liver when liver qi is deficient. This principle applies to other zang-organs.

*****

[03] 凡肝脏，自不可轻啖，自死者弥甚。

Interpretations

The liver of all animals should be eaten with caution, especially when these animals died of illness.

*****

[04] 凡心皆为神识所舍[1]，勿食之，使人来生复其报对矣。

Annotations

[1] *Fan Xin Jie Wei Shen Shi Suo Ṣhe*: The heart stores spirit and dominates mental activities (functions of the brain).

Interpretations

The heart of all animals stores spirit and controls mental activities. Do not eat it, otherwise they may return to revenge in the afterlife.

*****

[05] 凡肉及肝，落地不着尘土者[1]，不可食之。

Annotations

[1] *Fan Rou Ji Gan, Luo Di Bu Zhuo Chen Tu Zhe*: Spoiled or contaminated meat or liver may have an abnormally smooth surface and do not get stained with dust.

Interpretations

Do not eat animal meat or liver that do not get stained with dust when dropped to the ground.

*****

[06] 猪肉落水浮者〔1〕，不可食。

Annotations

[1] *Zhu Rou Luo Shui Fu Zhe*: *Zhu Rou* literally means pork. Here it refers to all types of meat. When placed into water, meat is supposed to sink to the bottom because its specific gravity is heavier than water; decayed meat may produce gas and float on top of the water.

Interpretations

Do not eat animal meat that floats on top of water.

*****

[07] 诸肉及鱼，若狗不食、鸟不啄者〔1〕，不可食。

Annotations

[1] *Gou Bu Shi, Niao Bu Zhuo*: Animals (dog, birds, etc.) have a better sense of smell than humans. The meat or fish they do not touch is not edible.

Interpretations

Do not eat meat or fish that dogs do not eat and birds do not peck.

*****

[08] 诸肉不干，火炙不动〔1〕，见水自动者〔2〕，不可食之。

Annotations

[1] *Zhu Rou Bu Gan, Huo Zhi Bu Dong*: Meat naturally dries up when exposed to air or shrinks when exposed to high heat. If not, this indicates the meat is decayed.

[2] *Jian Shui Zi Dong Zhe*: Decayed meat may produce gas and move in water.

Interpretations

Do not eat meat that fails to dry up when exposed to air or high heat. Do not eat meat that moves in water.

*****

[09] 肉中有如朱点〔1〕者，不可食之。

Annotations

[1] *Rou Zhong You Ru Zhu Dian*: Presence of red spots on meat indicates that animals died of pestilence.

Interpretations

Do not eat meat that has red spots.

*****

[10] 六畜肉〔1〕，热血不断〔2〕者，不可食之。

Annotations

[1] *Liu Chu Sheng*: Meat of six livestock—ox, horse, pig, goat, chicken and dog.

[2] *Re Xue Bu Duan*: Persistent bleeding (may indicate poisoning or pestilence).

Interpretations

Do not eat the meat of ox, horse, pig, goat, dog and chicken with persistent bleeding.

*****

[11] 父母及身本命肉〔1〕，食之，令人神魂不安。

Annotations

[1] *Ben Ming Rou*: Meat of one's own and parents' zodiac animals.

Interpretations

Eating meat of one's own or parents' zodiac animals may cause mental uneasiness.

*****

[12] 食肥肉及热羹，不得饮冷水。

Interpretations

Do not drink cold water after eating fatty meat and hot soup.

*****

[13] 诸五藏及鱼，投地尘土不污者，不可食之。

Interpretations

Do not eat organ meat or fish that do not stain dust when dropped to the ground.

*****

[14] 秽饭、馁肉、臭鱼，食之皆伤人。

Interpretations

Contaminated rice, decayed meat and spoiled fish are harmful to the body.

*****

[15] 自死肉、口闭者，不可食之。

Interpretations

Do not eat meat of animals that died of pestilence or poisoning with mouth closed.

*****

[16] 六畜自死，皆疫死，则有毒，不可食之。

Interpretations

When the six livestock die on their own, they usually die of pestilence. Do not eat their meat, for they are poisonous.

*****

[17] 兽自死，北首〔1〕及伏地〔2〕者，食之杀人。

Annotations

[1] *Bei Shou:* The head faces the north.

[2] *Fu Di*: Lying prone to the ground, mostly indicating a sudden death from a fatal illness.

Interpretations

Meat of dead animals with the head facing north and lying prone on the ground is harmful to the body.

*****

[18] 食生肉，饱饮乳，变成白虫〔1〕一作血蛊〔2〕。

Annotations

[1] *Bai Chong:* Tapeworms (in pork or beef).

[2] *Xue Gu*: Tympanites due to blood retention or parasites. It is characterized by abdominal bulging that resembles a drum, varicose abdominal veins, inability to eat food and a sallow, gray-dark complexion.

Interpretations

Ingestion of undercooked meat (pork or beef) and raw (unpasteurized) milk can cause tapeworms in the digestive and intestinal tract or tympanites.

*****

[19] 疫死牛肉，食之，令病洞下〔1〕；亦致坚积〔2〕，宜利药〔3〕下之。

Annotations

[1] *Dong Xia:* Severe diarrhea.

[2] *Jian Ji*: Abdominal masses due to parasites or food retention.
[3] *Li Yao*: Medicinals to promote bowel movements.

Interpretations

Ingestion of beef contaminated with pestilence can cause persistent diarrhea (with vomiting and abdominal pain) or abdominal masses that need to be treated with medicinals to promote bowel movements.

*****

[20] 脯〔1〕藏朱瓮〔2〕中有毒，及经夏食之，发肾病。

Annotations

[1] *Fu:* Dried meat.
[2] *Zhu Weng*: Rice cauldron.

Interpretations

Dried meat that stored in a rice cauldron may become poisonous in hot summer. Eating it may cause kidney problems.

*****

[21] 治自死六畜肉中毒方：黄柏屑，捣，服方寸匕。

Interpretations

A formula to treat poisoning from eating the meat of six livestock that died of pestilence: pound *Huang Bai* (Cortex Phellodendri Chinensis) into a powder and take a square-inch spoon.

*****

[22] 治食郁肉[1]漏脯[2]中毒方：郁肉，密器盖之，隔宿者是也。漏脯，茅屋漏下，沾着者是也。

烧犬屎酒服方寸匕。每服人乳汁亦良。

饮生韭汁三升[3]，亦得。

Annotations

[1] *Yu Rou:* Uncooked or cooked meat stored overnight in a tightly sealed container.

[2] *Lou Fu*: Air-dried meat that hang on a leaky, thatched hut and became wet.

[3] *Yin Sheng Jiu Zhi San Sheng*: Chinese chive juice. It acts to tonify the kidney, warm the spleen and stomach, move qi and remove toxins.

Interpretations

A method to treat poisoning from eating meat stored overnight in a tightly sealed container or air-dried meat that hang on a leaky, thatched hut and became wet: charred dog feces and take a square-inch spoon with rice wine. Drinking human breast milk also works. Another option is to drink 3 *shēng* of Chinese chives juice.

*****

[23] 治黍米中藏干脯[1]，食之中毒方：大豆浓煮汁，饮数升，即解。亦治狸肉、漏脯等毒。

Annotations

[1] *Shu Mi Zhong Can Gan Pu:* Dried meat stored in sorghum. The meat is easily spoiled because of the hot, unventilated environment.

Interpretations

A method to treat poisoning from eating dry, spoiled meat that stored in sorghum: drink several *shēng* of thick soybean juice. It also works for poisoning from eating wildcat meat or air-dried meat that hang on a leaky, thatched hut and became wet.

*****

[24] 治食生肉中毒方：掘地深三尺，取其下土[1]三升，以水五升，煮数沸，澄清汁。饮一升，即愈。

Annotations

[1] *Jue Di Shen San Chi, Qu Qi Xia Tu:* Dig three *chǐ* deep into the ground and take the earth to decoct with water.

Interpretations

A method to treat poisoning from eating uncooked meat: Dig three *chǐ* deep into the ground and take 3 *shēng* of the earth to decoct with 5 *shēng* of water. Bring it to boil several times and drink 1 *shēng* of the clear liquid. This often brings a quick recovery.

*****

[25] 治六畜鸟兽肝中毒方：水浸豆豉[1]，绞取汁，服数升愈。

Annotations

[1] *Shui Jin Dou Chi:* Fermented soybean. It acts to remove toxins and drain dampness.

Interpretations

A method to treat poisoning from eating the liver of six livestock, wild birds and beasts: Soak the fermented soybean (Semen Sojae Preparatum) in water, wring it to get the juice and drink several *shēng*. This often brings a quick recovery.

*****

[26] 马脚无夜眼者〔1〕，不可食之。

Annotations

[1] *Ye Yan:* It literally means night eyes—chess-sized, black hairless spots on the knee. When horses have them, they can travel at night, hence the name.

Interpretations

Do not eat the meat of a horse that has no night eyes.

*****

[27] 食酸马肉〔1〕，不饮酒则杀人。

Annotations

[1] *Suan Ma Rou:* Here it refers to a fine horse. Horse meat acts to strengthen the bones and sinews/muscles.

Interpretations

Eating the meat of a fine horse without drinking alcohol is harmful to the body.

*****

[28] 马肉不可热食，伤人心。

Interpretations

Eating hot horse meat is harmful to the heart (stomach).

*****

[29] 马鞍下肉[1]，食之杀人。

Annotations

[1] *Ma An Xia Rou:* The horse meat underneath the saddle. It is hard to be digested and harmful to the body.

Interpretations

Eating horse meat underneath the saddle is harmful to the body.

*****

[30] 白马黑头者，不可食之。
[31] 白马青蹄者，不可食之。

Interpretations

Do not eat the meat of white horses with a black head. Do not eat the meat of white horses with bluish hoofs.

*****

[32] 马肉豘肉共食，饱醉卧，大忌。

Interpretations

Do not eat horse meat together with pork. It's even worse to have a full stomach (hard to digest), drink a lot of alcohol and sleep afterwards.

*****

[33] 驴〔1〕马肉合猪肉食之，成霍乱〔2〕。

Annotations

[1] *Lú:* Donkey. Donkey meat acts to benefit qi and calm the mind.

[2] *Huo Luan*: A sudden attack of alternating vomiting with diarrhea. It is different from cholera (an infection of the small intestine by some strains of the bacterium Vibrio).

Interpretations

Do not eat donkey meat and horse meat together with pork, for it may cause severe vomiting and diarrhea.

*****

[34] 马肝及毛，不可妄食，中毒害人。

Interpretations

Do not eat horse liver and horsehair, for they are poisonous and harmful to the body.

*****

[35] 治马肝毒，中人未死方：雄鼠屎二七粒，末之，水和服，日再服。又方：人垢，取方寸匕，服之佳。

Interpretations

A formula to treat poisoning (not critical yet) from eating horse liver: Grind 14 (2×7) droppings of a male mouse into a fine powder, mix with water, and take in two divided doses.

Another effective option: Take a square-inch spoon of body dirt.

*****

[36] 治食马肉中毒欲死方：

香豉二两杏仁三两右二味，蒸一食顷，熟杵之服，日再服。

又方：煮芦根汁，饮之，良。

Interpretations

A formula for poisoning (critical) from eating horse meat: Steam 2 *liǎng* of *Xiang Chi* (Semen Sojae Praeparatum) and 3 *liǎng* of *Xing Ren* (Semen Armeniacae Amarum) for the time that takes to cook a meal, smash when they are thoroughly cooked and take in two divided doses.

Another effective option: Take medicinal juice of *Lu Gen* (Rhizoma Phragmitis).

*****

[37] 疫死牛，或目赤，或黄，食之大忌。

Interpretations

Do not eat the beef of cattle that died of pestilence. Their eyes appear red or yellow.

*****

[38] 牛肉共猪肉食之，必作寸白虫。

Interpretations

People who eat undercooked beef together with pork will contract tapeworms.

*****

[39] 青牛肠不可合犬肉食之。

Interpretations

Do not eat intestines of water buffalo together with dog meat.

*****

[40] 牛肺从三月至五月，其中有虫如马尾，割去勿食[1]，食则损人。

Annotations

[1] *Niu Fei...Ge Qu Wu Shi:* The time between March and May is a transitional period from spring to summer, which allows larval development of parasites. These parasitic larvae may enter the cattle's intestine and migrate to the lung.

Interpretations

Between March and May, the lungs of cattle may have worms that resemble a horse tail. Be sure to cut them and do not eat it. Eating it is harmful to the body.

*****

[41] 牛、羊、猪肉皆不得以楮木、桑木蒸炙食之，令人腹内生虫。

Interpretations

Do not steam or roast beef, mutton and pork over the wood from paper mulberry or white mulberry. Eating it may cause tapeworms in the abdomen.

*****

[42] 啖蛇牛肉〔1〕杀人，何以知之？啖蛇者，毛发向后顺〔2〕者，是也。

Annotations

[1] *Dan She Niu Rou*: Eating the beef of cattle that has been poisoned to death by ingesting a venomous snake.

[2] *Mao Fa Xiang Hou Shun*: The hair of the cattle that ingested a venomous snake point backwards.

Interpretations

Eating the beef of cattle that died of ingesting a venomous snake is harmful to the body. How can you know whether the cattle have ingested a venomous snake? Their hair pointed backwards.

*****

[43] 治啖蛇牛肉，食之欲死方：饮人乳汁一升，立愈。又方：以泔洗头，饮一升，愈。牛肚细切，以水一斗，煮取一升。暖饮之，大汗出者，愈。

Interpretations

A formula for a critical condition after eating the beef of cattle that died from ingesting a venomous snake: Drinking 1 *shēng* of human breast milk brings a quick recovery. Another option: Wash the head with rice-washed water and then drink 1 *shēng* of this water.

Cut the cattle's stomach into fine pieces, decoct in 1 *dòu* of water to get 1 *shēng*. Drink when it is warm to induce sweating. This will bring a full recovery.

*****

[44] 治食牛肉中毒方：甘草煮汁，饮之即解〔1〕。

Annotations

[1] *Gan Cao Zhu Zhi, Yin Zhi Ji Jie*: (with its glycyrrhizin and calcium salt,) *Gan Cao* (Radix et Rhizoma Glycyrrhizae) removes bacterial toxins or resolve poisoning from medicinals, food (such as snake or blowfish) or metabolites.

Interpretations

A formula for poisoning from eating beef: Decoct *Gan Cao* (Radix et Rhizoma Glycyrrhizae) and drink the juice.

*****

[45] 羊肉〔1〕其有宿热者〔2〕，不可食之。

Annotations

[1] *Yang Rou*: Meat of sheep or goat. It is warm in property and acts to warm the spleen and stomach, supplement qi, and reinforce the body. It is beneficial to abdominal pain due to deficiency cold; however, it's contraindicated for pregnant women or people with febrile diseases.

[2] *Su Re Zhe*: People with pre-existing febrile diseases.

Interpretations

Mutton is contraindicated for people with pre-existing febrile diseases.

*****

[46] 羊肉不可共生鱼[1]、酪食之，害人。

Annotations

[1] *Sheng Yu*: Here it refers to processed (pickled) fresh fish.

Interpretations

Mutton should not be eaten in together with processed fresh fish and dairy product, for this is harmful to the body.

*****

[47] 羊蹄甲中有珠子白[1]者，名羊悬筋，食之，令人癫。

Annotations

[1] *Zhu Zi Bai*: White spots in the toenails.

Interpretations

White spots in toenails of a goat is called suspended ligament. Eating it can cause paroxysmal mental disorder.

*****

[48] 白羊黑头，食其脑，作肠痈。

Interpretations

Eating the brain of a white goat with a black head may cause intestinal abscess.

*****

[49] 羊肝共生椒〔1〕食之，破人五脏。

Annotations

[1] *Sheng Jiao*: Pricklyash peel. It acts to warm the spleen and stomach and resolve dampness.

Interpretations

Eating goat liver together with pricklyash peel damages the internal organs.

*****

[50] 猪肉共羊肝和食之，令人心闷。

Interpretations

Eating pork together with goat liver may cause stomach stuffiness and distension.

*****

[51] 猪肉以生胡荽〔1〕同食，烂人脐。

Annotations

[1] *Sheng Hu Sui*: Fresh parsley. It acts to release the exterior, induce skin eruption and promote digestion.

Interpretations

Eating pork together with fresh parsley does harm to the umbilicus.

*****

[52] 猪脂〔1〕不可合梅子食之。

Annotations

[1] *Zhu Zhi*: Lard.

Interpretations

Do not eat lard together with green plums.

*****

[53] 猪肉和葵食之，少气。

Interpretations

Eating pork together with Chinese mallow consumes qi.

*****

[54] 鹿人不可和蒲白作羹，食之发恶疮。

Interpretations

Deer meat cannot be cooked into broth with cattail. Eating this may cause sores or ulcers.

*****

[55] 麋脂〔1〕及梅、李子，若妊妇食之，令子青盲〔2〕，男子伤精。

Annotations

[1] *Mi Zhi*: Milu fat. Milu, also known as the Père David's deer, is a species within the deer family. It is informally named *Si Bu Xiang* in Chinese (literally means like none of the four), because it has the antlers of a deer but not a deer, the head of a horse but not a horse, the body of a donkey but not a donkey, and the hooves of a cow but not a cow".

[2] *Qing Mang*: An eye condition due to yin deficiency of the liver and kidney. It causes poor vision and blindness; however, the appearance of the eyes is normal.

Interpretations

If a pregnant woman eats Milu fat together with mume and plums, the child will have poor eyesight. If eaten by a man, this will damage his semen.

*****

[56] 獐肉不可合虾〔1〕及生菜、梅、李果食之，皆病人。

Annotations

[1] *Xia*: Shrimp. It acts to tonify kidney yang, promote lactation and help to remove toxins.

Interpretations

Do not eat the meat of water deer together with shrimp, lettuce, mume and plums, for this may cause illness.

*****

[57] 痼疾人不可食熊肉〔1〕，令终身不愈。

Annotations

[1] *Xiong Rou*: Bear meat. It is sweet and greasy. Although it reinforces the body, bear meat also causes pathogenic factors to retain in the body.

Interpretations

Patients with chronic intractable diseases must not eat bear meat, or they will never recover for the rest of their life.

*****

[58] 白犬自死，不出舌者〔1〕，食之害人。

Annotations

[1] *Bai Quan Zi Si, Bu Chu She Zhe*: The *Yi Zong Jin Jian* (Golden Mirror of the Medical Tradition) states, "The tongue of a dead dog is always protruding; if not, the dog has been poisoned to death. In this case, eating dog meat is harmful to the body".

Interpretations

Eat the meat of a dead white dog without sticking out its tongue is harmful to the body.

*****

[59] 食狗、鼠余〔1〕，令人发瘘疮〔2〕。

Annotations

[1] *Gou, Shu Yu*: Leftovers by dogs or mice. The food touched by dogs or mice is contaminated.

[2] *Lou Chuang*: Axillary or cervical lymph node tuberculosis.

Interpretations

Eating the leftovers by dogs or mice can cause axillary or cervical lymph node tuberculosis.

*****

[60] 治食犬肉不消，心下坚，或腹胀，口干大渴，心急发热，妄语如狂〔1〕，或洞下方：杏仁一升，合皮，熟研用。以沸汤三升，和取汁。分三服，利下肉片，大验。

Annotations

[1] *Wang Yu Ru Kuang*: talk nonsense.

Interpretations

A method to treat poor digestion of dog meat with abdominal fullness, distension and hardness, a dry mouth, excessive thirst, heartburn, abdominal pain, talking nonsense, or persistent diarrhea: Boil 1 *shēng* of *Xing Ren* (Armeniacae Semen) with the peel and then smashed. Mix the smashed *Xing Ren* in 3 *shēng* of boiling water, take in three divided doses. A better efficacy can be achieved by passing of stools that contain dog meat pieces.

*****

[61] 妇人妊娠，不可食兔肉〔1〕、山羊肉及鳖、鸡、鸭，令子无声音。

Annotations

[1] *Tu Rou*: Rabbit meat. It fortifies the spleen and stomach and benefits qi.

Interpretations

Women during pregnancy should not eat rabbit meat, goat meat, turtle, chicken and duck, for these will make the child mute.

*****

[62] 兔肉不可合白鸡肉食之，令人面发黄。
[63] 兔肉着干姜食之，成霍乱。

Interpretations

Eating rabbit meat together with the meat of white chick causes a yellowish complexion (because of indigestion).

Eating (undercooked) rabbit meat with dried ginger causes severe vomiting and diarrhea.

*****

[64] 凡鸟[1]自死，口不闭、翅不合者，不可食之。

Annotations

[1] *Niao*: Birds. The *Jin Gui Yao Lüè Zhi Jie* (Direct Interpretation of the 'Essentials from the Golden Cabinet') states, "The mouth and wings of a dead bird are always closed; if not, they have been poisoned to death."

Interpretations

Do not eat the meat of birds that died with an open mouth and spreading wings.

*****

[65] 诸禽肉，肝青者，食之杀人。

Interpretations

Eating the meat of poultry with a dark-bluish liver is harmful to the body.

*****

[66] 鸡有六翮、四距者，不可食之。

Interpretations

Do not eat the meat of a chicken with six wings and four feet.

*****

[67] 乌鸡白首者，不可食之。

Interpretations

Do not eat the meat of black chickens with a white head.

*****

[68] 鸡不可共葫蒜食之，滞气。一云鸡子。

Interpretations

Do not eat chicken meat together with garlic, for it may cause flatulence or bloating. Another text mentions "do not eat eggs with garlic".

*****

[69] 山鸡不可合鸟兽肉食之。

Interpretations

Do not eat pheasant meat together with the meat of other birds or animals.

*****

[70] 雉肉久食之，令人瘦。

Interpretations

Eating pheasant meat for a long period may cause weight loss.

*****

[71] 鸭卵不可合鳖肉食之。

Interpretations

Do not eat duck eggs together with turtle meat (both are cold in nature, eating in combination is harmful to the body).

*****

[72] 妇人妊娠，食雀肉[1]，令子淫乱无耻。

Annotations

[1] *Que Rou*: Sparrow meat. It increases libido. Since in spring or summer, a male sparrow copulates with several female sparrows, here it assumes (not true) that eating sparrow meat causes the child to be licentious.

Interpretations

Eating sparrow meat during pregnancy may cause the child to be licentious.

*****

[73] 雀肉不可合李子食之。

Interpretations

Do not eat sparrow meat (warm and heat) together with plums (sour and astringent).

*****

[74] 燕肉勿食，入水为蛟龙所啖。

Interpretations

Do not eat the edible-nest swiftlets, or one will be eaten by the aquatic dragon.

*****

[75] 鸟兽有中毒箭死者，其肉有毒，解之方：大豆煮汁及盐汁〔1〕服之，解。

Annotations

[1] *Yan Zhi*: It literally means salty water. It is written *Lan Zhi* (Herba Polygoni Hydropiperis) in other texts.

Interpretations

A formula for eating the meat of birds or animals that have been killed by a poisoned arrow: decoct soybean and drink together with the juice of Herba Polygoni Hydropiperis.

*****

[76] 鱼头正白，如连珠至脊上，食之杀人。
[77] 鱼头中无腮者，不可食之，杀人。

[78] 鱼无肠胆者，不可食之。三年阴不起，女子绝生。

Interpretations

Fish with pure white spots on the head that extend to the spine is poisonous.

Fish with no cheeks in the head are not edible.

Fish with no intestines or gallbladder are not edible. Eating it causes three years of impotence and infertility in women.

*****

[79] 鱼头似有角者，不可食之。

Interpretations

Fish with an overgrowth that resembles a horn on the head are not edible.

*****

[80] 鱼目合者，不可食之。

Interpretations

Fish with closed eyes are not edible.

*****

[81] 六甲〔1〕日，勿食鳞甲之物。

Annotations

[1] *Liu Jia*: The six combinations beginning with the first Heavenly stem of the sixty combinations of the ten Heavenly Stems and the twelve

Earthly Branches, namely, *Jia Zi*, *Jia Yin*, *Jia Chen*, *Jia Wu*, *Jia Shen*, and *Jia Xu*.

Interpretations

On the six Jia days, do not eat food with scales or shells.

*****

[82] 鱼不可合鸡肉食之。

[83] 鱼不得合鸬鹚肉食之。

Interpretations

Do not eat fish together with chicken or cormorant meat.

*****

[84] 鲤鱼鲊，不可合小豆藿[1]食之；其子不可合猪肝食之，害人。

[85] 鲤鱼不可合犬肉食之。

Annotations

[1] *Xiao Dou Huo*: Leaves of red beans. They act to secure the kidney and astringe urine.

Interpretations

Do not eat salted carp together with leaves of red beans. Do not eat carp eggs together with pork liver.

Do not eat carp together with dog meat.

*****

[86] 鲫鱼[1]不可合猴、雉肉食之，一云不可合猪肝食。

Annotations

[1] *Ji Yu*: Crucian carp. It acts to fortify the spleen and resolve dampness.

Interpretations

Do not eat crucian carp together with monkey or pheasant meat. It is also said that crucian carp must not be eaten together with pork liver.

*****

[87] 鳀鱼合鹿肉生食，令人筋甲缩。

Interpretations

Eating raw anchovy together with deer meat causes contracture of the fingers.

*****

[88] 青鱼鲊，不可合生葫荽及生葵并麦中食之。

Interpretations

Do not eat salted black carp together with fresh parsley, raw mallow and wheat-contained sauce.

*****

[89] 鳅、鳝不可合白犬血食之。

Interpretations

Do not eat mudfish and eel together with the blood of a white dog.

*****

[90] 龟〔1〕肉不可合酒果子食之。

Annotations

[1] *Gui*: Tortoise. Its meat nourishes yin and tonifies blood.

Interpretations

Do not eat tortoise meat together with fruits or alcohol.

*****

[91] 鳖目凹陷者，及厌下有王字形者，不可食之。
[92] 其肉不得合鸡、鸭子食之。

Interpretations

Do not eat the meat of turtles with sunken eyes and lines in the shape of a Chinese character "王" on the underbelly. In addition, do not eat turtle meat together with chicken or duck eggs.

*****

[93] 龟、鳖肉不可合苋菜食之。

Interpretations

Do not eat turtle or tortoise meat together with amaranth.

*****

[94] 虾无须及腹下通黑，煮之反白者，不可食之。

Interpretations

Do not eat shrimps with no antennae and a black line on the underbelly that turns white when cooked.

*****

[95] 食脍饮乳酪，令人腹中生虫为瘕。

Interpretations

Eating pieces of raw fresh fish and drinking raw (unpasteurized) milk causes one to be infected with parasitic worms.

*****

[96] 脍食之，在心胸间不化，吐复不出，速下除之，久成症病，治之方：橘皮一两大黄二两朴硝二两右三味，以水一大升，煮至小升。顿服即消。

Interpretations

A formula for fast removal of undigested raw fresh fish that cannot be expelled through vomiting:

橘皮	*jú pí*	1 *liǎng*	Pericarpium Citri Reticulatae
大黄	*dà huáng*	2 *liǎng*	Radix et Rhizoma Rhei
芒硝	*máng xiāo*	2 *liǎng*	Natrii Sulfas

Decoct the three ingredients in 2 *shēng* of water to get 1 *shēng*. Drink up at a draught.

*****

[97] 食脍多不消，结为症病，治之方：马鞭草[1]右一味，捣汁饮之，或以姜叶[2]汁饮之一升，亦消。又可服吐药吐之。

Annotations

[1] *Ma Bian Cao* (Herba Verbenae): The whole plant of verbena. It acts to move blood, break masses, remove toxins and kill parasites.

[2] *Jiang Ye*: Fresh ginger leaves. It removes fish toxins.

Interpretations

A method for ingestion of raw fresh fish: Pound *Ma Bian Cao* (Herba Verbenae) and drink the juice. Alternatively, pound the fresh ginger leaves and drink 1 *shēng* of the juice. Another option is to take medicinals that produce nausea and vomiting.

*****

[98] 食鱼后食毒，两种烦乱[1]，治之方：橘皮浓煎汁服之，即解。

Annotations

[1] *Liang Zhong Fan Luan*: The first word *Liang* is believed to be a wrong spelling of *Mian*, meaning facial puffiness.

Interpretations

A method for facial puffiness, vexation and restlessness due to fish poisoning (or allergic reactions): Decoct *Ju Pi* (Pericarpium Citri Reticulatae) into thick juice and drink it.

*****

[99] 食鯸鮧鱼[1]中毒方：芦根煮汁服之，即解。

Annotations

[1] *Hou Yi Yu:* Pufferfish. Its internal organs, such as liver, ovary and blood contain highly toxic tetrodotoxin.

Interpretations

A method for pufferfish poisoning: Decoct *Lu Gen* (Rhizoma Phragmitis) and drink the juice.

*****

[100] 蟹目相向，足班目赤者，不可食之。

Interpretations

Do not eat the meat of crabs that have red, crossed eyes and legs with macule lines.

*****

[101] 食蟹中毒治之方：紫苏煮汁饮之三升。紫苏子捣汁饮之，亦良。又方：冬瓜[1]汁饮二升，食冬瓜亦可。

Annotations

[1] *Dong Gua:* White gourd. It acts to clear heat, promote urination and remove toxins.

Interpretations

A method for crab poisoning: Decoct *Zi Su* (Folium Perillae) and drink 3 *shēng* of the juice. Drinking the juice of *Zi Su Zi* (Fructus Perillae) is also effective. Alternatively, drink 2 *shēng* of the white gourd juice or eat white gourd.

*****

[102] 凡蟹未遇霜，多毒[1]，其熟者，乃可食之。

Annotations

[1] *Fan Xie Wei Yu Shuang, Duo Du:* Crabs before the Frost's descent (the 18th solar term on the traditional Chinese lunar calendar) are poisonous because they eat black henbane (a poisonous plant). After the Frost's descent, crabs start to eat rice and are therefore less poisonous.

Interpretations

Crabs before the Frost's descent are often poisonous; do not eat them until cooked.

*****

[103] 蜘蛛落食中，有毒，勿食之。

Interpretations

If a spider drops on food, the food becomes toxic. Do not eat it.

*****

[104] 凡蜂、蝇、虫、蚁等多集食上，食之致瘘。

Interpretations

Eating the food bitten by bees, flies, worms or ants may cause fistulas.

果实菜谷禁忌并治第二十五
Chapter 25 Fruits, Vegetables and Grains—Contraindications and Treatment

Overview

This chapter discusses the contraindications of fruits, vegetables and grains and prevention and treatment of food poisoning.

*****

[01] 果子生食生疮。

Interpretations

Eating unripe fruit may cause sores or ulcers.

*****

[02] 果子落地经宿，虫蚁食之者，人大忌食之。

Interpretations

Do not eat fruits that have fallen on the ground overnight, for they may have eaten by worms or ants (and become contaminated).

*****

[03] 生米停留多日，有损处，食之伤人。

Interpretations

Eating uncooked rice that has been stored for days and shown contaminated signs is harmful to the body.

*****

[04] 桃子〔1〕多食令人热，仍不得入水浴，令人病淋沥〔2〕寒热病。

Annotations

[1] *Tao Zi:* Peach. It acts to move blood, resolve masses, regenerate fluids and moisten the intestines.

[2] *Ling Li*: Here it refers to persistent fever and chills.

Interpretations

Overeating of peaches may cause heat. It's advisable not to bathe with cold water, or it may cause lingering of fever and chills.

*****

[05] 杏酪〔1〕不熟伤人。

Annotations

[1] *Xing Lao:* Almond paste/crisp, a processed almond product. It acts to moisten the five-zang organs and alleviate coughing.

Interpretations

Eating undercooked almond paste/crisp is harmful to the body.

*****

[06] 梅多食，坏人齿。

Interpretations

Overeating green plums is harmful to the teeth.

*****

[07] 李不可多食，令人胪胀。

Interpretations

Overeating plums may cause abdominal distension.

*****

[08] 林檎不可多食，令人百脉弱。

Interpretations

Overeating Chinese pearleaf crabapple may cause general weakness.

*****

[09] 橘、柚〔1〕多食，令人口爽〔2〕不知五味。

Annotations

[1] *Ju, You*: Orange and grapefruit. Oranges act to regulate qi, harmonize the stomach, moisten the lung and generates fluids. Grapefruits act to promote digestion and resolve phlegm. They both have significant contents of vitamin C.

[2] *Kou Shuang*: Poor sense of taste.

Interpretations

Overeating oranges and grapefruits may weaken one's sense of taste.

*****

[10] 梨〔1〕不可多食，令人寒中。金疮、产妇亦不宜食。

Annotations

[1] *Li*: Pears. They act to clear heat, resolve phlegm, generate fluids and moisten dryness.

Interpretations

Overeating pears may cause deficiency cold of the spleen and stomach. People with incise wounds or new mothers after childbirth should not eat pears.

*****

[11] 樱桃、杏〔1〕多食，伤筋骨。

Annotations

[1] *Yin Tao, Xing*: Cherry and apricot. Cherries act to fortify the spleen and benefit the kidney. Apricots act to generate fluids, moisten the lung and resolve phlegm.

Interpretations

Overeating cherries and apricots may impair the sinews and bones.

*****

[12] 安石榴不可多食，损人肺。

Interpretations

Overeating pomegranates may impair the lung.

*****

[13] 胡桃〔1〕不可多食，令人动痰饮。

Annotations

[1] *Hu Tao*: Walnuts. They act to tonify kidney essence.

Interpretations

Overeating walnuts may cause phlegm fluid.

*****

[14] 生枣多食，令人热渴气胀。寒热羸瘦者，弥不可食，伤人。

Interpretations

Overeating raw jujubes may cause restless, a hot sensation, thirst and abdominal distension. Thin, weak people or people with fever and chills should not eat raw jujubes; they may do harm to these people.

*****

[15] 食诸果中毒治之方：猪骨烧过右一味，末之，水服方寸匕。亦治马肝、漏脯等毒。

Interpretations

A formula for fruit poisoning: Grind boiled pig bone into a fine powder and drink a square-inch spoon with water. It can also be used to treat poisoning from horse liver and contaminated air-dried meat.

*****

[16] 木耳[1]赤色及仰生者，勿食。菌仰卷及赤色者，不可食。

Annotations

[1] *Mu Er*: Black (wood ear) fungus. They act to move and tonify blood and stop bleeding.

Interpretations

Black fungi that are red in color and growing curled up are not edible. Mushrooms that are growing curled up and red in color are not edible.

*****

[17] 食诸菌中毒，闷乱欲死，治之方：人粪汁饮一升；土浆饮一二升；大豆浓煮汁饮之。服诸吐利药，并解。

Interpretations

A formula for stomach stuffiness, distension and upset after eating poisonous mushrooms: Drink 1 *shēng* of liquefied human feces; drink 1 or 2 *shēng* of decocted earth water; drink thick, decocted soybean juice. At the same time, take formulas that induce nausea, vomiting and diarrhea to remove toxins out of the body.

*****

[18] 食枫柱菌而哭不止，治之以前方。

Interpretations

The aforementioned formula can also be used for unexplained and unstoppable laughing and crying after eating poisonous mushrooms that grow on maple trees.

*****

[19] 误食野芋，烦毒欲死，治之方。以前方。

Interpretations

The aforementioned formula can also be used for life-threatening conditions after eating highly poisonous wild taro.

The root of wild taro is called *Kui Yu* in Shandong Province. When people plant taro and do not harvest for three years, these taro turn into wild and highly poisonous.

*****

[20] 蜀椒闭口〔1〕者有毒，误食之，戟人咽喉〔2〕，气病欲绝。或吐下白沫，身体痹冷。急治之方：肉桂煎汁饮之，多饮冷水一二升。或食蒜，或饮地浆，或浓煮豉汁饮之，并解。

Annotations

[1] *Shu Jiao Bi Kou*: Pricklyash peel is pungent in taste and heat in property. It is toxic. A closed seedpod increases its toxicity. Eating it by mistake may irritate the throat.

[2] *Ji Ren Yan Hou*: Irritate the throat. Other symptoms of poisoning include throwing up white foam, qi blockage, and cold limbs.

Interpretations

Eating poisonous pricklyash with a closed seedpod may irritate the throat, block qi and result in throwing up white foam and cold limbs. An emergency formula: Drink decocted juice of cinnamon bark, along with 1 or 2 *shēng* of cold water. Alternatively, eat garlic, drink decocted earth water, or drink thick, decocted juice of soybeans. All these methods help to remove toxins.

*****

[21] 正月勿食生葱，令人面生游风〔1〕。

Annotations

[1] *You Feng*: It literally means wandering wind affecting the face—an acute skin condition characterized by red rashes.

Interpretations

Do not eat uncooked scallions in the first month of the lunar year, for it may cause red rashes on the face.

*****

[22] 二月勿食蓼，伤人肾。

Interpretations

Do not eat water pepper in the second month of the lunar year, for it may damage kidney yang.

*****

[23] 三月勿食小蒜，伤人志性。

Interpretations

Do not eat single clove garlic in the third month of the lunar year, for it may affect one's mental activities.

*****

[24] 四月、八月勿食胡荽，伤人神。

Interpretations

Do not eat parsley in the fourth and eighth month of the lunar year, for it may affect one's spirit.

*****

[25] 五月勿食韭[1]，令人乏气力。

Annotations

[1] *Jiu*: Chive. It warms kidney yang. The *Jin Gui Yao Lüè Zhi Jie* (Direct Interpretation of the 'Essentials from the Golden Cabinet') states, "Chives taste good in spring but bad in summer. The spleen dislikes bad taste. Since the spleen controls muscles, eating bad-taste food causes general weakness".

Interpretations

Do not eat chives in the fifth month of the lunar year, for it may cause general weakness.

*****

[26] 五月五日勿食一切生菜，发百病。

Interpretations

Do not eat any raw vegetables on the fifth day of the fifth month of the lunar year, for it may cause a variety of diseases.

*****

[27] 六月、七月勿食茱萸，伤神气。

Interpretations

Do not eat Chinese cornel dogwood in the sixth and seventh month of the lunar year, fir it may impair one's spirit.

*****

[28] 八月、九月勿食姜，伤人神。

Interpretations

Do not eat fresh ginger in the eighth and ninth month of the lunar year, for it may impair one's spirit.

*****

[29] 十月勿食椒〔1〕，损人心，伤心脉。

Annotations

[1] *Jiao*: Black pepper. It acts to warm the spleen and stomach and regulates qi.

Interpretations

Do not eat black pepper in the tenth month of the lunar year, for it may damage one's heart (stomach) and blood vessels.

*****

[30] 十一月、十二月勿食薤，令人多涕唾。

Interpretations

Do not eat long stamen onion bulb in the eleventh and twelfth month of the lunar year, for it may generate phlegm.

*****

[31] 四季〔1〕勿食生葵〔2〕，令人饮食不化，发百病。非但食中，药中皆不可用，深宜慎之。

Annotations

[1] *Si Ji*: The last month of the four seasons, i.e., March, June, September and December.

[2] *Sheng Kui:* Leaves of cluster mallow.

Interpretations

Do not eat leaves of cluster mallow in March, June, September and December, for it may cause poor digestion and result in a variety of diseases. In addition, cluster mallow should be used with caution as a medicinal ingredient.

*****

[32] 时病差未健，食生菜，手足必肿。

Interpretations

For patients who haven't fully recovered from febrile diseases (poor functioning of the spleen and stomach), eating raw vegetables may cause limb swelling.

*****

[33] 夜食生菜，不利人。

Interpretations

Eating raw vegetables at night is not beneficial to health.

*****

[34] 十月勿食被霜生菜，令人面无光，目涩，心痛，腰疼或发心疟〔1〕。疟发时手足十指爪皆青，困委。

Annotations

[1] *Xin Nüè*: The heart-associated malaria. The *Huang Di Nei Jing* (Yellow Emperor's Internal Classic) states, "Symptoms of malaria affecting the heart include severe restlessness, severe chills and mild fever".

Interpretations

In the tenth month of the lunar year, do not eat raw vegetables that have been exposed to frost, for it may cause lusterless complexion, dry eyes, pain in the chest and low back, and in severe cases, heart-associated malaria. At the onset of this condition, patients may present with bluish discoloration of fingernails and listlessness.

*****

[35] 葱韭初生芽者，食之伤人心气。

Interpretations

Eating scallions and chives during their early sprouting may damage the gastrointestinal function.

*****

[36] 饮白酒，食生韭，令人病增。

Interpretations

Drinking liquor and eating raw chives may aggravate one's pre-existing conditions.

*****

[37] 生葱不可共蜜食之，杀人，独颗蒜弥忌。

Interpretations

Do not eat raw scallion together with honey, for it is harmful to the body. Single clove garlic is especially contraindicated.

*****

[38] 枣合生葱食之，令人病。

Interpretations

Eating jujube with raw scallion may cause one to be sick.

*****

[39] 生葱和雄鸡、雉、白犬肉食之，令人七窍经年流血。

Interpretations

Eating raw scallion together with the meat of roosters, pheasant or white dogs may cause bleeding from the seven orifices (mouth, nose, eyes and ears) for years.

*****

[40] 食糖、蜜后，四日内食生葱、韭，令人心痛。

Interpretations

Eating raw scallions or chives within four days of eating sugar or honey may cause gastric or abdominal pain.

*****

[41] 夜食诸姜、蒜、葱等，伤人心。

Interpretations

Eating fresh ginger, garlic and scallions at night may damage one's heart (mind).

*****

[42] 芜菁根[1]多食，令人气胀。

Annotations

[1] *Wu Jing Gen*: Turnip root. It acts to increase the appetite, down-regulate qi, resolve dampness and remove toxins.

Interpretations

Overeating turnip root may cause abdominal bloating.

*****

[43] 薤不可共牛肉作羹食之，成瘕病〔1〕。韭亦然。

Annotations

[1] *Jia Bing*: Abdominal masses due to qi stagnation. They come and go and have no fixed locations.

Interpretations

Do not cook meat broth with long stamen onion bulb and beef, for they may cause (poor digestion) and abdominal masses. Do not use chives either.

*****

[44] 莼〔1〕多病，动痔疾。

Annotations

[1] *Chun*: Water shield. Its leaves act to clear heat and promote urination.

Interpretations

Overeating water shields may cause hemorrhoids.

*****

[45] 野苣〔1〕不可同蜜食之，作内痔。

Annotations

[1] *Ye Ju*: The whole plant or root of endive. In summer, eating endive helps to clear heat, cool blood and remove toxins. Decocted juice is used to wash hemorrhoids. However, when eaten together with honey, it may cause internal hemorrhoids.

Interpretations

Do not eat endive together with honey, for it may cause internal hemorrhoids.

*****

[46] 白苣不可共酪同食〔1〕，作虫。

Annotations

[1] *Bai Ju*: The stalk or leaves of lettuce. It removes toxins and alleviates thirst.

Interpretations

Do not eat lettuce together with raw (unpasteurized) milk, for it may generate parasitic worms.

*****

[47] 黄瓜食之〔1〕，发热病。

Annotations

[1] *Huang Gua*: Cucumber. It clears heat and promotes urination. The *Shi Liao Ben Cao* (Materia Medica for Dietary Therapy) states, "Cucumber is cold in property, do not eat too much. It stirs wind and causes chills and fever". The *Jin Gui Yao Lüè Zhi Jie* (Direct Interpretation

of the 'Essentials from the Golden Cabinet') states, "Cucumber causes chills and fever. Patients with deficiency heat or after febrile diseases cannot not it".

Interpretations

Overeating cucumber may cause heat.

*****

[48] 葵心不可食，伤人，叶尤冷。黄背赤茎者，勿食之。

Interpretations

Mallow's heart is toxic and inedible. It is harmful to the body. Its leaves are even colder in property. Do not eat mallow with yellow leaves but red stalks (because they are poisonous).

*****

[49] 胡荽久食之，令人多忘。

Interpretations

Eating parsley for a long period may cause poor memory.

*****

[50] 病人不可食胡荽及黄花菜。

Interpretations

Sick people should not eat parsley or day lily.

*****

[51] 芋[1]不可多食，动病。

Annotations

[1] *Yu*: Taro. It reinforces the body and dissipate masses. However, excessive ingestion may cause poor digestion and abdominal distension.

Interpretations

Do not overeat taro, for it may trigger the pre-existing conditions.

*****

[52] 妊妇食姜，令子余指[1]。

Annotations

[1] *Yu Zhi*: Here it refers to the extra (sixth) finger/toe.

Interpretations

Eating ginger during pregnancy may cause the child to have an extra finger/toe.

*****

[53] 蓼多食，发心痛。

Interpretations

Overeating water pepper may cause stomachache.

*****

[54] 蓼和生鱼食之，令人夺气，阴欬疼痛。

Interpretations

Eating water pepper together with salted fresh fish may consume qi and cause clitoral pain.

*****

[55] 芥菜不可共兔肉食之，成恶邪病。

Interpretations

Do not eat mustard leaf together with rabbit meat, for it may cause intractable diseases.

*****

[56] 小蒜多食，伤人心力。

Interpretations

Overeating single clove garlic may damage one's heart (spirit).

*****

[57] 食躁式躁方：豉浓煮汁饮之。

Interpretations

A formula for vexation (vomiting) after eating certain vegetables: Decoct fermented soybean and drink the thick juice.

*****

[58] 钩吻[1]与芹菜相似，误食之，杀人。解之方：《肘后》云：与茱萸食芥相似。荠苨八两右一味，水六升，煮取二升。分温两服钩吻生地旁无它草，其茎有毛，以此别之。

Annotations

[1] *Gou Wen*: The whole plant of yellow jasmine. It is highly toxic and can only be used externally.

Interpretations

Yellow jasmine is similar to celery. Eating it by mistake can be life threatening. The *Zhou Hou Bei Ji Fang* (Emergency Formulas to Keep Up One's Sleeve) states, "Yellow jasmine is similar to evodia leaf". A rescue formula: Decoct 8 *liǎng* of *Ji Ni* (Adenophora hunanensis Nannf.) in 6 *shēng* of water to get 2 *shēng* and take in two divided doses. Identification of yellow jasmine: It grows on soil where no other herbs grow and its stalk is hairy.

*****

[59] 菜中有水莨菪〔1〕，叶圆而光，有毒。误食之，令人狂乱，状如中风。或吐血。治之方：甘草煮汁服之，即解。

Annotations

[1] *Shui Liang Dang*: The whole plant of celery-leaved buttercup. It is a toxic grass.

Interpretations

The celery-leaved buttercup has smooth, round leaves. It is toxic. Eating this grass may cause mental derangement that resembles wind stroke. Some may experience vomiting of blood. A method for this condition: Decoct licorice and drink the juice.

*****

[60] 春秋二时，龙带精[1]入芹菜中，人偶食之为病，发时手青、腹满，痛不可忍，名蛟龙病，治之方：硬糖二三升右一味，日两度服之，吐出如蜥蜴三五枚，差。

Annotations

[1] *Long Dai Jing*: Parasitic ovum. Long originally refers to an aquatic dragon. Here it means a lizard-like parasite.

Interpretations

In spring and autumn, people may eat celeries that have parasitic ova and experience abdominal fullness and pain, and in severe cases, bluish discoloration of the hands and feet. This is called "aquatic dragon disease". A formula to treat this condition: Take hard sugar twice a day. Patients recover after throwing up 3–5 lizard-like worms.

*****

[61] 食苦瓠[1]中毒治之方：黍穰煮汁，数服之，解。

Annotations

[1] *Ku Hu*: Calabash. It is mildly toxic and can promote urination, resolve edema and induce vomiting.

Interpretations

A formula for poisoning of eating calabash: Decoct sorghum stalks and drink the juice for several times.

*****

[62] 扁豆，寒热者不可食之。

Annotations

[1] *Bian Dou*: Lablab. It fortifies the spleen and resolves dampness. The *Jin Gui Yao Lüè Jin Shi* (Modern Interpretation of the 'Essentials from the Golden Cabinet') states, "Patients with malaria cannot eat lablab, for it may aggravate the malaria or trigger relapse".

Interpretations

Patients with fever and chills cannot eat lablab.

*****

[63] 久食小豆，令人枯燥。

Interpretations

Eating red beans for a long period may cause skin dryness.

*****

[64] 食大豆屑，忌啖猪肉。

Interpretations

Soybean flakes cannot be eaten together with pork.

*****

[65] 大麦久食，令人作癣。

Interpretations

Eating barley for a long period may cause lassitude.

*****

[66] 白黍米不可同饴蜜食，亦不可合葵食之。

Interpretations

Do not eat white broomcorn millet together with malt sugar or mallow.

*****

[67] 荍麦面多食之，令人发落。

Interpretations

Too much intake of buckwheat flour may cause hair loss.

*****

[68] 盐多食，伤人肺。

Interpretations

Too much salt intake is harmful to one's lung.

*****

[69] 食冷物，冰人齿。

Interpretations

Eating cold food make one's teeth cold.

*****

[70] 食热物，勿饮冷水。

Interpretations

Do not drink cold water immediately after eating hot food.

*****

[71] 饮酒，食生苍耳，令人心痛。

Interpretations

Eating raw cocklebur fruit while drinking alcohol may cause epigastric pain.

*****

[72] 夏月大醉汗流，不得冷水洗着身，及使扇，即成病。

Interpretations

After profuse sweating from heavy drinking, do not bathe in cold water or use a fan, for it may cause illnesses.

*****

[73] 饮酒大忌炙腹背，令人肠结。

Interpretations

Performing moxibustion on the back or abdomen is highly contraindicated after drinking alcohol, for it may cause intestinal or gastric dryness.

*****

[74] 醉后勿饱食，发寒热。

Interpretations

Do not eat too much when you're drunk, for it may cause fever and chills.

*****

[75] 饮酒，食猪肉，卧秫稻穰中则发黄。

Interpretations

Drinking alcohol, eating pork and sleeping on sorghum or rice straw may cause jaundice.

*****

[76] 食饴，多饮酒，大忌。

Interpretations

Heavy drinking is highly contraindicated with eating malt sugar.

*****

[77] 凡水及酒照见人影动者，不可饮之。

Interpretations

Do not drink water or liquor that cannot reflect or mirror the move of people.

*****

[78] 醋合酪食之，令人血瘕〔1〕。

Annotations

[1] *Xue Jia*: Retention of stagnant blood.

Interpretations

Eating vinegar with raw milk may cause retention of stagnant blood.

*****

[79] 食白米粥，勿食生苍耳，成走疰。

Interpretations

Do not eat rice congee together with raw cocklebur fruit, for it may cause deep multiple abscesses.

*****

[80] 食甜粥已，食盐即吐。

Interpretations

Intake of salt after eating sweet congee may cause vomiting.

*****

[81] 犀角筯[1]搅饮食，沫出，及浇地坟起者[2]，食之杀人。

Annotations

[1] *Xi Jiao Zhu*: Chopsticks made from rhinoceros horn.

[2] *Jiao Di Qi Fen Zhe*: Bubbles erupt when the food is poured to the ground. This is caused by toxins reacting with the soil.

Interpretations

Presence of white foams when stirring food with chopsticks made from rhinoceros or eruption of bubbles when the food is poured to the ground indicates the food is deadly toxic.

*****

[82] 饮食中毒，烦满，治之方：苦参〔1〕三两 苦酒一升半右二味，煮三沸，三上，三下。服之，吐食出即差，或以水煮亦得。

又方：犀角汤〔2〕亦佳。

Annotations

[1] *Ku Shen*: Radix Sophorae Flavescentis (light yellow sophora root). It acts to clear heat and promote urination. Modern studies have shown that it works for cardiac arrhythmias due to poisoning.

[2] *Xi Jiao Tang* (Rhinoceros Horn Decoction): A formula to clear heat, calm the mind, cool blood and remove toxins.

Interpretations

A formula for anguish and restlessness due to poisoning: Decoct 3 *liǎng* of *Ku Shen* and 1.5 *shēng* of rice vinegar and bring it to boil 3 times. Drink up at a draught. Patients recover after vomiting of the food. Alternatively, decoct it in water. Another option is *Xi Jiao Tang* (Rhinoceros Horn Decoction).

*****

[83] 贪食，食多不消，心腹坚满痛，治之方：盐〔1〕一升水三升右二味，煮令盐消。分三服，当吐出食，便差。

Annotations

[1] *Yan*: Salt. It acts to soften hardness, remove toxins and induce vomiting.

Interpretations

A formula for abdominal harness, distension, fullness and pain due to poor digestion of excessive food intake: Decoct 1 *shēng* of salt in 3 *shēng* of water until the salt dissolves. Take the decoction in three divided doses. Patients recover after vomiting of the undigested food.

*****

[84] 矾石〔1〕生入腹，破人心肝，亦禁水。

Annotations

[1] *Fan Shi*: Alumen. It is often used externally. Oral administration may irritate gastric mucosa and cause reflex vomiting.

Interpretations

Swallowing alum without water damages the stomach and liver. Do not take alum with water either.

*****

[85] 商陆〔1〕以水服，杀人。

Annotations

[1] *Shang Lu*: Radix Phytolaccae (pokeberry root). It is bitter in taste and cold in property. A small dose of pokeberry root removes water retention; however, a large dose is toxic.

Interpretations

Taking *Shang Lu* (Radix Phytolaccae) with water is harmful to the body.

*****

[86] 葶苈子，傅头疮〔1〕。药成入脑，杀人。

Annotations

[1] *Ting Li Zi, Fu Tou Chuang*: Semen Lepidii (pepperweed seed) can be taken orally to disperse the lung and move water. It can also be applied externally to treat head sores.

Interpretations

Ting Li Zi (Semen Lepidii) can be externally applied to treat scalp sores. Sores affecting the brain upon external application can be life-threatening.

*****

[87] 水银〔1〕入人耳及六畜等，皆死。以金银着耳边，水银则吐。

Annotations

[1] *Shui Yin*: Liquid metallic mercury. It is highly toxic and cannot be taken orally. It can be used topically to kill worms, but only in a small dose for a short period of time.

Interpretations

Mercury can cause a life-threatening condition if it enters human ears or ears of the six livestock. Place gold or silver jewelries on the sides of the ears to suck the mercury out.

*****

[88] 苦练〔1〕无子者，杀人。

Annotations

[1] *Ku Lian*: Fructus Meliae (Chinaberry): It is bitter in taste and cold in property. It is toxic and acts to regulate qi and kills worms.

Interpretations

Seedless Chinaberries are highly toxic to the body.

*****

[89] 凡诸毒，多是假毒以投无知时，宜煮甘草、荠苨汁饮之，通除诸毒药。

Interpretations

For all kinds of poisoning without known causes, decoct the leaves of *Gan Cao* (Radix et Rhizoma Glycyrrhizae) and *Qi Ni* (Adenophora trachelioides) and drink it.

Index

www.ingramcontent.com/pod-product-compliance
Lightning Source LLC
LaVergne TN
LVHW021055220926
848484LV00021B/945
* 9 7 8 1 9 4 5 5 5 2 0 6 9 *